Hemodialysis Technology

Contributions to Nephrology

Vol. 137

KARGER

Hemodialysis Technology

Volume Editors

Claudio Ronco *Vicenza*
Giuseppe La Greca *Vicenza*

113 figures, 28 in color, and 31 tables, 2002

KARGER

Basel · Freiburg · Paris · London · New York ·
New Delhi · Bangkok · Singapore · Tokyo · Sydney

Contributions to Nephrology
Founded 1975 by Geoffrey M. Berlyne

Claudio Ronco
Department of Nephrology
St. Bortolo Hospital
I–36100 Vicenza (Italy)

Giuseppe La Greca
Department of Nephrology
St. Bortolo Hospital
I–36100 Vicenza (Italy)

Library of Congress Cataloging-in-Publication Data

Hemodialysis technology/volume editors, Claudio Ronco, Giuseppe La Greca.
p.; cm. – (Contributions to nephrology, ISSN 0302–5144; vol. 137)
Includes bibliographical references and index.
ISBN 3805574231 (hard cover : alk. paper)
1. Hemodialysis–Equipment and supplies. I. Ronco, C. (Claudio), 1951– II. La Greca, G.
III. Series.
[DNLM: 1. Renal Dialysis–instrumentation. 2. Renal Dialysis–methods. WJ 378 H48857 2002]
RC901.7.H45 H453 2002
617.4′61059–dc21

2002021536

Drug Dosage. The authors and the publisher have exerted every effort to ensure that drug selection and dosage set forth in this text are in accord with current recommendations and practice at the time of publication. However, in view of ongoing research, changes in government regulations, and the constant flow of information relating to drug therapy and drug reactions, the reader is urged to check the package insert for each drug for any change in indications and dosage and for added warnings and precautions. This is particularly important when the recommended agent is a new and/or infrequently employed drug.

www.karger.com
Printed in Switzerland on acid-free paper by Reinhardt Druck, Basel
ISSN 0302–5144
ISBN 3–8055–7423–1

Contents

XI Preface
Ronco, C.; La Greca, G. (Vicenza)

Opening Remark

1 The Role of Technology in Hemodialysis
Ronco, C.; La Greca, G. (Vicenza)

Vascular Access

13 Vascular Access Use and Outcomes: Results from the DOPPS
Pisoni, R.L. (Ann Arbor, Mich.)

20 How to Achieve a High Rate (90%) of Native Arteriovenous Fistulae
Konner, K. (Cologne)

31 Diagnostic Methods for Vascular Access: Access Flow Measurements
Leypoldt, J.K. (Salt Lake City, Utah)

38 Temporary Vascular Access for Hemodialysis Treatment. Current Guidelines and Future Directions
Weijmer, M.C.; ter Wee P.M. (Amsterdam)

46 Prosthetic Devices for Vascular Access
Quarello, F.; Forneris, G.; Pozzato, M. (Turin)

54 Effect of Hemodynamic Conditions on Arteriovenous Fistula for Hemodialysis Access
Ene-Iordache, B.; Bruno, S.; Remuzzi, A. (Ranica); Remuzzi, G. (Ranica/Bergamo)

60 Quality Assurance and Continuous Quality Improvement in the Management of Vascular Access
Bosch, J.P.; Walters, B.A.J. (Fort Lauderdale, Fla.)

Dialysis Membranes

70 **Membranes for Dialysis.** Composition, Structure and Function
Clark, W.R. (McGaw Park, Ill./Indianapolis, Ind.); Gao, D. (Lexington, Ky.); Ronco, C. (Vicenza)

78 **Methods of Sterilisation and Their Effects on Membrane Performance and Safety**
Gavioli, G. (Mirandola); Gennari, M. (Munich) Bruns, S. (Glandorf)

85 **Nano-Controlled Membrane Spinning Technology: Regulation of Pore Size, Distribution and Morphology of a New Polysulfone Dialysis Membrane**
Bowry, S.K. (Bad Homburg)

95 **Vitamin E-Modified Dialyzers**
Galli, F. (Perugia)

106 **Modified Cellulose Triacetate Membranes**
Masuda, T. (Osaka)

111 **The AN69ST Dialysis Membrane.** A New Approach for Reducing Systemic Heparinization
Renaux, J.-L.; Atti, M. (Lyon)

Hemodialyzers

120 **Flow Distribution and Cross Filtration in Hollow Fiber Hemodialyzers**
Ronco, C.; Brendolan, A.; Crepaldi, C.; Gastaldon, F. (Vicenza); Levin, N.W. (New York, N.Y.)

129 **Optimal Use of Hemodialyzers**
Leypoldt, J.K.; Cheung, A.K. (Salt Lake City, Utah)

138 **Sterilization Procedures and Biocompatibility**
Rodríguez-Benot, A.; Santamaría, R.; Martín-Malo, A.; Aljama, P. (Córdoba)

146 **Computerized Selection of Membranes and Hemodialyzers**
Ronco, C. (Vicenza); Ghezzi, P.M. (Cuneo) Hoenich, N.A. (Newcastle/New York, N.Y.); Delfino, P. (Cuneo)

Adsorbents

158 **Adsorbents: From Basic Structure to Clinical Application**
Ronco, C.; Bordoni, V. (Vicenza); Levin, N.W. (New York, N.Y.)

165 **Biocompatibility of Sorbent Systems**
Hoenich, N.A. (Newcastle upon Tyne)

170 **Sorbent Augmented Dialysis Systems**
Winchester, F.J. (New York, N.Y.); Ronco, C. (Vicenza); Salsberg, J.; Yousha, E.; Brady, J.A. (New York, N.Y.); Cowgill, L.D. (Davis, Calif.); Choquette, M.; Albright, R.; Clemmer, J. (New York, N.Y.); Davankov, V.; Tsyurupa, M.; Pavlova, L.; Pavlov, M. (Moscow); Cohen, G.; Hörl, W. (Vienna); Gotch, F. (San Francisco, Calif.,); Levin, N.W. (New York, N.Y.)

181 **Use of Adsorbents in ARF Therapy**
Tetta, C. (Mirandola); Bellomo, R. (Melbourne); Formica, M.; Livigni, S.; Mariano, F. (Turin); Wratten, M.L. (Mirandola); Carraro, G. (Padua); Ronco, C. (Vicenza)

Dialytic Techniques

189 **Low Flux Dialysis?** Still a Role
Hoenich, N.A. (Newcastle upon Tyne)

193 **High-Flux Hemodialysis and Hemodiafiltration.** Impact on Outcome
Locatelli, F.; Pozzoni, P.; Manzoni, C.; Di Filippo, S. (Lecco)

201 **On-Line Hemodiafiltration.** Gold Standard or Top Therapy?
Passlick-Deetjen, J. Pohlmeier, R. (Bad Homburg)

212 **New Options for On-Line Hemodiafiltration**
Tetta, C. (Mirandola); Ghezzi, P.M. (Cuneo); De Nitti, C.; Fiorenzi, A.; Cianciavicchia, D.; Gervasio, R. (Mirandola)

221 **On-Line Hemofiltration.** Old Concept – New Approach
Ledebo, I. (Lund)

227 **The Ideal Hemodialysis Machine**
Polaschegg, H.-D. (Köstenberg)

Dialysis Machines, Monitoring and Biofeedback

233 **Blood Volume Monitoring Systems and Biofeedback**
Santoro, A.; Mancini, E. (Bologna)

245 **Blood Temperature Monitor: A Novel Tool in the Management of Dialysis-Induced Hypotension**
van der Sande, F.M.; Kooman, J.P.; Leunissen, K.M.L. (Maastricht)

254 **Optimization of Convection on Hemodiafiltration by Transmembrane Pressure Monitoring and Biofeedback**
Pedrini, L.A.; De Cristofaro, V.; Pagliari, B.; Filippini, M.; Ruggiero, P. (Sondrio)

260 **Potassium Profiling in Acetate-Free Biofiltration**
Santoro, A.; Mancini, E. (Bologna); Fontanazzi, F.; Paolini, F. (Medolla)

268 **On-Line Clearance: Advanced Methodology to Monitor Adequacy of Dialysis at No Cost**
Gotch, F.A. (San Francisco, Calif.)

272 **Dry Weight Determination**
Levin, N.W. (New York, N.Y.); Folden, T.; Zhu, F. (New York, N.Y.), Ronco, C. (Vicenza)

Data Acquisition and Management

279 **Information Technology Applied to Hemodialysis**
Ronco, C. (Vicenza); Levin, N.W. (New York, N.Y.); Milan, M. (Vicenza)

287 **Practical Approach to Data Collection in a European Dialysis Network**
Hegbrant, J. (Lund/Denver, Colo.); Alper, A. (Denver, Colo.); Bosch, J.P. (Stockholm/Denver, Colo.)

293 **Data Management and Quality Assurance for Dialysis Network**
Marcelli, D.; Moscardó, V.; Steil, H.; Day, M.; Kirchgessner, J.; Mitteregger, A.; Orlandini, G.; Gatti, E. (Bad Homburg)

300 **Continuous Quality Improvement for a Hemodialysis Network**
Bosch, J.P.; Walters, B.A.J. (Fort Lauderdale, Fla.)

311 **Pre-End-Stage Renal Disease and Dialysis Programs: The View of the Manager**
Donald, L.L. (New York, N.Y.)

Dialysis Quality and Composition

317 **Water Treatment for Hemodialysis**
Cappelli, G.; Inguaggiato, P.; Ferramosca, E.; Albertazzi, A. (Modena)

325 **Dialysate Purity: A Must**
Ramírez, R.; Carracedo, J.; Martín-Malo, A.; Rodríguez, M.; Aljama, P. (Córdoba)

332 **On-Line Fluid Preparation**
Lonnemann, G. (Langenhagen)

338 **Sodium Content and Profiling**
Locatelli, F.; Colzani, S.; Pozzoni, P.; Manzoni, C.; Di Filippo, S. (Lecco)

344 **Dialysate/Infusate Composition and Infusion Mode in On-Line Hemodiafiltration**
Pedrini, L.A.; De Cristofaro, V.; Pagliari, B.; Ruggiero, P. (Bergamo)

350 **Dialysate/Infusate Calcium and Magnesium**
Vitale, C.; Marangella, M.; Ramello, A. (Turin)

357 **Dialysate/Infusate Buffer Modulation in Dialysis**
Feriani, M. (Mestre-Venezia)

Chronic Inflammation

364 **Chronic Inflammation: An Overview**
Levin, N.W. (New York, N.Y.); Ronco, C. (Vicenza)

371 Oxidant Stress in Hemodialysis Patients
Galli, F.; Floridi, A.; Buoncristiani, U. (Perugia)

379 End-Stage Renal Disease: A Slowly Progressive Systemic Inflammatory Response Syndrome
Ronco, C. (Vicenza); Levin, N.W. (New York, N.Y.)

386 LDL Modification during Hemodialysis. Markers for Oxidative Stress
Sevanian, A.; Asatryan, L. (Los Angeles, Calif.)

Anemia Management

396 Erythropoietin Therapy in Europe: Results from the DOPPS
Pisoni, R. (Ann Arbor, Mich.)

403 Clinical Experience with Darbepoetin-Alfa (Aranesp®)
Locatelli, F.; Del Vecchio, L.; Marai, P. (Lecco)

408 Once-Weekly Epoetin-Beta in Renal Anemia: The Clinical Evidence
Albertazzi, A. (Modena)

412 Iron Therapy in Hemodialysis Patients: How and When?
Crepaldi, C.; Bordoni, V.; Carta, M.R. (Vicenza)

426 Carnitine as Adjuvant Therapy in the Management of Renal Anemia
Cianciaruso, B.; Torraca, S.; De Blasio, A.; Fiorillo, M.; Marino, R. (Naples)

431 Erythropoietin Therapy and the Cardiovascular System
Santoro, A. (Bologna)

436 Author Index
438 Subject Index

Preface

Replacement of renal function by dialysis is a well-established form of treatment. The number of patients suffering from end-stage renal disease is continuously increasing and the combined challenge today is both to provide dialysis for all individuals who need it, and to provide a quality of therapy such as to improve medium and long-term outcomes. In this setting, hemodialysis technology can be of help for clinicians who prescribe the treatment and the nurses and technicians who deliver the prescribed therapy. Dialysis, however, is a rapidly changing field. The knowledge that physicians have in terms of machinery and disposables is estimated to last for a maximum of 5 years and if no refresher or educational courses are attended, large areas of ignorance can be expected. On the other hand, the knowledge of nurses and technicians who daily operate with new machines and the most recent devices has the risk of remaining superficial and mechanical if adequate information is not provided in terms of theory and the principles behind the practical procedures. For this reason, we feel that both for physicians and nurses this course can represent an invaluable occasion of education and information. The course is integrated in a program of continuous medical education generated by the Department of Nephrology of St. Bortolo Hospital in Vicenza, accredited with CME credits both by the Italian Ministry of Health and the UEMS (Union Européenne des Médecins Spécialistes). The course includes all the aspects related to the hemodialysis technology from the most basic to the most sophisticated.

An outstanding group of experts in the field discuss aspects related to vascular access and new forms of monitoring of access function. Anticoagulation strategies and antimicrobial treatment are debated with special emphasis on temporary catheters and prosthetic devices.

Membrane composition and structure, methods of sterilization and performance are discussed by a mixture of experts and manufacturers leading to a perfect integration of science, theory and manufacturing procedures. The same synthesis is achieved in the sessions related to hemodialyzers, adsorbent devices, dialysis techniques and machines. A new interest has also arisen in the possibility of computer-assisted data collection and managing. For this reason, experts in the field of electronic management of data together with managers of large dialysis networks are involved in the discussion of quality assurance and continuous quality improvement programs.

Special attention is given to dialysate and water purity since this is the starting point for newer dialytic techniques such as on-line hemodiafiltration. This is of paramount importance since chronic inflammation seems to represent one of the factors involved in long-term dialysis outcomes. In this view, the results obtained from the IDOPPS study are incorporated into the discussion of different practice patterns and anemia management could not be neglected. Finally, future trends are explored including automatic sensors and biofeedback monitors.

The format of the course is the one traditionally scheduled for the Vicenzanephrocourses. Every year a new event takes place but the topics (traditionally peritoneal dialysis, critical care nephrology and hemodialysis technology) are repeated only every 3 years. This year all the topics are presented by the most important and regarded experts in the field. In this course, the partnership between the academic world and industry is transparent and perfectly integrated. The final common target is the improvement of outcomes through the research and development of new technology. We are grateful to all the institutions, companies and individuals who made the event possible.

Claudio Ronco
Giuseppe La Greca

Ronco C, La Greca G (eds): Hemodialysis Technology.
Contrib Nephrol. Basel, Karger, 2002, vol 137, pp 1–12

The Role of Technology in Hemodialysis

Claudio Ronco, Giuseppe La Greca

Department of Nephrology, St. Bortolo Hospital, Vicenza, Italy

The Birth of Modern Hemodialysis

The birth of modern dialysis can be identified with a series of discoveries made in the 1960s. Based on the experience of Kolff [1] and other investigators [2], in the 1960s in acute renal failure, Scribner et al. [3] started the application of hemodialysis on a large scale in chronic renal failure. External arteriovenous (A-V) shunts were used as a vascular access [4]. Kiil plate dialyzers were employed [5] and dialysis machines including systems for dialysate preparation and delivery were developed in Seattle [6]. Subsequently, the shunt was modified into a silastic-teflon structure [7] until 1966 when the internal A-V fistula was proposed by Brescia and Cimino [8]. During the same years, bicarbonate was substituted with acetate in the dialysis bath [9] and both central delivery and single station dialysis systems were developed [9]. By the late 1960s, hollow fiber artificial kidneys were also manufactured and dialysis started to be performed out of hospital in self-care centers or even at home [10, 11]. Dialysis for chronic renal failure was no longer experimental. The problem of logistically organizing dialysis for all who needed it was the real challenge. The solution was in part offered by new technological advances that made dialysis more reliable and widely applicable.

The Search for Reliable Standards

The evolution of biomaterials and technology made dialysis easier and simpler in the 1970s leading to a dramatic growth in the number of patients on chronic renal replacement therapy. With the advent of internal A-V fistulas, by the end of the decade the external shunt was almost abandoned. However, this evolution brought the need for other technological advancements. Kiil dialyzers could originally be used without a blood pump because of their low internal resistance and the possibility of utilizing the A-V pressure gradient available in the external shunt. With the use of A-V fistulas and the increasing utilization of dialyzers with higher resistance, the blood pump became mandatory. With the advent of the pump-driven circulation, safety alarms and devices also became necessary in the new dialysis machines to prevent air embolism or other accidents. This, however, ensured a constant blood flow throughout the session with a consequent stability of treatment performance. As a further progress, dialysate delivery systems became more accurate utilizing controls in conductivity and temperature. Most of central delivery systems were transformed to single stations for hemodialysis to better meet single patient needs. Ultrafiltration control, however, was still very naive utilizing simple clamps on the venous or the dialysate outlet line.

Early Concepts of Adequacy and Prescription

In 1971, the Seattle group outlined the square meter hour hypothesis [12] and 1 year later, the same group suggested the middle-molecule hypothesis [13]. The use of a more open membrane to better remove larger solutes was proposed in France at the same time [14].

Approaching the mid-1970s, the dialysis duration was progressively reduced and the treatment schedule was set at three sessions/week [15]. In Italy, Cambi et al. [16] introduced the concept of short dialysis while in Germany, Quellhorst et al. [17] demonstrated the importance of ultrafiltration to remove middle molecular weight solutes. In the US, Henderson et al. [18] pointed out the mechanisms of convective transport across highly permeable membranes.

The square meter hour hypothesis and the middle molecule theory profoundly influenced dialysis strategies and generated much discussion on dialysis duration and dialyzer surface area [19]. The increasing number of treated patients also brought consequent organizational needs, to accommodate all patients who required renal replacement by hemodialysis. These needs together with the social requirement for full patient rehabilitation led to a progressive decrease in dialysis duration reaching an average schedule of 4–6 h per session 3 times a week. By the end of the decade, while the target of achieving reliable therapy and safe devices was reached, clinical tolerance was still an issue. As a consequence further steps in technology were made to solve some of the problems. Bicarbonate was proposed as a buffer instead of acetate whose negative effects had clearly been demonstrated [20]. Bicarbonate had originally been abandoned because of the ease of contamination in large central delivery systems. The use of bicarbonate was made possible by newer machines with the instantaneous preparation of fresh bicarbonate solution from acidic and basic concentrates [21].

Rapid Hemodialysis and the Search for Efficiency

The search for full patient rehabilitation and reduction of treatment time in the mid 1980s culminated in the advent of rapid hemodialysis. The National Cooperative Dialysis Study and its mechanistic analysis [22] had pointed out that a minimum dose of dialysis is necessary to reduce the risk of morbidity and treatment failure. Therefore, to effectively reduce treatment time without major clinical consequences, a parallel increase in the efficiency of treatment was definitely needed. Modifications in the available machines made it possible to achieve significantly higher performances. The feasibility of ultrashort hemodialysis sessions was demonstrated in different papers [23–25] and the satisfactory results were rapidly communicated to the scientific community. However, a precise warning was made concerning the technical requirements necessary to perform high-efficiency hemodialysis [26]. Blood flows higher than the standard 250 ml/min were required to achieve higher clearances. For this purpose, adequate large bore needles, calibrated pumps and precise pressure monitors in the circuit were needed. Because negative pressure in the prepump segment could reach 300 mm Hg, concerns were expressed about the capability of vascular accesses to tolerate blood flows up to 400–500 ml/min. However, thanks to the emerging Doppler flow measurements, studies were able to demonstrate that these flows are commonly present in mature A-V fistulas and no damage was induced by the use of high blood flows in the extracorporeal circuit [27]. Dialysis machines required accurate calibration of dialysate flow delivery, concentrate proportioning systems, deaeration and temperature of dialysate. Since high surface area dialyzers were employed, bicarbonate became mandatory as a buffer [28]. The increasing use of highly permeable membranes made ultrafiltration control systems indispensable to perform a well-tolerated hemodialysis session. Ultrafiltration was controlled in different machines by closed volumetric loops, single pass open volumetric chambers, ultrasonic flow meters, gravimetric balance or by Coriolis principle-based flowmeters [29]. All systems displayed a remarkable accuracy such that perfect fluid balance could be obtained in highly efficient rapid sessions.

Evolution of Techniqes, Membranes and Dialyzers

Classic cellulosic membranes such as Cuprophan were typically low-flux membranes (i.e. permeability to water in the range of 5–6 ml/h $\times$ mm Hg $\times$ m^2)

strongly hydrophilic and remarkably thin so as to permit an optimal utilization in diffusive treatments such as hemodialysis.

On the other hand, classic high-flux synthetic membranes were originally fully hydrophobic, strongly asymmetric and had a thick wall. They were principally employed in convective therapies such as hemofiltration due to their high hydraulic permeability (i.e. 30–40 ml/h $\times$ mm Hg $\times$ m^2) and their high sieving coefficients.

Only recently synthetic membranes have been designed with reduced wall thickness and mixed hydrophobic-hydrophilic structure. This has permitted their use in new techniques such as high-flux hemodialysis and hemodiafiltration [30] in which diffusion and convection are conveniently combined.

Today's dialysis is basically divided into two categories: low-flux dialysis and high-flux dialysis. Low-flux dialysis includes the standard hemodialysis technique in which dialyzers with low hydraulic permeability are utilized. Blood and dialysate flows are at 250 and 500 ml/min, respectively, and the average duration is 4 h. When the dialyzer surface area is increased, blood and dialysate flows are increased up to 400 and 800 ml/min, respectively; the treatment is defined as high-efficiency hemodialysis. In this treatment the clearance for small molecules is remarkably increased and the treatment time can generally be shortened, but the clearance for middle-large molecules is still very low due to the sieving characteristics of the membrane.

When high-flux membranes are utilized, three different approaches can be chosen: (1) hemofiltration is a fully convective treatment in which large amounts of ultrafiltrate are produced and replaced by a clean substitution fluid. No dialysis fluid is present. This technique offers the advantage of excellent clearances for large molecules. The treatment, however, has only been applied in Europe because of the need for large quantities of substitution fluid in commercially prepared bags. (2) Hemodiafiltration is a form of therapy in which diffusion and convection are conveniently combined. Dialysate is circulated countercurrent to blood but the amount of ultrafiltration exceeds the programmed patient weight loss and, therefore, the final fluid balance is achieved by the infusion in the venous line of appropriate amounts of substitution fluid. Several forms of hemodiafiltration including acetate-free hemodiafiltration, paired filtration dialysis and others have been proposed to obtain specific efficiency targets or particular forms of solute transport [31–33]. Due to high costs related to replacement solutions, new approaches have been proposed in Europe leading to on-line hemofiltration and hemodiafiltration [34]. Part of fresh dialysate is diverted from its line to the dialyzer, it is filtered and it is finally used as a replacement solution. These on-line treatments have the advantage of reduced costs and unlimited production of substitution fluid. On the other hand, the microbiological and chemical purity of the on-line produced fluid is essential. (3) High-flux dialysis is a technique in which highly permeable dialyzers are utilized in conjunction with an accurate ultrafiltration control. Because of the nature of the hollow fiber dialyzer, correct water balance is achieved thanks to an internal filtration in the proximal part and backfiltration in the distal part of the filter [35]. In this way, part of the advantages of hemodiafiltration are maintained with a simpler and easier layout of the technique [35]. Again, dialysate purity is a key issue in this treatment since it may affect the entire biocompatibility of the system [36].

During the evolution of techniques and membranes, the shape of hemodialyzers has remained basically unchanged. This has sometimes represented a problem of performance and control when highly permeable membranes began to be utilized. Accurate ultrafiltration control systems almost completely solved the problems of excessive ultrafiltration. Other problems of performance are today appearing due to the higher viscosity of blood in patients treated with recombinant human erythropoietin, and to the higher dialysate flows employed in highly efficient treatments. The first problem is substantially dealing with an inadequate distribution of the blood flow within the fiber bundle, presenting maximal velocity of the flow in the central region and minimal velocity in the peripheral fibers [37]. Such a problem may result in very low wall shear rates in peripheral fibers with easy clotting and poor capacity for solute transport in that region of the dialyzer where, in turn, dialysate flow is maximal. This problem has been partially overcome by the application of special blood flow distributors that permit today a rather homogeneous distribution of the flow in the blood compartment. Special diagnostic techniques have been developed to study this phenomenon [38]. Similar diagnostic procedures have also been utilized for studying the distribution of flow in the dialysate compartment [39]. In standard dialyzers, there was a poor penetration of dialysate in the central part of the bundle, while the maximal velocity of dialysate was experienced in the external part of the bundle. Special construction technology based on the use of spacing filaments external to fibers or the application of a peculiar 'moiré' structure (microondulation) keeping the fibers separated permit the distribution of the dialysate flow to be more homogeneous, leading to a more efficient exchange between blood and dialysate [39]. Further studies are designed today to create newer shapes and new configurations in the dialyzer for the future [40] aiming at increasing performance and reliability. A full family of membranes has been created in recent years with a wide possibility of choice. The most interesting aspects are related to the selectivity of these membranes, their high sieving coefficients, their high biocompatibility and finally the application of nanotechnology to the spinning procedure for a precise construction process resulting in improved performances.

From Treatment Personalization to Biofeedback

Personalization: Prescribing a Treatment for Each Individual

Since the beginning of renal replacement therapy, different approaches have been tried out to identify a minimal or adequate 'dose' of treatment. This concept highlights that each patient has individual needs and specific requirements in terms of blood purification. Individual tolerance may also vary even in the presence of similar treatments. In detail, a need for treatment individualization and personalization has emerged clearly over the years.

Several studies have demonstrated that nutritional status and morbidity of patients undergoing chronic hemodialysis are correlated with the amount of dialysis delivered [41–44]. The mechanistic analysis of the National Cooperative Dialysis Study [22] led Gotch and Sargent to identify Kt/V as an index of dialysis dose. The role of kinetic analysis in the determination of urea generation rate (G), protein catabolic rate and urea distribution volume (V) has then become crucial to identify a personalized prescription of dialysis therapy [45–48]. The measure of these parameters has become a tool to uncover possible discrepancies between original prescription and effective delivery of dialysis. Several factors are known to influence such discrepancy; among them, the effective calculation of treatment time, effective blood flow, vascular access recirculation, double pool kinetics and effective dialyzer clearance are the most widely recognized [49–51]. The use of urea kinetics to measure dialysis delivery has, however, faced a series of problems due to the sporadic nature of the measurement and the complexity of kinetic formulas. The last aspect has been claimed to be the main cause for under-use of urea kinetics in quality assurance programs. On the other hand, monthly measurement of Kt/V is not sufficient to describe what kind of treatment and dialysis dose the patient is receiving on a regular basis. As regards clinical tolerance, variations in blood pH or serum potassium and other electrolytes have demonstrated that the patient's values may vary significantly throughout the session. In other words, what is adequate at the beginning of dialysis in terms of ultrafiltration, dialysate conductivity and buffer concentration may not be adequate in the subsequent hours of treatment. For all these reasons, a further step was tested some years ago proposing the concept of treatment profiling [52].

Profiling the Session to Meet Individual Actual Needs

The advent of computers in hemodialysis profoundly modified the way in which dialysis machines were conceived. The dialysis machine, till now based on hydraulic components with minimal electronic controls, began to be equipped with electronic hardware and software. In other words it became possible to modify dialysis treatment parameters throughout the session according to specific preset instructions [51]. Thus, ultrafiltration could be programmed at a variable rate in different moments of the session setting for example maximal rates at the beginning and minimal values in the last minutes. These instructions were contained in specific software and were physically actuated via hardware with the regulation of the transmembrane pressure and the ultrafiltration control system. The same approach could be tried for dialysate conductivity, by increasing dialysate sodium concentration in the last part of the session when hypotension is more likely to occur and the process of plasma volume refilling may be slowed down when the patient is approaching dry body weight. Unfortunately, the assumption that the patient should better tolerate high ultrafiltration at the beginning of the session and higher conductivity at the end of the treatment, which should help prevent hypotension appeared inconsistent and this approach failed to achieve the desired targets. It was clear that the basic reason for failure was the 'blind' preset profile of dialysis parameters that was based on assumptions and empirical observations and not on objective signals and data collected from the patient via an accurate monitoring system. The need for on-line signals emerged clearly [52].

Monitoring in Dialysis

During dialysis, assessment of the patient is normally limited to the occasional measurement of body weight and blood pressure, with therapeutic intervention only upon the appearance of symptoms or side effects. A more perceptive monitoring of the patient from a biochemical and physical standpoint might enable early recognition of signs of intolerance where action needs to be taken.

The development of dialysis technology and the extensive application of electronics and information technology have paved the way for the realization of systems and devices dedicated to real-time and continuous measurement of chemical-physical signals coming from the dialysis patient [53–60]. The meaning of monitoring can be easily seen in the subsequent possibility to analyze the collected data, to evaluate their acceptability and to plan any possible intervention to modify conditions that are not considered acceptable. In these years, clinical demands and technological progress have given rise to a series of on-line monitoring systems. On-line monitoring is today possible for different parameters such as conductivity, urea kinetics, blood volume changes, thermal balance and access recirculation [52–54, 60–65].

The Biofeedback Approach

For a certain period of time, on-line monitoring devices were considered as toys rather than real tools for routine clinical application. The purpose of these biosensors was to identify as early as possible inadequate performances of the treatment or physiological abnormalities induced by the treatment with consequent patient discomfort and dialysis-related side effects. The problem was corrected by the nurse or the physician after a careful evaluation of the collected signals and after a remarkable latency often leading to intervention carried out too late to prevent the problem. To imitate what happens in nature where rapid feedbacks occur in response to physiological signals, an automatic biofeedback loop has also been proposed for hemodialysis [65]. In an attempt to prevent the occurrence of dialysis hypotension, signals coming from biosensors such as blood volume changes and conductivity measures have been integrated in a multi-input controller able to provide via software a series of output signals that result in variations of treatment parameters. Corrections are practically actuated by changes in the rate of ultrafiltration and in the dialysate inlet conductivity. Instead of waiting for late authorized feedback operated by the nurse, the multi-input-multi-output controller tends to reach the selected target of intradialytic weight loss and maximal tolerance by a continuous compromise between ultrafiltration, conductivity and effective weight loss. This type of automatic biofeedback has been utilized in multiple sessions demonstrating a significant capacity of reducing the incidence of hypotension during treatment. Biofeedback loops could also be used to modify blood flow rates in response to inadequately predicted Kt/V by a urea sensor. Variations in absolute body temperature at the end of dialysis or the effective thermal balance in a session can be obtained by modifying the dialysate inlet temperature according to on-line blood temperature monitoring. Plasma sodium concentrations at the end of a dialysis session can be targeted and the wanted results can be obtained by accurate variations in dialysate conductivity operated as a feedback to the conductivity sensor. These and other implementations may be expected as a further impact of technology on the continuous search for reliability, efficiency and clinical tolerance.

Present and Future Issues

The question arising today is whether these new technologies should be considered as tools or toys, whether they will have an impact on outcomes and finally whether we will be able to afford the application of these devices to all our patients with the consequent complex financial issues.

We are today certainly more limited in our modern hemodialysis by the nature of the human physiology than by the available tools and materials. However, new discoveries tend to be immediately applied to the edge of dialysis research to find a more effective and reliable renal replacement. It is true that today dialysis is no longer experimental, but it is also true that we cannot content ourselves simply by making the patient survive. We need to go further by improving long-term clinical outcomes and the quality of life of our patients. In this sense we should not forget our mission as physicians and we should consider technology an important aid but not a substitute for good clinical practice and humanity.

Our patients are getting sicker and older. The expenditure for healthcare is increasing despite efforts to constrain the budgets. The demand for high-quality medical care is increasing at a time when resources appear to be limited. The additional cost for high technology requires strong evidence of utility and efficacy. Once this hurdle has been overcome, the cost of technology may be absorbed by a lower rate of hospitalization or other positive outcome measures. The application on a large scale of a single device will also permit to reduce production and distribution costs.

We are always struggling to move ahead from where we are. It is hard to say whether we will be able to do it, but certainly we cannot afford to go back.

References

1 Kolff WJ: Dialysis in the treatment of uremia. Arch Intern Med 1954;94:142–147.
2 Bywaters EGL, Joeckes BM: The artificial kidney: Its clinical application in the treatment of traumatic anuria. Proc R Soc Med 1948;41:411–420.
3 Scribner BH, Buri R, Caner JEZ, Hegstrom R, Burnell JM: The treatment of chronic uremia by means of intermittent hemodialysis: A preliminary report. Trans Am Soc Artif Intern Organs 1960;6:114–120.
4 Quinton WE, Dillard D, Scribner BH: Cannulation of blood vessels for prolonged hemodialysis. Trans Am Soc Artif Intern Organs 1960;6:104–108.
5 Kiil F, Amundsen B: Development of a parallel flow artificial kidney in plastics. Acta Chir Scand Suppl 1960;253:142–149.
6 Scribner BH, Caner JEZ, Buri R, Quinton WE: The technique of continuous hemodialysis. Trans Am Soc Artif Intern Organs 1960;6:88–94.
7 Ramirez O, Swartz C, Onesti G, Mailloux L, Brest AN: The winged in-line shunt. Trans Am Soc Artif Intern Organs 1966;12:220–223.
8 Brescia MJ, Cimino JE, Appel K, Hurwitz BJ: Chronic hemodialysis using venipuncture and a surgically created arterio-venous fistula. N Engl J Med 1966;275:1089–1091.
9 Mion CM, Hegstrom RM, Boen ST, Scribner BH: Substitution of sodium acetate for bicarbonate in the bath fluid for hemodialysis. Trans Am Soc Artif Intern Organs 1964;10:110–114.
10 Scribner BH, Babb AL: Chronic hemodialysis in Seattle 1960–1966. Part II. Dial Transplant 1982;11:324–330.
11 Merrill JP, Schupak E, Cameron E, Hampers CL: Hemodialysis in the home. Trans Am Soc Artif Intern Organs 1965;11:7–12.
12 Babb AL, Popovich RP, Christopher TG, Scribner BH: The genesis of the square meter-hour hypothesis. Trans Am Soc Artif Intern Organs 1971;17:81–86.
13 Babb AL, Farrell PC, Uvelli DA, Scribner BH: Hemodialyzer evaluation by solute molecular spectra. Trans Am Soc Artif Intern Organs 1972;18:98–103.
14 Funck-Brentano JL: Experience with a new open membrane. Proc Clin Dial Transplant Forum 1971;1:56–63.

15 Gurland HJ, Brunner FP, Chantler C, Jacobs C, Scharer K, Selwood NH, Spies G, Wing AJ: Combined report on regular dialysis and transplantation in Europe. Part VI. Proc Eur Dial Transplant Assoc 1976;13:3–9.

16 Cambi V, Savazzi G, Arisi L, Bignardi L, Bruschi L, Rossi E, Migone L: Short dialysis schedule (SDS) – Finally ready to become routine? Proc Eur Dial Transplant Assoc 1974;11:112–118.

17 Reiger J, Quellhorst E, Lowitz HD, Kong RG, Scheler F: Ultrafiltration for middle molecules in uremia. Proc Eur Dial Transplant Assoc 1974;11:158–165.

18 Henderson LW, Colton CK, Ford CA: Kinetics of hemodiafiltration: Clinical characterization of a new blood cleansing modality. J Lab Clin Med 1975;85:355–361.

19 Babb AL, Strand MJ, Uvelli DA, Multinovic J, Scribner BH: Quantitative description of dialysis treatment: A dialysis index. Kidney Int 1975;7(suppl 2):S23–S27.

20 Scribner BH: Substitution of bicarbonate for acetate in the dialysate for the care of a critically ill patient. Dial Transplant 1977;6/3:26–30.

21 Ward RA, Wathen RL, Williams TE: Effects of long-term bicarbonate hemodialysis (BHD) on acid-base status. Trans Am Soc Artif Intern Organs 1982;28:295–301.

22 Gotch F, Sargent JA: A mechanistic analysis of the National Cooperative Dialysis Study (NCDS). Kidney Int 1985;28:526–531.

23 Rotellar E, Martinez E, Samsò JM, Barrios J, Simò R, Mulero JF, Perez D, Bandres S, Pinol J: Why dialyze more than six hours a week? Trans Am Soc Artif Intern Organs 1985;31: 538–541.

24 Miller JH, von Albertini B, Gardner PW, Shinaberger JH: Technical aspects of high flux hemodiafiltration for adequate short (under 2 hours) treatment. Trans Am Soc Artif Intern Organs 1984; 30:377–380.

25 Keshaviah P, Collins A: Rapid high efficiency hemodialysis. Trans Am Soc Artif Intern Organs 1986;32:17–21.

26 Ronco C, Fabris A, Chiaramonte S, De Dominicis E, Feriani M, Brendolan A, Bragantini L, Milan M, Dell'Aquila R, La Greca G: Comparison of four different short hemodialysis techniques. Int J Artif Organs 1988;3:169–174.

27 Ronco C, Fabris A, Chiaramonte S, De Dominicis E, Feriani M, Brendolan A, Bragantini L, Milan M, Dell'Aquila R, La Greca G: Impact of high blood flows on vascular stability in hemodialysis. Nephrol Dial Transplant 1990;1(suppl 5):109–114.

28 Tolchin DO: Acetate metabolism and high efficiency hemodialysis. Int J Artif Organs 1979;2:1–6.

29 Ronco C, Fabris A, Feriani M, Chiaramonte S, Brendolan A, Bragantini L, Milan M, Dell'Aquila R, Conz P, Frigato G, Borra M, von Albertini B, La Greca G: Technical and clinical evaluation of a new system for ultrafiltration control during hemodialysis. Trans Am Soc Artif Intern Organs 1988;3:613–615.

30 Bosch JP, von Albertini B, Ronco C: Hemofiltration and hemodiafiltration; in Glassock RJ (ed): Current Therapy in Nephrology and Hypertension, ed 2. Toronto, BC Decker, 1987, pp 258–263.

31 Santoro A, Spongano M, Ferrari G, Zucchelli P: Analysis of the factors influencing bicarbonate balance during acetate free biofiltration. Kidney Int 1993;43(suppl 41):S184–S187.

32 Ghezzi PM, Frigato G, Fantini GF, et al: Theoretical model and first clinical results of the paired filtration dialysis. Life Support Syst 1983(suppl 1):271–278.

33 Feriani M, Ronco C, Biasioli S, Bragantini L, La Greca G: Effect of dialysate and substitution fluid buffer on buffer flux in hemodiafiltration. Kidney Int 1991;39:711–717.

34 Canaud B, Imbert E, Kaaki M, Assounga A, Nguyen QV, Stec F, Garred LJ, Bostrom M, Mion C: Clinical and microbiological evaluation of a postdilutional hemofiltration system with inline production of substitution fluid. Blood Purif 1990;8:160–170.

35 Ronco C: Backfiltration in clinical dialysis: Nature of the phenomenon, mechanisms and possible solutions. Int J Artif Organs 1990;13:11–21.

36 Ronco C, Brendolan A, Crepaldi C: Water and dialysate treatment for hemodialysis; in Bosch JP (ed): Hemodialysis; High Efficiency Treatments. New York, Churchill Livingstone, 1993, pp 41–61.

37 Ronco C, Ghezzi PM, Brendolan A, Crepaldi C, La Greca G: The haemodialysis system: Basic mechanism of water and solute transport in extracorporeal renal replacement therapies. Nephrol Dial Transplant 1998;13(suppl 6):3–9.

38 Brendolan A, Ronco C, Ghezzi PM, Scabardi M, La Greca G: Hydraulic and flow-dynamic characteristics of PMMA dialyzers. Contrib Nephrol. Basel, Karger, 1998, vol 125, pp 41–52.
39 Ronco C, Scabardi M, Goldoni M, Brendolan A, Crepaldi C, La Greca G: Impact of spacing filaments external to hollow fibers on dialysate flow distribution and dialyzer performance. Int J Artif Organs 1997;20:261–266.
40 Ronco C, Orlandini G, Brendolan A, Lupi A, La Greca G: Enhancement of convective transport by internal filtration in a modified experimental hemodialyzer. Kidney Int 1998;54:979–985.
41 Lowrie EG, Laird NM, Parker TF, Sargent JA: Effect on the hemodialysis prescription on patient morbidity. N Engl J Med 1981;20:1176–1181.
42 US Renal Data System: USRDS 1991 Annual Data Report. Bethesda, National Institutes of Health, National Institute of Diabetes and Digestive and Kidney Diseases, 1991, pp D.1–E.62.
43 Acchiardo SR, Hatten KW, Ruvinsky MS, Dyson B, Fuller J, Moore LW: Inadequate dialysis increases gross mortality rate. ASAIO J 1992;38:M282–M285.
44 Levin NW, Gotch FA, Daugirdas JT, Teschan PE, Collins AJ, Keshaviah P: What is the role of Kt/V urea in chronic dialysis. Semin Dial 1990;3/2:73–74.
45 Jindal KK, Manuel A, Goldstein MB: Percent reduction of the blood urea concentration during hemodialysis (PRU), a simple and accurate method of estimate Kt/V urea. Trans Am Soc Artif Intern Organs 1987;33:286–288.
46 Daugirdas JT: Rapid methods of estimating Kt/V: Three formulas compared. ASAIO Trans 1990; 36:M362–M364.
47 Garred LJ, Canaud BC, McCready WG: Optimal hemodialysis: The role of quantification. Semin Dial 1994;1/4:236–245.
48 Schneditz D, Polaschegg HD, Levin NW, et al: Caridopulmonary recirculation in dialysis. An underrecognized phenomenon. ASAIO J 1992;38:M194–M196.
49 Sargent JA: Shortfalls in the delivery of dialysis. Am J Kidney Dis 1990;15:500–510.
50 Depner TA: Assessing adequacy of hemodialysis: Urea modeling. Kidney Int 1994;45:1522–1535.
51 Peticlerc T, Man NK, Goureau Y, Jepenne G, Funck-Brentano JL: Optimization of sodium dialysate concentration by plasma water conductivity monitoring; in Nosé Y, Kjellestrand C, Ivanovich P (eds): Progress in Artificial Organs. New York, Isao Press, 1985.
52 Locatelli F, Di Filippo S, Manzoni C: Monitoring sodium removal and delivered dialysis by conductivity. Int J Artif Organs 1995;18:716–721.
53 Santoro A: On-line monitoring (editorial). Nephrol Dialysis Transplant 1995;10:615–618.
54 Keshaviah P, Ebben J, Luhving D, Emmerson P: Clinical evaluation of new on-line monitor of dialysis adequacy. J Am Soc Nephrol 1992;3:374.
55 Thomaseth K: PANSYM: A symbolic equation generation for mathematical modeling, analysis and control of metabolic and pharmacokinetic systems. Comput Methods Programs Biomed 1994; 42:99–112.
56 Thavarungkul P, Makanson H, Holst O, Mattianson B: Continuous monitoring of urea in blood during dialysis. Biosens Bioelectron 1991;6:323–328.
57 Lindsay R, Heidenheim P, Abunadar P, McCarthy G: On-line urea kinetic modeling: Preliminary results. Nephrol Dial Transplant 1993;8:995–996.
58 Depner T, Collins A, Jindal K, et al: Multicenter clinical validation of an on-line urea monitor (abstract). J Am Soc Nephrol 1993;4:343–347.
59 Garred LS, Amour NRST, McCready WG, Canaud BC: Urea kinetic modelling with a prototype urea sensor in the spent dialysate stream. ASAIO J 1993;39:M337–M341.
60 Stiller S, Wirt UD, Waterbar F, Gladziwa U, Dashnamurty KV, Mann H: Less symptomatic hypotension using BV-controlled ultrafiltration. Trans Am Soc Artif Int Organs 1991;37:139–141.
61 Ronco C, Bellomo R: Central circulation, peripheral circulation and recirculation. Blood Purif 1997;15:334–345.
62 Ronco C, Brendolan A, Crepaldi C, Frisone P, Ghiotto F, Zamboni S, Gastaldon F, La Greca G: On-line urea monitoring: A further step towards adequate dialysis prescription and delivery. Int J Artif Organs 1995;9:534–543.
63 Depner TA: Techniques for prospective detection of venous stenosis. Adv Ren Replace Ther 1994;1:119–130.

64 Krivitski NM: Theory and validation of access flow measurement by dilution technique during hemodialysis. Kidney Int 1995;48:244–250.
65 Santoro A, Mancini E, Paolini F, Cavicchioli G, Bosetto A, Zucchelli P: Blood volume regulation during hemodialysis. Am J Kidney Dis 1998;32:739–748.

Dr. Claudio Ronco, Department of Nephrology,
St. Bortolo Hospital, I–36100 Vicenza (Italy)
Tel. +39 0444 993869, Fax +39 0444 920693, E-Mail cronco@goldnet.it

Ronco C, La Greca G (eds): Hemodialysis Technology.
Contrib Nephrol. Basel, Karger, 2002, vol 137, pp 13–19

Vascular Access Use and Outcomes: Results from the DOPPS

Ronald L. Pisoni

University Renal Research and Education Association (URREA), Ann Arbor, Mich., USA

The Dialysis Outcomes and Practice Patterns Study (DOPPS) is an international prospective, longitudinal study examining the relationships between dialysis unit practices and outcomes for hemodialysis (HD) patients [1]. Since 1996, the 7 countries of France, Germany, Italy, Japan, Spain, the United Kingdom, and the United States (US) have participated in DOPPS, each for a minimum of 2 years. These countries have contributed longitudinal mortality data for >50,000 HD patients, and detailed patient data for nearly 20,000 patients at >300 dialysis units. Beginning in 2002, DOPPS is further extending to the countries of Australia, Belgium, Canada, New Zealand and Sweden. DOPPS is designed to provide nationally representative patient samples by randomly selecting dialysis units within each country to achieve a representative distribution of dialysis units by geographic region and unit type. The international scope of DOPPS provides representation for ~80% of the world's in-center HD practice. The large size of DOPPS coupled with its study design provides an especially powerful approach for investigating HD practices that yield the best outcomes for HD patients. The following is a brief summary of some recent findings concerning vascular access (VA) use and outcomes from DOPPS.

Prevalence of VA Use in Europe and US

An analysis of prevalent VA use in DOPPS has indicated a high use of native arteriovenous fistulae (AVF) in the five European DOPPS countries of

France, Germany, Italy, Spain and the UK (referred to as EUR). Within EUR, prevalent AVF use varies from 67% in the United Kingdom to 90% in Italy [2]. In contrast, AVF are used by only 25% of US patients, with synthetic and bovine grafts serving as the predominant access type for 58% of US HD patients. There has been a small increase in AVF use in the US from 24 to 27% for the years 1997–2000, but these levels remain below the 40% target level recommended in the 1997 NKF-DOQI guidelines for AVF use [3].

Results from DOPPS indicate that AVF versus graft use is not dictated by the ability to achieve a predetermined targeted blood flow rate. In the US, with its substantial use of grafts and AVF, the same median prescribed blood flow rate of 400 ml/min is observed for patients dialyzing with an AVF or a graft [Port et al., unpubl. results]. Furthermore, lower blood flow rates can be used for AVF with excellent results as indicated in EUR where AVF are typically used at blood flow rates of approximately 300 ml/min.

Estimates of the prevalence of catheter use indicate that catheters account for 17% of VA use in the US compared with 8% in EUR [2]. Tunneled catheters comprise 69% of catheters in EUR and 59% of catheters in the US among prevalent patients.

VA Use among New HD Patients in EUR and US

Countries exhibiting high AVF use for prevalent patients also display high AVF use for new HD patients when initiating dialysis. In EUR, approximately 65% of new ESRD patients start HD with an AVF compared with 15% in the US [2]. Furthermore, only 2–3% of incident patients start HD with a synthetic graft in EUR, whereas 24% of new HD patients start HD with a synthetic graft in the US. An interesting finding in comparing access use in EUR and the US was that AVF use was less likely for patients treated in dialysis units in which surgery trainees either assisted or performed permanent VA placements (adjusted odds ratio = 0.61, p = 0.04) [2]. This latter result suggests that graft placement may be emphasized to a greater extent in surgical training settings or that trainees are not adequately prepared to create functioning AVF in a diverse patient population.

US HD patients have a greater level of comorbidity than HD patients in EUR [4]. However, subgroup analyses restricted to patients of similar comorbidity and other analyses adjusted for differences in patient mix strongly suggest that the much higher use of grafts in the US compared with EUR is largely due to differences in VA preferences by practitioners rather than dictated by patient characteristics [2, 5].

AVF and Graft Survival: AVF Survival in EUR and US

For new ESRD patients starting HD with a graft or AVF, case-mix-adjusted survival curves have indicated better access survival for AVF than for grafts (risk ratio of AVF vs. graft failure = 0.56, $p < 0.001$). This result is similar to that found in other studies [2]. Furthermore, for incident patients using AVF, an adjusted risk ratio of 0.49 ($p < 0.001$) was observed for AVF failure in EUR versus the US. The reasons for the 2-fold greater longevity of AVF in EUR compared with the US are not known at the present time.

Facility Characteristics Yielding High AVF Use

The continuing higher use of synthetic grafts compared with AVF in the US has occurred despite numerous studies indicating better survival for AVF than for grafts [2], a severalfold greater number of procedures associated with grafts compared with AVF [6], and case-mix-adjusted annual costs shown to be marginally higher for grafts than AVF [7]. Some common themes learned from facilities successful in placing AVF at a high rate in a broad range of patients [8, 9] have been: (1) a strong commitment to AVF as the permanent access of first choice for nearly all patients, which is facilitated by a multidisciplinary health care structure well trained in placement, referral, needling and maintenance of AVF, (2) applying a highly skilled surgical technique with variations in procedure to successfully accommodate differences in patient vasculature and comorbidity, and (3) devising a system of care that minimizes delays in AVF placement during the pre-ESRD period.

High Catheter Use among New ESRD Patients when Starting HD

Catheter use is very common among new ESRD patients, with 60% of US patients and 31% of EUR patients starting HD with a catheter [2]. Part of the explanation for this high catheter use among incident patients is that 16% of EUR and 26% of US incident patients first present to a nephrologist less than 30 days prior to ESRD. However, a striking statistic is that 46% of US patients and 25% of EUR patients start HD with a catheter and have not had a permanent VA created prior to starting HD. For this large group of patients who start HD with a catheter but have not had a permanent access created prior to starting HD, more than half (55%) had seen a nephrologist for >1 month prior to starting HD [2].

Table 1. Factors affecting ability of dialysis units to increase the proportion of new ESRD patients starting HD with a native AVF

Proportion of patients seen by a nephrologist >4 months prior to ESRD
Early referral of patients for access surgery
Creation of AVF soon after referral for surgery (e.g. <2 weeks)
Availability of skill among dialysis staff to successfully needle AVF in a relatively short time period (e.g. 25–60 days)
Surgical technique and success rate: fraction of first AVF placements that successfully mature into functioning accesses

The high use of catheters among incident patients can have detrimental consequences for future permanent access survival. Recent studies indicate that prior catheter use is associated with a 1.4- to 2.1-fold higher risk of failure for subsequently used grafts or AVF, and that the side and location of the temporary access relative to the permanent access are important factors associated with survival of subsequently used permanent VAs [2, 10, 11; Rayner et al., unpubl. results]. Improved VA outcomes may be achieved for new ESRD patients if the proportion of patients starting HD with a functioning AVF is increased. Five important factors relevant to increasing the fraction of new ESRD patients starting with an AVF are listed in table 1.

Proportion of Patients Seen by a Nephrologist > 4 Months Prior to ESRD

In order for a new ESRD patient to start HD with an AVF, the patient must present to the nephrologist early enough so the nephrologist can accurately establish the patient's state of renal insufficiency, refer the patient for access placement, and allow sufficient time for access maturation prior to the projected date of ESRD onset. Patient responses in DOPPS have indicated that 80% of incident patients in EUR and 68% in the US have seen a nephrologist more than 4 months prior to ESRD [2]. At least 4 months of pre-ESRD care are generally required in order for a large fraction of new patients to have an opportunity to initiate HD with AVF. This is to accommodate (1) the wide variation in the time necessary for access maturation depending upon the nature of a patient's vasculature, and (2) the considerable imprecision associated with predicting the onset of ESRD.

Creation of AVF Soon after Referral for Surgery

A striking variation, ranging from less than 2 weeks to as long as 4 months, has been observed among EUR and US DOPPS facilities regarding the time from referral to permanent access creation [2]. Incident patients treated in facilities in which permanent VA were created ≤2 weeks from date of referral had a 1.76 higher adjusted odds ratio of starting HD with a permanent VA ($p = 0.002$). Therefore, units which minimize the time between referral and permanent access creation enhance the probability for a new ESRD patient to begin HD with a permanent VA.

Development of Skill to Successfully Needle AVF in a Relatively Short Time Period

Rayner et al. [unpubl. results] have found that for new ESRD patients, the median time for first cannulation of AVF varies from 25 to 98 days across the different countries in DOPPS. Furthermore, countries with a low median time for first needling of AVF do not show worse adjusted AVF survival rates than countries with long median needling times. These results indicate that dialysis practice in some settings has evolved to successfully cannulate AVF in a relatively short time period. This skill allows patients within these dialysis units a greater opportunity to start dialysis with a functioning AVF rather than with a catheter. This ability to successfully cannulate AVF in a short time period is advantageous to dialysis units because it provides flexibility in not having to refer patients quite as early for AVF creation and it can allow units to successfully accommodate patients who may first present to the nephrologist 2–3 months prior to ESRD. However, facilities with long median needling times (>100 days) are placed in the position of having to refer the majority of patients for AVF creation at least 4 months prior to ESRD in order to have 65–70% of all new ESRD patients starting HD with an AVF.

Surgical Success Rate: Fraction of First AVF Placements That Successfully Mature into Functioning Accesses

As Konner [12] and others have recently reported, there are many important aspects of creating an AVF for a broad range of patients. The physical examination, vasculature mapping and expertise in surgically creating different types of AVF are critical in creating AVF that will successfully function for a diverse patient population. The surgical success rate impacts the probability of new ESRD patients being able to start HD with a functioning AVF.

Patients in Facilities with High Catheter Use Have Higher Hospitalization and Mortality Risks

Catheters often are viewed as a temporary access for HD patients until an AVF or graft is ready for use. However, recent results from DOPPS suggest that in some facilities, central vein catheters are routinely used for dialysis in a large proportion of patients. In EUR and US DOPPS, 15% of facilities displayed high catheter use in which 28–52% of prevalent patients within these facilities were dialyzing with a catheter. Part of this high prevalence of catheter use within these units is due to the extended use of tunneled central vein catheters. Part of this high prevalence of catheter use within these units is due to the extended use of tunneled central vein catheters. Whereas untunneled temporary catheters are used for only brief periods of time ranging from 0 to 2 months, tunneled catheters are used for many months in numerous instances [13].

Adjusted rates for VA infection in DOPPS have been found to be 7-fold higher for catheters compared with AVF or grafts [14]. When outcomes of hospitalization and mortality were examined, patients treated in high-catheter-use facilities were found to have substantially higher adjusted risks for infectious hospitalizations, all-cause hospitalization and mortality [13]. The higher risk of hospitalization for infections is likely due to the higher rates of infection associated with catheters compared with AVF or grafts. The reasons for higher all-cause hospitalization and mortality in facilities with high catheter use are being evaluated further. These findings of higher morbidity agree with the observation of a higher risk of mortality with catheters than with permanent AV access [15].

Conclusion

Large differences are seen across countries and facilities concerning VA practice. AVF are recognized as the preferred VA for most HD patients in the majority of dialysis practices. Some important factors associated with successful implementation of AVF for a large fraction of patients have been described. However, the high use of catheters among new ESRD patients continues to be seen across countries with the possible detrimental effect of an association with higher morbidity and decreased survival of subsequently used permanent AV accesses. Organizational and facility practices observed in DOPPS have been important in understanding approaches for increasing AVF use for ESRD patients starting HD therapy.

Acknowledgment

Funding for DOPPS was provided by a scientific educational grant from Kirin-Amgen.

References

1 Young EW, Goodkin DA, Mapes DL, Port FK, Keen ML, Chen K, Maroni BL, Wolfe RA, Held PJ: The Dialysis Outcomes and Practice Patterns Study (DOPPS): An international hemodialysis study. Kidney Int 2000;57(suppl 74):S74–S81.

2 Pisoni RL, Young EW, Dykstra DM, Greenwood RN, Hecking E, Gillespie B, Wolfe RA, Goodkin DA, Held PJ: Vascular access use in Europe and the United States: Results from the DOPPS. Kidney Int 2002;61:305–316.
3 Schwab S, Besarab A, Beathard G, Brouwer D, Etheredge E, Hartigan M, Levine M, McCann R, Sherman R, Trerotola S: National Kidney Foundation DOQI: Clinical practice guidelines for hemodialysis vascular access. Am J Kidney Dis 1997;30(suppl 3):S150–S189.
4 Goodkin DA, Mapes DL, Held PJ: The Dialysis Outcomes and Practice Patterns Study (DOPPS): How can we improve the care of hemodialysis patients? Semin Dial 2001;14:157–159.
5 Goodkin DA, Chen K, Held PJ, Keen ML, Mapes DL, Maroni BJ, Port FK, Wolfe RA, Young EW, Pisoni RL: Factors influencing type of permanent vascular access at start of hemodialysis. Proceedings of the 8th Annual Clinical Nephrology Meeting, National Kidney Foundation, Washington, D.C., 1999, pp 187–188.
6 Hakim R, Himmelfarb J: Hemodialysis access failure: A call to action. Kidney Int 1998;54: 1029–1040.
7 Collins A, Chen S, Ebben J, Ma J: Bridge catheters as transitional devices for vascular access: A cost-effectiveness study. J Am Soc Nephrol 1999;10:203A.
8 Allon M, Bailey R, Ballard R, Deierhoi MH, Hamrick K, Oser R, Rhynes VK, Robbin ML, Saddekni S, Zeigler ST: A multidisciplinary approach to hemodialysis access: Prospective evaluation. Kidney Int 1998;53:473–479.
9 Kalman PG, Pope M, Bhola C, Richardson R, Sniderman KW: A practical approach to vascular access for hemodialysis and predictors of success. J Vasc Surg 1999;30:727–733.
10 Rodriguez JA, Ferrer E, Olmos A, Codina S, Borrellas J, Piera L: Analysis of the survival of permanent vascular access ports. Nefrologia 2001;21:260–273.
11 Schwab SJ, Beathard G: The hemodialysis catheter conundrum. Hate living with them, but can't live without them. Kidney Int 1999;56:1–17.
12 Konner K: A primer on the av fistula – Achilles' heel, but also Cinderella of haemodialysis. Nephrol Dial Transplant 1999;14:2094–2098.
13 Pisoni RL, Young EW, Combe C, Leavey SF, Greenwood RN, Hecking E, Canaud BJ, Locatelli F: Higher catheter use within facilities is associated with increased mortality and hospitalization: Results from DOPPS. J Am Soc Nephrol 2001;12:299A.
14 Combe C, Pisoni RL, Port FK, Young EW, Canaud B, Mapes DL, Held PJ: Dialysis Outcomes and Practice Patterns Study: Données sur l'utilisation des cathéters veineux centraux en hémodialyse chronique. Néphrologie 2001;22:379–384.
15 Dhingra RK, Young EW, Hulbert-Shearon TE, Leavey SF, Port FK: Type of vascular access and mortality in U.S. hemodialysis patients. Kidney Int 2001;60:1443–1451.

Ronald L. Pisoni, PhD, University Renal Research and Education Association,
315 W. Huron Suite 360, Ann Arbor, MI 48103 (USA)
Tel. +1 734 665 4108, ext. 223, Fax +1 734 665 2103, E-Mail rlpisoni@urrea.org

Ronco C, La Greca G (eds): Hemodialysis Technology.
Contrib Nephrol. Basel, Karger, 2002, vol 137, pp 20–30

How to Achieve a High Rate (90%) of Native Arteriovenous Fistulae

Klaus Konner

Krankenhaus Merheim, Medical Faculty University of Cologne, Germany

In the last few years there has been a revival with regard to the discussion of the problem of vascular access for hemodialysis treatment.

The predominance of graft insertions for vascular access during the last 25 years resulted in a remarkably increased rate of surgical revisions and/or interventional procedures to extend the life span of vascular access [1]. Many authors reported on primary PTFE bridge fistulae even in up to 80% of diabetic patients [2, 3]. The impact on patients' morbidity and mortality as well as on expenditures is well documented [4].

The NKF-DOQI Clinical Practice Guidelines for Vascular Access [5] stated that 'primary AV fistulae should be constructed in at least 50% of all new patients elected to receive hemodialysis as their initial form of renal replacement therapy. Ultimately, 40% of prevalent patients should have a native AV fistula'.

Recently published data from the Dialysis Outcomes Practice Patterns Study (DOPPS) try to analyze differences in strategies and outcomes between Europe and the United States, a major contribution to the new discussion in this field [6].

The following remarks on an arteriovenous (AV) fistula rate exceeding 90% are based on a single-center experience where one nephrologist (KK) is responsible for the creation of vascular access including preoperative clinical examination, diagnostic and interventional radiological interventions, surgical procedures and access revisions. In addition, ultrasonographic evaluations are done in close cooperation with nephrologists working in this institution. Thus, all decisions with regard to nephrological, surgical and radiological aspects of vascular access are made by one physician. These results are, therefore, not representative of Germany and of Europe.

Decades ago, immediately after the publication of the ingenious method of Brescia and Cimino in 1966, only young patients were elected for maintenance hemodialysis and received an AV fistula at the wrist [7]. Diabetes for example was considered a contraindication to dialysis treatment [8]. Since then, the number of diabetic and elderly patients has increased worldwide, especially type II diabetes has become more frequent in the aging dialysis population [9, 10].

The objective now is to develop a strategy that will make it possible to realize the NKF-DOQI goal.

Some ideas on how to plan and create native AV fistulae and on how to maintain long-term fistula function as prerequisite for adequate dialysis therapy will be discussed. The data presented are based on my own personal experience in planning, constructing and maintaining native AV fistulae.

Study Results

Seven-hundred and forty-eight patients underwent construction of a primary AV fistula as the first vascular access from 1993 to 1998 with a follow-up through December 1999. There was no patient with a primary graft insertion as the first access. No patient was transferred to another surgeon for initial access operation. Statistical and survival analyses were performed by Prof. Friedrich K. Port and his team at the Kidney Epidemiology and Cost Center, University of Michigan, Ann Arbor, Mich., USA.

Of the 748 patients, 24% were diabetics with an average age of 63 years; the nondiabetic group was 5 years younger than the diabetic one. A forearm access was created in 24% of the 181 diabetic patients. The other 76% diabetics received a primary elbow access. In contrast, 62% of the 567 nondiabetics had a forearm fistula as the primary vascular access. So, the preferred access for diabetic patients was the elbow perforating vein fistula and for nondiabetics the forearm AV fistula. Two hundred and thirty-six first surgical and 7 interventional revisions were performed during the 1- to 7-year follow-up period including 80 complete failures. PTFE prosthetic graft material was used in only 17 cases at the time of the first revisions.

Analyzing the number of access events per patient-year at risk, a mean value of 0.18 is found for all interventions. Unexpectedly, a lower thrombosis rate was observed for diabetic than nondiabetic patients. Fistula thrombosis occurred at an annual rate of 0.03–0.06 (average of 0.05 events) per patient-year at risk, i.e. one thrombotic event per 20 patient-years at risk.

Diabetic patients suffered significantly more often from peripheral ischemia, particularly those with nonperforating vein elbow accesses. Early thrombosis within 4 weeks following initial access placement was observed in

4% of patients with a forearm fistula; elbow fistulae amounted to 1 and 2%, respectively. It seems remarkable that no early thrombosis was seen in diabetics with forearm and perforating vein elbow fistulae.

Exclusion from AV access creation occurred in patients who had a clinical contraindication for the creation of any AV access because of peripheral ischemia or congestive heart failure. This affected only a very small minority of patients, who had to be treated exclusively with a central venous access. Retrospectively, the exact number of such exclusions could not be determined for the population of this study. So, we evaluated prospectively the frequency of these contraindications to an AV access during the year 2000. Among the 153 patients who were approaching or had started hemodialytic therapy and were referred and evaluated for initial access creation, we found 9 patients (5.9%) who had a clinical contraindication for an AV access (AV fistula or AV graft), 8/100 in the nondiabetic and 1/53 in the diabetic group; they started hemodialysis using a permanent atrial catheter. In addition, 31 patients were accepted for peritoneal dialysis therapy during 2000.

Planning for AV Fistula

An early referral of patients suffering from chronic renal failure to a nephrologist is a mandatory requirement, although currently far from being realized. In any case, it should in turn result in an early referral to the vascular surgeon to obtain an early and final plan for initial access creation.

The choice of the right or left arm depends exclusively on the quality of the vessels involved. To give preference to the nondominant arm with poor vessels is a mistake. Early selection of the location of the first AV fistula – wrist, forearm, elbow region or upper arm – allows a precise preservation of veins. Blood samples should exclusively be taken from the dorsum of the hand, whenever possible. It is, by far, the best solution to instruct the patients themselves to cooperate to achieve this goal.

Preoperative investigations are basically clinical findings. It is mandatory for the nephrologist to obtain a specific medical history of peripheral ischemia, hypertension, stroke, diabetes, pace-maker implantation, coronary/carotid/aortic/peripheral vascular surgery, amputation and smoking. Careful clinical examination includes palpation of the arterial and venous vasculature preferably using a blood pressure cuff for congestion with variable pressures. Auscultation can reveal stenotic arterial bruits. Blood pressure should be assessed in both arms to exclude stenoses of the arterial inflow into the arm – a valuable screening technique.

In addition, ultrasonographic techniques demonstrate the morphology of the great veins and provide essential data on the diameter and flow rates of the brachial artery as well as the diameter and flow direction of the radial and ulnar arteries. Ultrasound should be considered a mandatory preoperative procedure today. The Allen test can be used as a bedside, screening technique when ultrasonography is not available. In our practice, the selection of the location to place the first AV fistula is in most patients based on the results of clinical examination and ultrasonographic findings.

Venography is indicated particularly in obese patients or in patients requiring an upper arm AV fistula due to the absence or exhaustion of veins in the forearm. When venography is performed the central veins should be evaluated for stenosis or occlusion. At the moment, CO_2 is the preferred contrast medium in the predialytic period.

It is our goal to develop a plan at an early point of chronic renal failure, a conception of how and where to create the first AV fistula. This is an individual decision, a tailored solution dependent on the patient's individual vascular pattern. So, later on, a timely construction of the primary vascular access could be achieved more easily using a well-preserved venous vasculature.

It can be assumed that (vascular) surgeons are grateful to care for a well-examined patient.

Constructing the AV Fistula

A well-functioning vascular access at the start of hemodialysis treatment saves costs of hospitalization and avoids large-bore central venous catheters for temporary access with all their potential complications, thus improving later access survival, as recently shown by Pisoni et al. [6].

Timing of the initial AV fistula creation: in patients with poor vessels, the first operation should be performed 3 or 4 months prior to the expected start of hemodialysis therapy taking into account a prolonged period of maturation, a second-step superficialization of an arterialized basilic vein or an occasionally secondary insertion of graft material. In patients with good, suitable arteries and veins, referral to the vascular surgeon for access creation within 1 or 2 months before the first hemodialysis session will be adequate.

There is a substantial need for focussing on the creation of primary vascular accesses using exclusively native veins. So, primary graft insertion will be a rare exception. The first anastomosis should be constructed as far in the periphery as possible using a 'healthy' artery and a 'healthy' vein – a rare event nowadays in face of the rising proportion of patients with arterial damage due to diabetes, hypertension and age. In addition, poor venous vasculature is common in this population due to a large series of cannulations for blood samplings and infusions during multiple hospitalizations.

Daily practice and a series of failures in our early experience showed us that a stiff and calcified radial artery with a narrowed lumen and loss of distensibility is not suitable for construction of an AV anastomosis. Here, arterial dilatation during maturation – prerequisite of the high fistula blood flow rates needed for adequate dialysis therapy – is missing. Since clinical experience reveals that arterial calcification decreases from the periphery to the axilla, one should avoid using the damaged peripheral radial artery and go for the proximal segment of the radial/ulnar artery or the brachial artery in the elbow region. It became evident that the problem is not the diameter of the artery, but the quality of the arterial wall. 'Healthy' arteries although with a small diameter are regularly and successfully used for access creation, e.g. in children.

Generally, the selection of the site and type of the initial AV anastomosis should take the patient's individual vascular pattern into account. Standardization prevents creativity and success.

Thus, any 'healthy' segment of the radial artery in the forearm can be used, depending on the availability of a suitable vein. Within the potential elbow accesses special attention should be given to the perforating vein fistula, an anastomosis of the perforating vein mostly to the brachial artery. My personal modification of the original technique published by Gracz et al. of Chicago, Ill., USA in 1977 preserves the deep venous system and provides a limited length of the anastomosis with only 3–5 mm [11]. So, the risk of peripheral ischemia in diabetic and elderly patients can be reduced substantially [12].

The subcutaneously fixed superficialized basilic vein is a true alternative to the use of grafts [13, 14]. In our experience with more than 200 procedures since 1985, it is sufficient to use the first 10 cm just proximal the elbow, thus preserving the cephalad part of the vein for future procedures, maybe in a few cases for the insertion of an upper arm loop graft. Adequate dialysis therapy can be achieved with a short but well-functioning segment of the subcutaneously placed basilic vein. In these patients the use of the button-hole cannulation technique may be considered. The main long-term risk of this technique is proximal venous stenosis, in most cases suitable for correction by angioplasty, in some cases with an additional stent insertion.

What is the role of graft material in this strategy which clearly prefers native vessels? It is a basic misunderstanding that a graft has to be inserted because a patient has unsuitable vessels for the creation of an AV fistula. If vessels are found that can be sutured to a 6-mm graft, then a direct anastomosis between the native artery and the native vein should be possible except in two situations: (1) very proximally located sites for anastomoses when an AV anastomosis cannot provide a satisfactory cannulation area and (2) the artery and vein are not close together to construct an anastomosis without any tension of the vessels involved.

In principle, the use of graft material should be avoided, particularly in diabetic patients because of three risk factors: (1) high blood flow rates increase the risk of peripheral ischemia and/or steal syndrome, (2) the increased graft infection rate in the diabetic uremic patient due to a well-known impaired immunological status, and (3) a higher rate of thrombotic events due to poor arterial inflow and venous outflow conditions.

For revisions, however, PTFE can occasionally be inserted successfully as an AV bridge graft or in a venovenous position or as a patch for repair of a stenosis in selected cases with a native AV fistula.

Two additional aspects of PTFE use should be mentioned: (1) the conversion of a PTFE bridge graft into a native AV fistula, preferably done in case of graft thrombosis; this procedure benefits from the predilated, mature arteries and veins [15], and (2) in case of exhaustion or absence of peripheral venous vasculature or if only the basilic and brachial veins in the upper arm are found, both hidden in the depth of the medial aspect of the upper arm in an obese patient, a two-stage procedure described by Keoghane et al. [16] can be successfully used. First, an AV anastomosis is constructed easily, but without any chance to cannulate one of these hidden veins. Maturation is evaluated ultrasonographically by measuring the increase in brachial artery blood flow volume. One or 2 months later, when arterial as well as venous dilatation has developed with a blood flow rate of 500 to 800 ml/min, a bridge graft in an AV position can successfully be inserted [16]. Alternatively, subcutaneous superficialization of the basilic or even one of the brachial veins can then be achieved in some of these patients, thus avoiding the use of graft material even in difficult cases.

In conclusion, constructing an AV anastomosis for vascular access using native vessels requires detailed information on the quality and suitability of arteries and veins for optimal selection of the site and side of the first AV anastomosis based on careful clinical investigation and ultrasonographic studies; in addition, surgical skill and a meticulous technique, experience, patience and creativity are mandatory. Hemodynamic patterns deriving from the physiology and pathology of such high AV blood flow rates should be respected. An essential contribution to this new strategy of preferring the elbow region for initial vascular access in patients suffering from peripheral arterial damage was recently published by Bonucchi et al. [17].

The use of graft material in the creation of initial vascular access should be reduced to extremely difficult vascular conditions.

Complete identification with all procedures and outcomes represents a challenge to be successful and to aim for the highest personal standards. Analysis of failures in the past contributes to a continuous learning curve.

Maintaining the AV Fistula

An essential point in access surveillance is continuity in education and practice. All members of the dialysis staff, nurses, technicians and doctors, are involved.

Diagnosis of vascular access dysfunction is primarily a clinical diagnosis: an initial clinical suspicion is followed by inspection, palpation and auscultation. Poststenotic venous segments will collapse following elevation of the arm beyond the level of the heart. A stenosis showing this phenomenon should undergo revision by surgery or by interventional radiological techniques. A single, isolated finding is not representative; it is better to compare the results of subsequent evaluations.

Intermittent dialysis therapy routinely provides hemodynamic data such as arterial and venous pressure – in native AV fistulae highly dependent on the site of cannulation – and bleeding time required to achieve hemostasis following removal of the cannulae. If available, recirculation can be tested in case of a suspected proximal stenosis.

Signs for early dysfunction are monitored closely. In 60–80% of all patients diagnosis of fistula dysfunction is confirmed or excluded by clinical parameters. If any uncertainty remains or more precise information is needed, further diagnostic steps are taken to decide on the best surgical or interventional procedure.

Increasing experience in ultrasound evaluations provides essential information on arterial diameter, characteristics of the structure of the arterial wall and on arterial flow rates as well as on flow patterns. Repeated measurements over time confirm the value of the results obtained; the trend observed provides the best information.

Furthermore, ultrasonography is indicated to monitor brachial artery flow rates to estimate fistula maturation preoperatively in all cases of planned subcutaneous superficialization of the basilic vein in the upper arm. In patients suffering from fistula-induced peripheral ischemia or steal syndrome, variable digital compression of different draining veins and/or side branches using ultrasonographical control can simulate the result of a planned surgical procedure such as ligation of venous branches or even closure of the anastomosis. An interesting aspect was recently published by Weitzel et al. [18] from Ann Arbor, Mich., USA: he found ultrasonographically that diastolic retrograde access blood flow develops before access recirculation can be observed. This intelligent idea is mainly useful in AV grafts, but can be helpful in native AV fistulae that have one main draining vein [18].

Surgeons mostly prefer angiographic visualization of vessels. The character of a stenosis determines the choice of the best technique for surgical revision or interventional procedures. In any peripheral angiography, central veins should be checked. The best peripheral revision is unsuccessful in case of an undetected central stenosis or occlusion. It is mandatory to reduce the amount of contrast agent as much as possible. Roentgenograms should not be 'nice', but informative.

It contradicts common experience to consider angiography and ultrasonography as competitors. We should benefit from the different indications and advantages of both techniques.

Early diagnosis of fistula dysfunction leads to early correction of the underlying anatomical finding. Timely and elective revision is the most effective tool to reduce thrombosis rate either surgically or by interventional techniques, thus avoiding potential risks of central-venous catheterization, hospitalization in most cases, high costs and emergency hemodialysis treatments. It also saves potential vasculature and prolongs the life span of vascular access. The overriding goal of this strategy is to look after the failing fistula and to minimize the need for emergency procedures for the failed fistula.

In our study, this approach has led to the finding that 47.5% of first revisions were done electively. In fact, 9% of the first revisions had been planned at the time of initial placement, including subcutaneous transposition of the basilic vein to enlarge cannulation sites or insertion of a graft loop. In our outcome analyses we counted such initially planned revisions as events. First revisions as emergency procedures, mainly thrombotic events, amounted to 43.5%.

Two additional aspects may be mentioned. First, a series of articles was published recently on 'venous ligation' to improve the function of maturing AV fistulae, mainly achieved by using interventional techniques [19]. In my opinion, flow patterns can neither be planned nor predicted. Obviously, venous ligation in case of venous hypertension is a clear indication e.g. ligation of the distal venous limb in a side-to-side anastomosis at the level of the elbow.

Delayed maturation is mainly caused by impaired arterial inflow maybe due to (1) surgical errors, (2) stenosis along the feeding artery, (3) stiffness (calcification) of the arterial wall, and (4) hypotension.

Here, the solution is not ligation of venous side branches. The best way to improve the quality of arterial inflow is to create a new anastomosis with a 'healthy' arterial segment, mostly in a more cephalad location. On the other hand, side branches should be preserved; they can be helpful in revisions as patch material or as autografts for repair of stenoses.

Second, the superficialization of the basilic vein along the upper arm is a well-accepted and successful technique, but the length of the subcutaneous placement should be restricted to 10–12 cm; the cephalad segment of the basilic vein should remain untouched. The main complication, stenoses along the proximal segment of the superficialized basilic vein, is today best and most successfully treated by angioplasty. The risk of any venous transposition is the transformation of the venous wall into a stiff and narrow scar tube. So, venous transposition is not the best solution in any case. The best results by far are obtained using predilated veins.

Interventional or Surgical Repair?

This competition is totally unnecessary. The best results are obtained by the most experienced specialists. Not the discipline itself is better or worse; success depends on the person doing the job, on his dedication, and on his experience in taking account of the limits of the techniques used.

Finally, I would like to make two remarks. First, excellent surgery is more curative than the majority of interventional procedures; second, the more centrally located sites of revision are a genuine field for interventional procedures [20].

Any decision should be aimed to help the patient.

Conclusions

The results of the present study indicate that AV fistulae can be created as the initial permanent access in the vast majority of incident ESRD patients.

The methods of achieving this goal with native AV fistulae are simple. One aim is the early referral of the pre-ESRD patient to the nephrological team as well as early referral to the vascular surgeon. Preservation of peripheral venous vasculature is mandatory. Careful clinical and ultrasonographic preoperative evaluation for early selection of the side and site of primary access leads to an early, but final plan. Absolute priority is given to native veins.

Special attention should be paid to focussing on the quality of the vessels involved for the initial AV fistula construction. To the exclusively used parameter of venous and arterial diameter [11] the quality of the wall of the vessels involved should be added. Here, the distensibility and the compliance of the artery play a key role, particularly in face of the dramatically increasing proportion of elderly and diabetic patients. The restricted use of graft material is assumed to contribute substantially to better outcomes in first vascular access procedures.

A meticulous, variable and dedicated surgical approach includes the perforating vein fistula technique [11] subcutaneous superficialization of the basilic vein and the two-step procedure as published by Keoghane et al. [16]. Paying attention to the individual vascular pattern helps avoid standardization.

Continuous surveillance preferring clinical parameters will lead to an early diagnosis of AV fistula dysfunction. Early, elective surgical or interventional revision of the failing, not the failed vascular access can reduce the rate of thrombotic events clearly exceeding the DOQI goal. There is no competition between surgery and interventional procedures. What really counts is success.

These factors will improve patient's quality of life: fewer hospitalizations, fewer central-venous catheters and fewer surgical or interventional vascular access procedures, resulting in a substantial reduction of expenditures.

The future belongs to the interdisciplinary team. One single strategy should be developed and practiced by the nephrologist, the surgeon and the radiologist. There is no place for competition. The nephrologist has the main responsibility; hemodialysis patients are nephrological patients. Successful cooperation for good results will be welcomed by our patients.

References

1 Sands JJ, Miranda CL: Prolongation of hemodialysis access survival with elective revision. Clin Nephrol 1995;44:329–333.

2 Windus DW, Jendrisak MD, Delmez JA: Prosthetic fistula survival and complications in hemodialysis patients: Effects of diabetes and age. Am J Kidney Dis 1992;19:448–452.

3 Leapman SB, Boyle M, Pescovitz MD, Milgrom ML, Jindal RM, Filo RS: The arteriovenous fistula for hemodialysis access: Gold standard or archaic relic? Am Surg 1996;62:652–656.

4 Dhingra RK, Young EW, Hulbert-Shearon TE, Leavey SF, Port FK: Type of vascular access and mortality in U.S. hemodialysis patients. Kidney Int 2001;60:1443–1451.

5 National Kidney Foundation: K/DOQI Clinical Practice Guidelines for Vascular Access, 2000. Am J Kidney Dis 2001;37(suppl 1):S137–S181.

6 Pisoni RL, Young EW, Dykstra DM, Greenwood RN, Hecking E, Gillespie B, Wolfe RA, Goodkin DA, Held PJ: Vascular access use in Europe and the United States: Results from the DOPPS. Kidney Int 2002;61:305–316.

7 Brescia MJ, Cimino JE, Appel K, Hurwich BJ: Chronic hemodialysis using venipuncture and a surgically created arteriovenous fistula. N Engl J Med 1966;275:1089–1092.

8 Ghavamian M, Gutch CF, Kopp KF, Kolff WJ: The sad truth about hemodialysis in diabetic nephropathy. JAMA 1972;222:1386–1389.

9 Young EW, Goodkin DA, Mapes DL, Port FK, Keen ML, Chen K, Maroni BL, Wolfe RA, Held PJ: The Dialysis Outcomes and Practice Patterns Study (DOPPS): An international hemodialysis study. Kidney Int 2000;57(suppl 74):S74–S81.

10 Woods JD, Turenne MN, Strawderman RL, Young EW, Hirth RA, Port FK, Held PJ: Vascular access survival among incident hemodialysis patients in the United States. Am J Kidney Dis 1997;30:50–57.

11 Gracz KC, Ing TS, Soung L-S, Armbruster KFW, Seim SK, Merkel FK: Proximal forearm fistula for maintenance hemodialysis. Kidney Int 1977;11:71–74.

12 Konner K: Primary vascular access in diabetic patients: An audit. Nephrol Dial Transplant 2000; 15:1317–1325.

13 Dagher FJ, Gelber RL, Ramos EJ, Sadler JH: Basilic vein to brachial artery fistula: A new access for chronic hemodialysis. South Med J 1976;69:1438–1440.

14 Oliver MJ, McCann RL, Indridason OS, Butterly DW, Schwab SJ: Comparison of transposed brachiobasilic fistulas to upper arm grafts and brachiocephalic fistulas. Kidney Int 2001;60: 1532–1539.

15 Nguyen VD, Griffith CN, Robinson KD: Graft-free hemodialysis (HD) practice is achievable despite high patients comorbid factors in a community based dialysis program (abstract A1536). J Am Soc Nephrol 2001;12:299A.

16 Keoghane SR, Kar Leow C, Gray DWR: Routine use of arteriovenous fistula construction to dilate the venous outflow prior to insertion of an expanded polytetrafluoro-ethylene (PTFE) loop graft for dialysis. Nephrol Dial Transplant 1993;8:154–156.
17 Bonucchi D, Cappelli G, Albertazzi A: Which is the preferred vascular access in diabetic patients? A view from Europe. Nephrol Dial Transplant 2002;17:20–22.
18 Weitzel WF, Khosla N, Rubin JM: Retrograde hemodialysis access flow during dialysis as a predictor of access pathology. Am J Kidney Dis 2001;37:1241–1246.
19 Arnold WP: Improvement in hemodialysis vascular access outcomes in a dedicated access center. Semin Dial 2000;13:359–363.
20 Konner K: Interventional strategies for haemodialysis fistulae and grafts: Interventional radiology or surgery? Nephrol Dial Transplant 2000;15:1922–1923.

Klaus Konner, MD,
Krankenhaus Merheim, Ostmerheimerstrasse 200, D–51109 Köln-Merheim (Germany)
Fax +49 221 899 11 44, E-Mail klaus.konner@uni-koeln.de

Ronco C, La Greca G (eds): Hemodialysis Technology.
Contrib Nephrol. Basel, Karger, 2002, vol 137, pp 31–37

Diagnostic Methods for Vascular Access: Access Flow Measurements

John K. Leypoldt

Research Service, VA Salt Lake City Health Care System and Departments of Internal Medicine and Bioengineering, University of Utah, Salt Lake City, Utah, USA

Thrombotic and infectious complications of the hemodialysis (HD) access are a major source of morbidity in chronic HD patients. Access stenosis often results in venous pressure increases in the dialysis circuit and decreases in flow through the access, and the presence of stenosis strongly increases the likelihood that thrombosis or failure of the access will occur. Although measurements of recirculation and pressure changes in the dialysis circuit have been used to evaluate access stenosis and thrombosis [1], measurements of the flow rate of blood though the access or the access flow rate is a preferred method for surveillance of the HD access [2].

The rationale for using the access flow rate to evaluate stenosis is based on the mechanics of fluid flow through conduits. The physics of laminar flow though a conduit with a circular cross section requires that the flow rate though the conduit is directly proportional to the radius of the cross section to the fourth power. Because of this fourth-power relationship, the access flow rate should be highly sensitive to decreases in radius of the cross section or to the degree of stenosis. For this reason, measurements of the blood flow rate through the HD access have long been of interest.

Methods for Measuring Access Flow

Several methods are available for measuring the access flow rate; these are listed in table 1. The most common techniques are based on the principle of indicator dilution. Early studies injected colored dyes [3] or radiolabeled

Table 1. Methods for determining the access flow rate

Indicator dilution
With reversal of dialysis lines
Ultrasound (saline) dilution [7–9]
Temperature dilution [10]
Ultrafiltration method [11]
Conductivity dilution [12]
Without reversal of dialysis lines
Saline dilution [14]
Glucose infusion [15, 16]
Doppler (duplex) ultrasound
Magnetic resonance imaging
Variable flow Doppler [17]

substances [4–6] into the access and measured the dilution of the injected substances downstream of the injection site. These methods were cumbersome and therefore not widely employed during routine HD. Doppler (duplex) ultrasound and magnetic resonance imaging methods also permit measurement of the access flow rate, but these methodologies are expensive, cannot be performed during routine HD treatments and may not be very accurate.

Ultrasound (Saline) Dilution – Reversed Dialysis Lines

Krivitski and colleagues [7–9] have developed a novel and practical approach for determining the access flow rate which requires reversal of the dialysis blood lines before injection of the indicator (saline). Reversal of the dialysis lines alters blood flow within the access and the HD circuit to facilitate the injection of the indicator in the arterial end of the access and its detection downstream. Moreover, reversal of the dialysis lines permits measurements to be made within the dialysis circuit instead of directly on the access. A key to this approach is accurate determination of the blood flow rate through the dialyzer since the access flow rate is directly proportional to this parameter. This approach will subsequently be referred to as the ultrasound dilution technique because the detector/sensor measures the velocity of ultrasound in the flowing blood.

Dilution Techniques – Reversed Dialysis Lines without Intravenous Injections

The need to inject saline into the dialysis lines when using the ultrasound dilution technique is inconvenient. Several approaches for using indicator dilution methods that do not require saline injections have been subsequently developed. Schneditz et al. [10] showed how changes in dialysate temperature with the dialysis lines in the normal and reversed configurations could be used to measure the access flow rate. Like the ultrasound dilution technique, this approach requires accurate assessment of the blood flow rate through the dialyzer. Subsequent studies by Yarar et al. [11] and Gotch et al. [12] showed how changes in the ultrafiltration rate or in dialysate conductivity with the dialysis lines in the normal and reversed configurations could be used to determine the access flow rate. These latter approaches do not require accurate determination of the dialyzer blood flow rate; rather, accurate assessment of the ultrafiltration rate and dialysate flow rate, respectively, are necessary. In a preliminary report, Lindsay et al. [13] have shown how the access flow rate can be determined from urea measurements with the dialysis lines in the normal and reversed configurations using an on-line dialysate urea monitor. This technique depends on an accurate assessment of dialyzer urea clearance by the dialysate urea monitor.

Dilution Techniques – No Reversal of Dialysis Lines

Recent work by Steuer et al. [14] has shown that the saline dilution principle can be used without reversal of the dialysis lines by using a novel transcutaneous or transdermal hematocrit sensor. The sensor is unique since it can detect changes in hematocrit in the blood flowing underneath the skin on which the sensor is placed. In preliminary reports, Magnasco et al. [15, 16] have described a related technique for determining the access flow rate which measures the dilution of a 10% glucose solution injected intravenously into the arterial side of the access using a syringe pump. This technique requires blood sampling distal to the injection site. Since reversal of the dialysis lines is not required when using these techniques, they can be used at any time and are not limited to evaluations during the HD procedure as are other techniques. These techniques can be considered direct descendants of the original indicator dilution approach used by Kult et al. [3].

Variable Flow Doppler – No Reversal of Dialysis Lines

Weitzel et al. [17] have developed a method for determining the access flow rate using Doppler velocity measurements which does not require reversal of the dialysis lines. Doppler signals that are proportional to flow velocity are measured for the access in between the arterial and venous needles at several different blood pump speeds. Extrapolation of these data to zero blood pump speed yields the access flow rate. This approach is unique since it does not rely on the principle of indicator dilution.

Clinical Guidelines for Access Flow Measurements during Access Surveillance

Before discussing the technical requirements for access flow measurements, it is important to keep in mind current guidelines for access surveillance. The recent NKF-K/DOQI guidelines [2] recommend a preference for access flow measurements during access surveillance; they recommend that access flow measurements be performed at least monthly during the first 1.5 h of treatment. Further, these guidelines recommend that a fistulogram be performed on a synthetic graft (1) when the access flow rate is less than 600 ml/min or (2) whose flow rate is less than 1,000 ml/min and has decreased by more than 25% over 4 months. Specific intervention protocols can vary and are not as well established for native arteriovenous (AV) fistulas; however, recent work suggests that fistulograms be performed if access flow rates in AV fistulas [18] decrease below 500 ml/min and if the access flow rate decreases by more than 20% from baseline values.

Technical Specifications for Access Flow Measurements

Accuracy

Reliable accuracy of access flow measurements is essential when evaluating whether a given flow rate is above or below a critical value. The ultrasound dilution technique has been shown to be accurate in a limited number of comparisons. For example, Depner and Krivitski [9] reported that the access flow rate determined by ultrasound dilution had a 9.2 ± 7.2% error when compared with that measured by a color duplex Doppler technique in 7 evaluations. Access flow rates determined by ultrasound dilution were also found to be in good agreement with measurements made by magnetic resonance angiography in 22 patients [19]. The accuracy of other methods for determining the access flow rate is difficult to assess because of the lack of a true gold standard. In practice, ultrasound dilution is the standard by which all other techniques are compared. The absolute accuracy of these techniques is not of critical importance (because intervention guidelines can be adjusted accordingly) and will not be discussed further.

Precision

Reliable precision of access flow measurements is key when assessing changes in the flow rate with time. The ultrasound dilution technique has been extensively tested and access flow measurements using the HD01 monitor (Transonic Systems, Ithaca, N.Y., USA) are precise. Based on studies in

25 patients, Depner and Kriviski [9] reported a mean (±SD) absolute error for duplicate measurements in close succession of the access flow rate to be 5.0 ± 3.8%. Using ultrasound dilution technology, Besarab [20] reported that 90% of all tested values were within 15% of each other (based on 4,000 measurements over 3 years); this also implies a coefficient of variation (CV) of approximately 5%.

The precision of other methods is less well defined but comparable. For example, Schneditz et al. [10] reported CVs of 7.3 and 8.6% from duplicate measurements of access flow rate by thermal dilution when measured early and late during the dialysis session in 11 patients. Yarar et al. [11] reported mean (median) CVs that averaged 13.4% (9.4%) or 9.4% (9.3%) from duplicate measurements using the ultrafiltration method during a given treatment session in 8 patients or in two consecutive sessions in 11 patients, respectively. Gotch et al. [12] reported a CV of 12% from observations on 14 patients using access flow measurements based on changes in dialysate conductivity.

The precision of dilution techniques which do not require reversal of the dialysis lines have also been reported to be analogous to those of other methods. Steuer et al. [14] reported a CV of 7.8% for duplicate measurements during the same treatment in 14 patients using the technique based on transcutaneous measurement of hematocrit. Recently, Weitzel et al. [21] reported a CV of 7% for the variable flow Doppler technique, but the precision of this approach becomes less reliable when the access flow rate exceeds 1,600 ml/min.

It should be emphasized that most of the above precision estimates are based on measurements in close succession during one treatment session; this estimate of precision primarily assesses that of the measuring instrument only. The true precision of access flow measurements from one treatment to another is difficult to assess since the overall variability is due to both the instrument and to other parameters that influence the access flow rate (see below). It is safe to assume that the precision of duplicate measurements from session to session is less than that reported in the literature based on duplicate measurements in close succession during a given treatment.

Concerns and Conclusions

There are two major concerns when using access flow measurements for access surveillance during routine HD. First, measured rates of access flow may be problematic in AV fistulas where considerable branching (or confluence) of vessels can occur. This concern has been described in some detail for the ultrasound dilution technique [22] and, in certain circumstances, may also cause inaccuracies in access flow rates when using techniques that do not require reversal of the dialysis lines. Second, significant variability in the access flow rate when measured either during a given treatment or between treatments can occur even when the anatomy of the access has not changed, and such additional variability in the access flow rate makes it difficult to determine trends for predicting access stenosis and thrombosis [23]. The magnitude of the variability in access flow rate is associated with variability of systemic hemodynamic parameters, especially blood pressure. For example, several investigators have shown an association between variability in access flow rate and variability in mean arterial pressure [24–27]. Recent work has also emphasized that the variability in mean arterial pressure during routine HD can be substantial [26]. The accuracy with which access stenosis and thrombosis can be predicted from routine access flow measurements remains controversial [28, 29].

We conclude that several devices are currently available for access surveillance using access flow measurements. Improvements in normalizing access flow measurements for changes in systemic hemodynamic variables (e.g. blood pressure) will likely improve their ability to predict access stenosis and thrombosis.

Acknowledgments

This work was supported by the office of Research and Development, Medical Research Service, Department of Veterans Affairs (USA) and the Dialysis Research Foundation (Ogden, Utah, USA).

References

1 Besarab A, Sullivan KL, Ross RP, Moritz MJ: Utility of intra-access pressure monitoring in detecting and correcting venous outlet stenoses prior to thrombosis. Kidney Int 1995;47:1364–1373.
2 National Kidney Foundation: K/DOQI Clinical Practice Guidelines for Vascular Access, 2000. Am J Kidney Dis 2001;37(suppl 1):S137–S181.
3 Kult VJ, Scheitza E, Grosswendt J, Klütsch K: Das reale Shuntvolumen subkutaner arteriovenöser Fisteln bei chronisch hämodialysierten Patienten. Z Kardiol 1973;62:158–164.
4 Gottlieb S, Garcia E, Cold SB, VanderWerf BA: Radiotracer method for nonsurgical measurement of blood flow in bovine graft arteriovenous fistulas. Proc Dial Transplant Forum 1976;6:107–108.
5 Kaye M, Lamaitre P, O'Regan S: A new technique for measuring blood flow in polytetrafluoroethylene grafts for hemodialysis. Clin Nephrol 1977;8:533–534.
6 O'Regan S, Lemaitre P, Kaye M: Hemodynamic studies in patients with expanded polytetrafluoroethylene (PTFE) forearm grafts. Clin Nephrol 1978;10:96–100.
7 Krivitski NM: Theory and validation of access flow measurement by dilution technique during hemodialysis. Kidney Int 1995;48:244–250.
8 Krivitski NM: Novel method to measure access flow during hemodialysis by ultrasound velocity dilution technique. ASAIO J 1995;41:M741–M745.
9 Depner TA, Krivitski NM: Clinical measurement of blood flow in hemodialysis access fistulae and grafts by ultrasound dilution. ASAIO J 1995;41:M745–M749.

10 Schneditz D, Fan Z, Kaufman A, Levin NW: Measurement of access flow during hemodialysis using the constant infusion approach. ASAIO J 1998;44:74–81.
11 Yarar D, Cheung AK, Sakiewicz P, Lindsay RM, Paganini EP, Steuer RR, Leypoldt JK: Ultrafiltration method for measuring vascular access flow rates during hemodialysis. Kidney Int 1999;56:1129–1135.
12 Gotch FA, Buyaki R, Panlilio F, Folden T: Measurement of blood access flow rate during hemodialysis from conductivity dialysance. ASAIO J 1999;45:139–146.
13 Lindsay RM, Sternby J, Olde B, Persson R, Thatcher ME, Sargent K: The measurement of access blood flow (Qa) using an on-line dialysate urea monitor (abstract). J Am Soc Nephrol 2000; 11:188A.
14 Steuer RR, Miller DR, Zhang S, Bell DA, Leypoldt JK: Noninvasive transcutaneous determination of access blood flow rate. Kidney Int 2001;60:284–291.
15 Magnasco A, Alloatti S, Bisso S, Paganini F, Solari P: Theory and in vitro validation of a new glucose-pump blood flow test (abstract). J Am Soc Nephrol 2001;12:296A.
16 Magnasco A, Alloatti S, Sanguineti P, Solari P: Access blood flow: Comparison of a new glucose-pump method and the Transonic device (abstract). J Am Soc Nephrol 2001;12:296A.
17 Weitzel WF, Rubin JM, Swartz RD, Woltmann DJ, Messana JM: Variable flow Doppler for hemodialysis access evaluation: Theory and clinical feasibility. ASAIO J 2000;46:65–69.
18 Tonelli M, Jindal K, Hirsch D, Taylor S, Kane C, Henbrey S: Screening for subclinical stenosis in native vessel arteriovenous fistulae. J Am Soc Nephrol 2001;12:1729–1733.
19 Bosman PJ, Boereboom FTJ, Bakker CJ, Mali WPT, Eikelboom BC, Blankestijn PJ, Koomans HA: Access flow measurements in hemodialysis patients: In vivo validation of an ultrasound dilution technique. J Am Soc Nephrol 1996;7:966–969.
20 Besarab A: Access monitoring methods. Blood Purif 2000;18:255–259.
21 Weitzel WF, Rubin JM, Leavey SF, Swartz RD, Dhingra RK, Messana JM: Analysis of variable flow Doppler hemodialysis access flow measurements and comparison with ultrasound dilution. Am J Kidney Dis 2001;38:935–940.
22 Krivitski NM, Depner TA: Development of a method for measuring hemodialysis access flow: From idea to robust technology. Semin Dial 1998;11:124–130.
23 Leypoldt JK: Standards for reproducible access flow measurements. Blood Purif 2002;20:20–25.
24 Schneditz D, Fan Z, Kaufman A, Levin NW: Stability of access resistance during haemodialysis. Nephrol Dial Transplant 1998;13:739–744.
25 Rehman SU, Pupim LB, Shyr Y, Hakim R, Ikizler TA: Intradialytic serial vascular access flow measurements. Am J Kidney Dis 1999;34:471–477.
26 DeSoto DJ, Ram SJ, Faiyaz R, Birk CG, Paulson WD: Hemodynamic reproducibility during blood flow measurements of hemodialysis synthetic grafts. Am J Kidney Dis 2001;37:790–796.
27 Besarab A, Lubkowski T, Vu A, Aslam A, Frinak S: Effects of systemic hemodynamics on flow within vascular accesses used for hemodialysis. ASAIO J 2001;47:501–506.
28 Paulson WD: Blood flow surveillance of hemodialysis grafts and the dysfunction hypothesis. Semin Dial 2001;14:175–180.
29 Krivitski NM, Gantela S: Access flow measurement as a predictor of hemodialysis graft thrombosis: Making clinical decisions. Semin Dial 2001;14:181–185.

John K. Leypoldt, PhD, Dialysis Program, University of Utah,
85 N. Medical Drive East Room 201, Salt Lake City, UT 84112–5350 (USA)
Tel. +1 801 585 3812, Fax +1 801 581 4750, E-Mail Ken.Leypoldt@hsc.utah.edu

Ronco C, La Greca G (eds): Hemodialysis Technology.
Contrib Nephrol. Basel, Karger, 2002, vol 137, pp 38–45

Temporary Vascular Access for Hemodialysis Treatment

Current Guidelines and Future Directions

Marcel C. Weijmer, Piet M. ter Wee

Department of Nephrology, Vrije Universiteit Medical Center, Amsterdam, The Netherlands

Temporary vascular access concerns access to the bloodstream with the use of a catheter to make adequate hemodialysis treatment possible. Catheters are frequently needed at the start of hemodialysis treatment and for bridging in case of failure of the permanent access or other renal replacement therapy. In current practice the use of temporary hemodialysis catheters is substantial. From the recent data of the Dialysis Outcomes and Practice Patterns Study (DOPPS), it is recognized that 15–50% of patients in Europe and 60% of patients in the US start hemodialysis treatment with a catheter for access [1]. However, the widespread application of catheters implies an enhanced exposure to catheter-related complications. Compared to patients with an arteriovenous fistula or graft, patients with a catheter had a relative risk for infection of 2.07 in a prospective study in 796 hemodialysis patients from seven outpatient centers [2]. A third of these patients had to be hospitalized because of their infection. The DOPPS reveals that 24% of all hospital admissions in the hemodialysis population are access-related. Therefore, developing new strategies to prevent catheter-related bacteremia and dysfunction is an important means to reduce patient morbidity and mortality and to reduce the rising costs of renal replacement therapy. Recently the National Kidney Foundation – Dialysis Outcome Quality Initiatives (NKF-DOQI) Clinical Practice Guidelines for Vascular Access have been updated and publicized [3]. In this article we discuss recent advances in temporary vascular access that can influence the NKF-DOQI guidelines and clinical practice in the future. We focus especially on catheter placement, catheter design and locking solutions.

Tunneled versus Temporary Catheters and Place of Insertion

The NKF-DOQI guidelines recommend that when it can be anticipated that a catheter will be needed for more than 3 weeks a tunneled cuffed catheter should be inserted. Even when a catheter is needed for less than 3 weeks, a tunneled cuffed catheter is acceptable. However, it was recognized that no randomized controlled trials are available to support these guidelines. Kairaitis and Gottlieb [4] showed that the risk of bacteremia, the most serious catheter-related complication, is high in temporary catheters [6.5/1,000 catheter days (cd)] and that 59% of all catheters had to be removed preliminarily because of a suspected complication. Oliver et al. [5] demonstrated in a study on 218 patients that a temporary uncuffed jugular catheter can be left in place for 3 weeks with an acceptable risk of bacteremia. Femoral catheters were associated with a high incidence of bacteremia when left in place for more than 1 week (10.7%). However, in this study occlusive dressings were applied and there was no strict protocol for the removal of catheters in case of exit site infection [5]. Still, no studies are available comparing temporary catheters and tunneled cuffed catheters. Because it is clearly demonstrated in the DOPPS that the incidence of catheter-related complications can vary widely between dialysis centers, an indirect comparison with data collected from studies performed in different hemodialysis centers can only be made with caution. Recently, we prospectively studied the outcomes of all inserted catheters that had been used consecutively for more than one hemodialysis in our department. The type of catheter, time of insertion, duration and place of insertion, and reason for removal were analyzed. In addition, all catheter-related infectious complications were evaluated. A total of 272 hemodialysis catheters were inserted in 149 patients (11,612 cd), 37 tunneled cuffed catheters, 83 temporary femoral catheters, 104 temporary jugular catheters and 48 temporary subclavian catheters). Of the temporary femoral catheters 28 (34%, 35.3/1,000 cd) had to be removed because of a complication, of the temporary jugular catheters 55 (53%, 17.1/1,000 cd), of the temporary subclavian catheters 24 (50%, 16.1/1,000 cd) and of the tunneled cuffed catheters 11 (30%, 1.8/1,000 cd). Infection rates for tunneled cuffed catheters (3.3/1,000 cd) were substantially lower compared to temporary jugular catheters (14.3/1,000 cd) and temporary femoral catheters (18.9/1,000 cd). From our data we estimated the patency rates for every day when a catheter was used to identify the safe period during which temporary catheters can be left in place. For every time period, removal because of infection or dysfunction was lower for tunneled cuffed catheters (range 1.7–5.0/1,000 cd) compared to temporary jugular (10.3–13.9), femoral (20.4–35.0) or subclavian catheters (16.8–28.5). Our data indicate that when a catheter is needed for more than 1 week, a tunneled cuffed catheter in the jugular vein is preferred. Insertion into the subclavian vein should be discouraged because it is associated with an important risk for subclavian vein thrombosis hampering the development of an adequate arteriovenous fistula or graft in the future. It is, therefore, remarkable that with the DOPPS it was shown that 46% of all temporary catheters used in the US in patients starting hemodialysis treatment are inserted into the subclavian vein.

Jugular Catheter Design

All studies analyzing the outcome of untunneled temporary jugular catheters included straight catheters pointing upward from the place of insertion. These catheters inserted into the internal or external jugular vein are not comfortable for the patient. Additionally, they cannot be fixated very well and have an upward directed skin port. For peritoneal dialysis catheters it has been demonstrated that an upward directed skin port is an important risk factor for exit site infection and peritonitis. Recently, we completed a clinical study with a temporary jugular catheter with a novel design (11.5 Fr, polyurethane, Raulerson®, Medcomp, Harleysville, PA., USA). This precurved catheter was inserted into the low jugular site and placed close to the upper border of the clavicle so the catheter bends over the clavicle and could be immobilized and fixated to the chest wall. Our primary intention was to reduce the discomfort in patients needing a temporary hemodialysis catheter in the jugular vein. We prospectively analyzed infectious complications and removals because of dysfunction. A comparison was made with tunneled cuffed catheters inserted during the same time period. A total of 58 precurved jugular catheters were inserted in 49 patients (1,813 cd) and 58 tunneled cuffed catheters in 48 patients (8,384 cd), mainly in the right jugular position. A comparison was also made with observational data on 104 upward pointing straight jugular catheters inserted in 77 patients (3,209 cd) in the period before the introduction of the precurved model. Nine precurved catheters (16%, 5.0/1,000 cd; $p < 0.01$ vs. straight catheters) had to be removed for a complication versus 18 tunneled catheters (31%, 2.1/1,000 cd; $p < 0.01$ vs. straight catheters) and 54 straight catheters (56%, 16.9/1,000 cd). There were no periods of bacteremia observed in patients with a precurved catheter and 1 skin port infection (0.6/1,000 cd). In tunneled catheters 15 periods of bacteremia (1.8/1,000 cd) and 11 periods of skin port infection (1.3/1,000 cd) were recorded. Seventeen periods of bacteremia (5.3/1,000 cd) and 29 periods of skin port infection (9/1,000 cd) occurred in patients with a straight jugular catheter. The cumulative hazard for bacteremia showed significantly lower rates for the catheter with the novel precurved design compared to the straight ($p < 0.001$) and even compared to tunneled cuffed catheters ($p < 0.01$). The same catheter care protocol was used and not changed at the time of the introduction of the new catheter. Furthermore, infection rates were similar for tunneled catheters inserted in the period when only straight temporary jugular catheters were used compared to the period after the precurved jugular catheter had been introduced. This finding makes a time bias as an explanation for the favorable outcome of the precurved model unlikely. We concluded that a well-positioned precurved hemodialysis catheter for temporary use is a safe option when a catheter is needed for access for a period of up to 3 months. The likely explanation for the low infection rates is that the fixation of a precurved catheter is better and that the skin port pointed forward to downward.

Tip Construction and Situation of the Catheter in the Blood Vessel

The geometry and tip design of catheters have been determined mainly by methods of trial and error. Multiple side holes were thought to be required for a sufficient inflow area, even in the case of obstruction of some side holes or when a catheter was situated close to the vessel wall. However, side holes can induce thrombosis because they often have an irregular surface [6]. Furthermore the diameter of the holes is not adapted to actual required flow rates. Despite the various types of catheters available, studies on the influence of tip construction on fluid dynamics are scarce. Recently, De Wachter et al. [7] presented a study on the hemodynamics of a dual lumen dialysis catheter with 5 arterial side holes and 3 venous ones (Gamcath®, Joka Kathetertechnik, Germany). A computer flow model was used simulating a flow of fluid of 300 ml/min through the catheter while situated in a 3-cm-wide tube also with a flow of fluid. The viscosity of blood could also be simulated. The sequential placement of the arterial holes was demonstrated to be the reason that mainly the first available hole is employed to draw the blood into a catheter. At the distal holes of the arterial side, a low flow zone was present, suggesting an increased risk for thrombus formation in clinical use. Also at the venous side the meaningfulness of the multiple side hole design was questioned. The first two side holes are greatly underemployed. At the most proximal venous side hole (closest to the hub), some of the blood is even drawn into the catheter due to the high difference in velocities between catheter and vein. Furthermore, locking solutions can easily dissolve from the tip when multiple side ports are brought into a catheter. They concluded that most currently available temporary catheters can be improved to optimize hemodynamics and reduce dysfunction. We are now using this computer model to analyze different catheter and tip designs to try to determine the optimal tip construction. Preliminary data reveal that open shotgun tips are preferred and more than one side hole is probably not necessary.

To further study whether longer femoral catheters could be advantageous and to study the influence of a tip construction, we compared three types of newly inserted femoral catheters in a clinical randomized trial. Patients were randomized either to a 20- or 24-cm catheter with a shotgun tip (Niagara® Bard, Salt Lake City, Utah, USA) or to a 20-cm tapered tip catheter (Gamcath®). Recirculation rates were measured at a Qb of 200, 250 and 300 ml/min with blood lines situated normally and after a reversal of pools. We could demonstrate a benefit concerning early failure rates for the shotgun tip. Furthermore, a 24-cm catheter showed lower recirculation rates and less primary dysfunction than a 20-cm catheter. Reversal of pools, often necessary for dysfunction, led to a mean increase of recirculation from 5 to 35%. In the same period, 20 consecutively inserted 15-cm dual lumen jugular catheters (Raulerson®) were analyzed for recirculation rates, revealing lower rates (<5%) than femoral catheters at all flows. A reversal of pools increased the recirculation to maximum values of 10% at 300 ml/min blood flow. These figures are comparable to tunneled cuffed jugular catheters.

Catheter Materials and Coating

In vitro data on the biocompatibility of the most regularly used polymers in catheter manufacturing, silicon and polyurethane, are conflicting. Likewise, in small randomized trials comparing tunneled cuffed catheters of different materials and construction, no clear benefit as regards one particular catheter was found. Recently, the largest trial to date with tunneled cuffed catheters was concluded by Richard et al. [8]. Ninety-four patients were randomly assigned to 38 Ash-split®, 39 Opti-flow® and 36 Tesio® catheters. There was no difference in hemodialysis flow rates, catheter-related infections or catheter survival. Insertion procedures for Ash-split® and Opti-flow® catheters were shorter (mean insertion time of Ash-split®: 29.4 min, of Opti-flow®: 29.6 min, of Tesio®: 41.5 min) and easier than for Tesio® catheters [8].

For temporary hemodialysis catheters there are no studies available comparing different catheter materials. We compared the patency of comparable temporary polyurethane catheters [Quinton Mahukar (Quinton, Seattle, Wash., USA, and Gamcath®) 15–20 cm, 11–11.5 Fr] and temporary silicon catheters (11.5 Fr, 20 cm, Medcomp Medical Components, Harleysville, Pa.,

USA) inserted at our department. There were no significant differences in the sites chosen for insertion (jugular, femoral or subclavian). The same catheter care protocol was applied. A total of 233 temporary polyurethane catheters were inserted in 134 patients (6,012 cd) and 51 temporary silicon catheters in 38 patients (2,464 cd). Of polyurethane catheters 49 (21%) had to be removed for a complication (8.2/1,000 cd), and of silicone 22 (43%; 8.9/1,000 cd).

In conclusion, to date there is no study that shows an advantage of silicon over polyurethane for the construction of hemodialysis catheters. On the other hand, silicon catheters are possibly more prone to construction failures because of the difficult manufacturing process necessary [9].

Promising progress is made with the coating of catheters. In intensive care patients catheters coated with antibiotics, silver or heparin reduce the number of infections substantially. However, only heparin-coated catheters are considered cost-effective in a recent review [10]. No studies have been reported on coated hemodialysis catheters. A problem with bonding of hemodialysis catheters is that they are often needed for a longer period of time and the substance impregnated or bonded on catheters can disappear over time.

Catheter Care and Measures to Prevent Catheter-Related Bacteremia and Thrombosis

It is known from in vitro studies that solutions containing antibiotics can prevent biofilm formation on foreign surfaces. However, the use of antibiotics in solutions for the interdialytic locking of catheters is associated with low systemic levels of the antibiotic resulting in the risk of development of bacterial resistance as well as hypersensitivity of the patient. Trisodium citrate (TSC) has been advocated for locking because it provides local anticoagulation and is thought to exhibit antimicrobial effects. Additional advantages of TSC are that it prevents unforeseen systemic anticoagulation and it is less expensive than heparin. We performed an in vitro analysis of increasing concentrations of TSC using two classical antimicrobial susceptibility tests and 5 microorganisms commonly found in catheter-related bacteremia. TSC was compared with heparin and a solution of TSC with gentamicin. We could demonstrate that TSC 30% was superior concerning bacterial and yeast killing. Ash et al. [11] reported their experience in a hemodialysis patient cohort of 70 patients with 60% tunneled cuffed catheters. After introduction of TSC 23–47% for catheter locking they observed a decline in the number of patients per month having a bacteremia from 4.5 to 0%. Urokinase utilization for catheter flow problems also decreased significantly. No clinically relevant side effects occurred during instillation of TSC into hemodialysis catheters. This is important, as concern has risen after a fatal accident as regards using TSC for locking catheters. In this particular case, however, a large amount of TSC was accidentally injected in a previously unstable patient with severe electrolyte disturbances.

The first antimicrobial locking solution containing taurolidine and TSC 4.4% is currently commercialized and preliminary studies show promising results. However, this solution is expensive and its cost-effectiveness warrants further investigation.

Conclusion

Recent developments in the temporary uncuffed hemodialysis catheter and its construction have revealed that catheters with improved flow characteristics and better patency rates which are easier to insert will become available in the future. The incidence of infectious complications that make it difficult to leave temporary jugular catheters in place for more than 3–4 weeks is likely to decrease. Antimicrobial locking solutions will probably replace the currently used heparin. It is likely that for temporary vascular access the importance of tunneled cuffed catheters which are more difficult to insert and more expensive will decrease.

References

1 Pisoni RL, Young EW, Dykstra DM, Greenwood RN, Hecking E, Gillespie B, Wolfe RA, Goodkin DA, Held PJ: Vascular access use in Europe and the United States: Results from the DOPPS. Kidney Int 2002;61:305–316.
2 Tokars JI, Light P, Anderson J, Miller ER, Parrish J, Armistead N, Jarvis WR, Gehr T: A prospective study of vascular access infections at seven outpatient hemodialysis centers. Am J Kidney Dis 2001;37:1232–1240.
3 NKF-K/DOQI Clinical Practice Guidelines for Vascular Access: Update 2000. Am J Kidney Dis 2001;37:S137–S181.
4 Kairaitis LK, Gottlieb T: Outcome and complications of temporary haemodialysis catheters. Nephrol Dial Transplant 1999;14:1710–1714.
5 Oliver MJ, Callery SM, Thorpe KE, Schwab SJ, Churchill DN: Risk of bacteremia from temporary hemodialysis catheters by site of insertion and duration of use: A prospective study. Kidney Int 2000;58:2543–2545.
6 Twardowski ZJ, Moore HL: Side holes at the tip of chronic hemodialysis catheters are harmful. J Vasc Access 2001;2:8–16.
7 De Wachter D, Deserranno D, Verdonck P: Hemodynamic characteristics of a temporary dual lumen catheter for hemodialysis. J Biomech, in press.
8 Richard HM 3rd, Hastings GS, Boyd-Kranis RL, Murthy R, Radack DM, Santilli JG, Ostergaard C, Coldwell DM: A randomized, prospective evaluation of the Tesio, Ash split, and Opti-flow hemodialysis catheters. J Vasc Interv Radiol 2001;12:431–435.
9 Weijmer MC, Kars SM, ter Wee PM: A scanning electron microscopy analysis of a spontaneous hemodialysis catheter fracture. Am J Kidney Dis 2001;38:858–861.

10 Marin MG, Lee JC, Skurnick JH: Prevention of nosocomial bloodstream infections: Effectiveness of antimicrobial-impregnated and heparin-bonded central venous catheters. Crit Care Med 2000; 28:3332–3338.

11 Ash SR, Mankus RA, Sutton JM, Criswell ER, Crull CC, Velasquez KA, Smeltzer BD, Ing TS: Concentrated sodium citrate (23%) for catheter lock. Hemodial Int 2000;4:22–31.

M.C. Weijmer, Department of Nephrology, Vrije Universiteit Medical Center,
PO Box 7057, NL–1007 MB Amsterdam (The Netherlands)
Tel. +31 20 4442673, Fax +31 20 4442675, E-Mail mc.weijmer@vumc.nl

Ronco C, La Greca G (eds): Hemodialysis Technology.
Contrib Nephrol. Basel, Karger, 2002, vol 137, pp 46–53

Prosthetic Devices for Vascular Access

Francesco Quarello, Giacomo Forneris, Marco Pozzato

Nephrology and Dialysis Unit, San Giovanni Bosco Hospital, Turin, Italy

The clinical application of hemodialysis started in 1960, when Scribner and Quinton developed an external shunt making the first stable access to circulation possible. A major improvement occurred in 1966 with the Cimino-Brescia arteriovenous fistula, currently still the gold standard for vascular access in hemodialysis. However, due to the rising percentage of ESRD patients with severe comorbid conditions, in the last decade an increasing use of central venous catheters (CVC) has been reported. The DOPPS study [1] reports a catheter use among prevalent and incident HD patients of 17 and 60% (USA) and 8 and 31% (Europe), respectively. In effect, CVC for hemodialysis can be a temporary solution for late referral patients who need quick dialysis treatment or can be used while arteriovenous fistulas or PTFE grafts are placed and need time to heal. For patients having run out of access sites because of poor vasculature, permanent catheters may prove the only alternative to establish access for dialysis.

Although central catheters provide an important advantage by allowing immediate access to blood, they are esthetically unsatisfactory for the patients and in the long-term carry high costs, because of a high incidence of thrombosis, dislodging and infection [2]. The most serious problem of tunneled catheters in hemodialysis is catheter-related bloodstream infection. In addition to the well-established risk factors for infection in dialysis population, an externalized catheter breaks the skin integrity and facilitates the adhesion and migration of bacteria into the circulation. Bloodstream infection is typically a cause for removal of the catheter and protracted systemic antibiotic therapy, a reason for hospitalization and the second highest cause of mortality in the USA hemodialysis population [3]. However, the frequent adoption of CVC, in spite of the fairly high complication rate, reflects the difficulty in coping with the traditional types of vascular access for hemodialysis.

In this setting a totally implanted device that minimizes the infection hazard has theoretical advantages. In the early 1980s a first attempt to transfer to hemodialysis the favorable experience made in oncology and parenteral nutrition with vascular access ports failed, due to the inability to support sufficiently high blood flow rates necessary without damage to red blood cell and platelet activation [4].

Recently, two new access devices, LifeSite (Vasca) and Dialock (Biolink), aimed at replacing the external catheter as a bridge or definitive access, became available for hemodialysis patients. At least theoretically, the advantages with respect to tunneled catheters consist of a lower risk of infection due to the subcutaneous location of the system, higher blood flows with a reduced rate of thrombosis, and an improvement of the image the patient has of him- or herself.

Prosthetic Devices

LifeSite Vasca

Device

The LifeSite Hemodialysis Access System (fig. 1) consists of a subcutaneous valve and a 12-Fr silicone cannula, usually implanted below the clavicle and tunneled in the right internal jugular vein (IJV). The distal tip is placed in the right atrium and has six side holes. The LifeSite requires the implantation of two separate valves equipped with a dimpled entrance in the center of the domed top, which facilitates the introduction of a standard 14-gauge needle. The valve is designed without a septum, in order to avoid failures associated with repetitive punctures. When the needles are inserted or removed, a mechanical pinch clamp opens or closes preventing any leakage. The system utilizes the buttonhole technique for puncture, forming a pain-free tissue tract. The channel for blood passage through the device is smooth without constriction or dead space. The skin over the valves is cleansed with a 4% chlorhexidine solution; then the valve and the buttonhole tract are sterilized using 0.2% oxychlorosene antimicrobial irrigation solution with a 25-gauge needle. The same procedure is repeated at the end of dialysis.

Clinical Experience with the LifeSite Vasca

Preliminary results were reported by Beathard and Posen [5] in 23 patients from two pilot studies in Canada and the USA. An increasing percentage of diabetic patients (47.8%) represents a high-risk group. No complication as a result of surgical implantation occurred, allowing the use of the device early after operation. A median duration of the device of 5.9 months and an incidence of

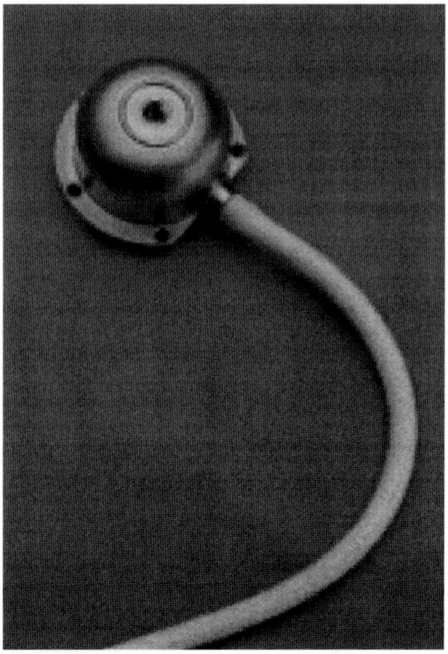

Fig. 1. LifeSite Hemodialysis Access System.

2.5 infectious episodes/1,000 patient-days are reported. A loss of 12 out of 23 valves (52.2%) results from infection episodes. The LifeSite allows high blood flow rates, averaging 348 ± 78 ml/min, without recirculation (Transonic Systems), even at the maximum Qb. Poor blood flows occurred occasionally, requiring only one catheter exchange to solve the problem. No postdialysis bleeding or difficulties with the buttonhole technique are reported. A very good acceptance by patients and dialysis staff has also been described.

A multicenter study comparing LifeSite valves and Tesio catheters reports better blood flows (358 vs. 331 ml/min; $p < 0.001$), fewer dialysis sessions needing urokinase (2.3 vs. 8.6/1,000 patient-days) and a higher survival rate at 1 year (74.2 vs. 48%; $p = 0.0617$) with the subcutaneous device [6].

The Dialock System

Device

The Dialock system (fig. 2) consists of a single titanium chamber (port) and two radiopaque, coil-reinforced, silicone catheters. The inlet side of the device has a trough-like design aimed at guiding the user to approach the two needle-accessible passageways. Within each passage a septum valve is opened at the time of needle insertion, which prevents the needle from slipping out of

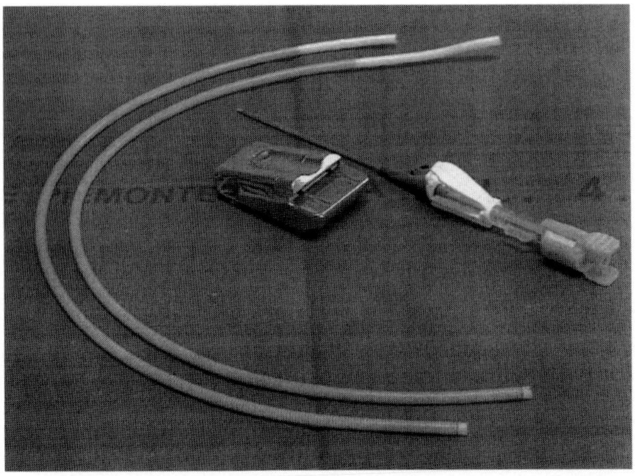

Fig. 2. Dialock Hemodialysis Access System with proprietary needle.

the port during dialysis and automatically closes when the needle is withdrawn at the end of dialysis.

The device is implanted in a subcutaneous pocket under the clavicle. The catheters are 40 cm long with inner and outer diameters of 3.6 mm (11 Fr) and 2.7 mm, respectively, tunneled from the base of the neck to the subcutaneous pocket. Their distal ends present a transversal incisure and lack the spiral hole pattern typical of many dialysis catheters. The connection to blood lines is obtained through trademark disposable cannula needles that pass through the skin and functionally convert the Dialock to a standard twin lumen catheter. The needle set consists of two square-tipped 15-gauge, stainless steel cannulas attached to PVC extension tubings with clamps and standard luer locks. Each cannula is temporarily converted to a noncoring needle by a stainless steel stylet.

Clinical Experience with the Dialock System

A preliminary study including 10 patients followed with this device for 7 ± 1.5 months on average reports a rate of bacteremia of 2.3 episodes/1,000 catheter-days; all resolved without port removal [7].

The work of Canaud et al. [8] refers to 10 hemodialysis patients with a total duration of use of 1,730 days (39–294) and 700 dialysis sessions performed. The authors report a mean blood flow of 307 ± 3.3 ml/min and a venous pressure of 195 ± 39 mm Hg. Dialysis performance was expressed by a KT/V index of 1.3 ± 0.028 and a recirculation rate of 6.6% measured by the stop-flow method. Three episodes of catheter-related bloodstream infection, successfully treated with antibiotic therapy, were reported. A good level of acceptance by both patients (70%) and nurses (80)% was reported. More comprehensive data from the USA and France on 23 patients accounted for an infection rate of 3 episodes/1,000 catheter-days [9].

More recently, in spite of a high incidence of pocket infections, a large German study [10] showed remarkable low figures (0.29 bacteremia episodes/1,000 catheter-days of use), employing a new catheter lock solution (currently available as Neutrolin, Biolink) instead of sodium citrate.

Dialock Turin Experience

Since February 2000 up to December 2001, 35 patients (18 males/17 females, mean age 61 ± 12 years), on regular dialysis treatment for 48 months on average (interval 0–273, median 13 months), received 35 implants at the San Giovanni Bosco Renal Unit. The systems were implanted by the nephrologist just below the clavicle; in all cases the IJV was cannulated (left IJV in 30 patients, right IJV in the remaining 5). In 6 late-referral patients (17%) the system was implanted as a first vascular access, because of poor viable vascular sites for the creation of an arteriovenous fistula. The overall observation period amounted to 400 patient-months; median duration of use was 348 ± 170 days (range 29–634 days). The median time to first use was 3.5 ± 4 days (range 0–19). No complications were observed during Dialock implantation, except for two small hematomas which spontaneously healed after 5 and 18 days, respectively. Because of poor blood flow, a surgical revision to adjust the length of the catheter was carried out in 16 patients. This procedure made it possible to restore the prescribed Qb (300 ml/min). Catheters have been replaced over a guidewire in 1 case, with a successful resolution of catheter-related bacteremia.

During the almost 2-year observation period 12 episodes of catheter-related bacteremias (0.9/1,000 catheter-days) were recorded in 9 patients. Two pocket infections were registered (0.16/1,000 catheter-days), and the patients fully recovered after a 2-week antibiotic course.

The system is still in use in 27 patients (77.2%), with a secondary survival rate of 85% at 1 year. In 5 cases the device had to be removed, due to central vein thrombosis (2 cases), sepsis (1 case), skin erosion with exposure of the port device (1 case) and unexplained persistent leukocytosis that turned to be a myelodysplasia (1 case). Three patients died of causes unrelated to the Dialock use.

In 1 case the relapse of a bacteremia episode was followed by an endocardial and vertebral spread of the infection (spondilodiscitis). Both infectious locations were eradicated by antibacterial therapy and replacement of both catheters, with normalization of all the cultures and radiological examinations. The device was salvaged, because there was inadequate vasculature to implant a graft or fistula.

During the 5,156 dialysis procedures that had been followed we observed a Qb lower than 250 ml/min in 7% of the sessions and the need for urokinase infusion in 4.3%, including the period preceding the surgical revisions.

Three patients were included in a program of long nocturnal dialysis (6 h 30 min) and felt more comfortable during sleep with their needles safely anchored over their chest. Another patient, on home hemodialysis for many years, could resume his treatment at home, interrupted as a result of several vascular access failures, after a short training period had been given to his spouse.

Dialock Italian Multicenter Study

In the 10 dialysis units* participating in the study 86 implants in 85 patients [41 males/44 females, mean age 66 ± 13 years (range 26–85), overall follow-up 796 patient-months] were carried out in the period from February 2000 to December 2001. In 24 patients (28%) the device has been implanted as a first vascular access. Sixty-six patients are still alive with a functioning system, with a technical survival rate of 82% at 1 year. Eight patients are dead as a result of causes not related to the vascular access, in 7 the device had been removed due to infection, in 4 as a result of thrombosis and in 1 because of rupture of the catheter. Twenty-three episodes of bacteremia have been observed in 14 patients (0.94/1,000 catheter-days). Oral anticoagulation was prescribed in 76% of the cases. Mean blood flow was 280 ± 36 ml/min, with an arterial pressure of –158 ± 27 and a venous pressure of 144 ± 27 mm Hg.

A blood flow lower than 250 ml/min was observed in 13.8% of the sessions (with urokinase use in 3.6%). Twenty-five surgical revisions due to catheter malposition/thrombosis or catheter/pocket bacterial colonization were performed in 24 patients.

Discussion

Even though arteriovenous fistulas with native vessels still continue to be the golden standard, the search for new venous access techniques for hemodialysis is still going on. The subcutaneous ports, introduced with the aim of reducing the complication rates of CVC and ameliorate the quality of

*M. Aloisi, P. Ferrandello (Pietrasanta), P. Altieri, O. Manca (Cagliari), F. Cavatorta, A. Zollo (Imperia), A. Salvadeo, F. Galli (Pavia), S. Di Giulio, A. Carnabuci (Roma), G. La Greca, C. Crepaldi (Vicenza), F. Quarello, M. Pozzato, G. Forneris (Turin), B. Ricciardi (Milazzo), F.P. Schena, G. Pertosa (Bari), S. Stefoni, L. Colì (Bologna).

life of dialysis patients, are indeed an important technical innovation in this field. Some of the most worrying fatal risks of CVC, such as air embolism and massive blood loss, can be prevented completely by totally implantable systems. Moreover, as far as preliminary experience is concerned, subcutaneous ports seem to allow a higher protection from external bacteria contamination. Preliminary experiences, including our own, have demonstrated the possibility of containing bacteremia rates at under 1 episode/1,000 catheter-days, consistently below other catheter studies, averaging 4 episodes/1,000 catheter-days [11, 12]. However, since severe infectious episodes can still occur, the possibility of reducing endoluminal contamination with an antibacterial catheter lock solution, as suggested by the bloodstream infection rate of 0.29 episodes/1,000 patient-days obtained by Sodemann et al. [10], could further improve the safety of the port and avoid the rare septic complications. As regards skin infection problems, quite relevant with external catheters, as evidenced by 3.94 episodes of exit site/tunnel infections/1,000 catheter-days in our experience [13], the maintenance of the skin barrier integrity has confirmed an almost complete protective ability of subcutaneous ports (0.16 episodes/1,000 catheter-days in our series). The high rate of dysfunctions in our experience with the Dialock probably reflects the initial difficulties with new catheters lacking the side holes at the distal end. This technical innovation probably limits catheter thrombosis but tends to lead to suction of the vessel wall. Therefore, the exact position of the catheter tip in the upper third of cardiac atrium seems to be highly critical.

Conclusion

With respect to tunneled dialysis catheters, subcutaneous ports represent a definite technical improvement and have proved to be a viable alternative in patients for whom a traditional vascular access with native vessels or grafts is not technically feasible. Worldwide preliminary clinical experiments suggest a significant reduction of infectious episodes, high survival rates, better quality of life and good acceptance by nurses and patients. Future technical developments for both current devices and the availability of new antimicrobial lock solution(s) will probably contribute to further reducing the already satisfactory low complication rates, in particular the catheter-related bloodstream infections.

However, to obtain a more precise pattern of indications of subcutaneous ports in hemodialysis patients and to better understand the limits and advantages of currently available devices a long-term widespread evaluation is still necessary.

References

1 Pisoni RL, Young EW, Dikstra DM, Greenwood RN, Hecking E, Gillespie B, Wolfe RA, Goodking DA, Held PJ: Vascular access in Europe and United States: Results from the DOPPS. Kidney Int 2002;61:305–316.

2 Schwab SJ, Beathard G: The hemodialysis catheter conundrum: Hate living with them, but can't live without them. Kidney Int 1999;56:1–17.

3 Feldman HI, Kobrin S, Wasserstein A: Hemodialysis vascular access morbidity. J Am Soc Nephrol 1996;7:523–535.

4 My H, Kepenekian G, Gallet M, Charpin B, Lopez M, Manchon J, Cibert J: Utilization in chronic hemodialysis of the 'implantable site' technique. Nephrologie 1994;15:173–174.

5 Beathard GA, Posen GA: Initial clinical results with the LifeSite Hemodialysis Access System. Kidney Int 2000;58:2221–2227.

6 Moran J: Clinical evaluation of subcutaneous access device (abstract). J Am Soc Nephrol 2000; 11:191A.

7 Levin NW, Yang PM, Hatch DA, Dubrow AJ, Caraiani NE, Ing TS, Gandhi VC, Alto A, Davila SM, Prosi FR, Polaschegg HD, Megerman J: Initial results of a new access for hemodialysis. Technical note. Kidney Int 1998;54:1739–1745.

8 Canaud B, My H, Morena M, Lami-Lacavalerie B, Leray-Moragues H, Bosc JY, Flavier JL, Chomel PY, Polaschegg HD, Prosl FR, Megerman J: Dialock®: A new vascular access device for extracorporeal renal replacement therapy. Preliminary clinical results. Nephrol Dial Transplant 1999;14:692–698.

9 Canaud B, Levin N, Ing T, My H, Dubrow AJ, Polaschegg HD, Prosl FR: Dialock®: Pilot trial of a new vascular port access device for hemodialysis. Semin Dial 1999;5:382–388.

10 Sodemann K, Polaschegg HD, Feldmer B: Two years' experience with Dialock and CLS™ (a new antimicrobial lock solution). Blood Purif 2001;19:251–254.

11 Marr KA, Sexton D, Conlon P, Schwab SJ, Kirkland K: bacteremia in patients with central venous catheter used for hemodialysis. Lack of efficiency of catheter salvage. Ann Intern Med 1997; 127:275–220.

12 Schwab SJ, Buller GL, McCnn RL, Bollinger RR, Stickel DL: Prospective evaluation of a Dacron cuffed hemodialysis catheter for prolonged use. Am J Kidney Dis 1988;11:166–169.

13 Quarello F, Forneris G: Prevention of hemodialysis catheter related bloodstream infection using an antimicrobial lock. Blood Purif 2002;20:87–92.

Francesco Quarello, MD, Divisione di Nefrologia e Dialisi, Ospedale San Giovanni Bosco, Piazza Donatore di Sangue, 3, I–10154 Torino (Italy)
Tel. +39 011 2402274, Fax +39 011 2402386, E-Mail fquarello@pobox.com

Ronco C, La Greca G (eds): Hemodialysis Technology.
Contrib Nephrol. Basel, Karger, 2002, vol 137, pp 54–59

Effect of Hemodynamic Conditions on Arteriovenous Fistula for Hemodialysis Access

Bogdan Ene-Iordache[a], *Simona Bruno*[a], *Andrea Remuzzi*[a], *Giuseppe Remuzzi*[a,b]

[a] Clinical Research Center for Rare Diseases, Aldo e Cele Daccò, Mario Negri Institute for Pharmacological Research, Ranica, and
[b] Nephrology and Dialysis Unit, Azienda Ospedaliera, Ospedali Riuniti di Bergamo, Italy

Vascular Access for Hemodialysis

Arteriovenous Fistula

Nowadays, providing and maintaining a vascular access (VA) for hemodialysis patients is becoming a crucial task, as the number of end-stage renal disease (ESRD) patients is continuously growing. With the VA morbidity growing faster than the ESRD population, the preservation of the VA function becomes even more crucial. Problems like delivering the dialysis dose, quality of life of the patients and financial costs represent difficult tasks to resolve. For example, it was estimated that morbidity and hospitalization related to VA complications amounted up to 25% of all-cause admissions for American dialysis patients, with an estimated annual hospital-related cost of over USD 1 billion [1].

Usually, VA for hemodialysis is provided by native arteriovenous fistulas (AVF) or synthetic arteriovenous grafts (AVG). Guidelines from the NKF-DOQI [2] recommend as a first alternative the native AVF and only when this is not possible the second choice should be the AVG. These guidelines are based on studies that showed a higher survival time for AVF when compared to AVG. There is substantial geographic variation in the distribution of VA types: while in Europe 81% of VA are AVF, the percentage of AVF in hemodialysis patients in the USA is only 21% [3]. In our dialysis unit the surgeons provide VA only by native AVF using end-to-end anastomosis as a first choice, and when this is surgically impossible, the alternative anastomosis type is side-to-side.

The surgical anastomosis between artery and vein induces a decrease of peripheral resistance and a high increase in blood flow due to the pressure gradient established between arterial and venous pressures. Afterwards, in a period of time that can be between 1 and 3 months, the higher amount of blood flow through the AVF induces vessel remodeling with an increase in the vessel lumen. This period is usually called 'maturation' of the fistula because during this time both the artery and vein dilate and the wall thickens, making repeated needle punctures possible as necessary during the dialysis sessions. In well-functioning AVF, this likely occurs as a result of a kind of a vicious cycle since the increase in the flow rate leads to an increase in the arterial diameter, and this results in an even higher blood flow and a further enlargement of the vessel lumen until an equilibrium is reached.

A primary failure occurs in 5–15% of all surgically created AVF that cannot develop and clot immediately after the surgery. In most cases, these 'early' failures are generally regarded as technical failures. Long-term failure is due to thrombosis associated with the presence of one or more stenoses. Usually, they are located at or near the venous anastomosis or elsewhere in the venous outflow tract [4]. They show the typical histology of intimal hyperplasia. Myointimal hyperplasia is a complex pathological process of the vascular system characterized by an abnormal proliferation of smooth muscle cells (SMC) of the vascular wall. Proliferating SMC migrate to the subendothelial area and form the hyperplastic region, which causes stenosis and obstruction of the vascular lumen. Intimal hyperplasia is higher at artery to vein or graft to artery and vein anastomoses in VA for hemodialysis. The vascular injury and the suture material that occupies the luminal surface of the anastomosis function as a nidus for platelet aggregation with the production of platelet-derived growth factor, which is mitogen to SMC and may promote proliferation and migration of SMC from the media into the anastomosis. The presence of a stenosis results in functional changes that include increase in resistance and pressure gradient over the stenosis, and a subsequent decline in access blood flow. Low flow causes intimal hyperplasia so that a vicious cycle is established: low flow generates obstructive neointima layers, which in turn further reduce the flow.

Hemodynamics of VA for Hemodialysis

Hemodynamics of AVF

Hemodynamic conditions have been extensively shown to play a major role in vascular remodeling and neointima formation. In human pathological conditions there is now a major consensus about the role of wall shear stress (WSS), the drag force exerted by flowing blood on the endothelium, as a pathogenetic factor for atherosclerosis. Location of arterial lesions at the carotid bifurcation [5] and within the abdominal aorta correlates with regions where WSS is low and oscillating. It is not clear yet how local hemodynamic conditions influence intimal hyperplasia, the major cause of failure for VA. It was observed that high WSS inhibits and low WSS favors development of intimal hyperplasia. Previous investigations have shown that areas of the circulation characterized by oscillation of WSS tend to develop intima hyperplasia and to favor atherosclerotic disease. To quantify this condition, it has been proposed that an oscillatory shear index (OSI) should be calculated, defined as the fraction of time cycle for which WSS is negative (i.e. in the opposite direction in respect to the main flow) [5]. Another condition that has been shown to influence vessel wall function is the elevated spatial shear stress gradient which can cause endothelial layer injury, and thus promoting SMC proliferation [6].

AVF involve complex hemodynamic conditions. The first factor influencing blood flowing in these vessels is the shunt between arterial and venous circulation that greatly increases the blood flow rate. Second, the nonuniform geometry of the anastomosis forces blood flow to change direction rapidly. If the anastomosis is end-to-end, blood flow is directed from the artery to the vein in a bending, U-shape-like structure. Side-artery-to-end-vein anastomosis has a Y-shape-like form, blood flow is directed from the artery to the vein, and there is also flow in the distal artery, which can be antegrade if the blood flows towards the hand, or retrograde if the blood flows backwards. As a result, blood flow conditions in these vessels are very different from the physiological state and can cause changes in the vascular wall responsible for vascular remodeling, narrowing or dilatation of the venous side and eventually for vessel occlusion. Intimal thickness is predominant in areas of low WSS, like the anastomotic floor and toe, also suggesting a determinant role of blood flow conditions in vessel wall injury.

Assessment of Hemodynamic Conditions in the AVF

To assess how hemodynamic forces affect the AVF, there is need for measurements or estimation of blood flow velocity and WSS along the three-dimensional vascular structure. There are mainly two methods to achieve these tasks: direct measurements (either in vivo or in vitro) and computer simulations.

Even if AVF have a higher primary failure rate than grafts, they have a lower subsequent failure rate requiring fewer procedures to maintain their long-term patency. Therefore, there is need for a test that, before hemodialysis access placement, could modify surgical management, increasing the number of AVF and predicting short- and long-term AVF outcomes. In other words, such a test should help the surgeon to choose the access site with the highest likelihood for success. The NKF-DOQI [2] guidelines provide recommendations with regard to diagnostic evaluation prior to permanent access selection that includes venography in patients who meet specified criteria. However, patients with residual renal function, in whom contrast studies are undesirable, may undergo alternative procedures such as Doppler ultrasound (US).

The literature to date suggests that routine preoperative US mapping can result in a change in surgical management, with a markedly increased number of AVF being placed and an improvement in the likelihood of selecting the most functional vessels preoperatively [7, 8]. Furthermore, data suggest that vessel size and blood flow are predictive of AVF outcome. In fact, AVF creation with a cephalic vein and/or radial artery smaller than 1.5–2.0 mm is likely to fail and may indicate that an upper arm AVF should be the primary access attempted [9]. Further studies are needed to evaluate the test properties of US in reducing the number of surgical procedures needed to achieve a successful long-term AVF or graft, and in predicting long-term outcomes.

Experimental measurements are performed using flow visualization techniques and laser Doppler anemometry in transparent silicone rubber of blood vessels. These are mounted in circuits that can simulate blood pulsatility using fluids with similar visco-elastic properties. Sivanesan et al. [10] performed an in vitro study of steady and pulsatile flow in a side-to-end AVF model with a 30° anastomotic angle and vein-to-artery diameter ratio of 1.6. They found that turbulence intensity is greater in the vein, within 10 mm of the suture line. The peak values of the WSS (~300 dyn/cm^2) were found in the anastomotic region, at the floor of the artery and on the outer wall of the vein [11], while distally on the vein the WSS returned within the physiological range. The flow characteristics in pulsatile flow were similar to those seen in steady flow with no significant changes over the cardiac cycle and this result is probably due to low pulsatility of the flow wave form in the AVF.

Computer simulations are performed using computational fluid dynamics (CFD) progressing, which allow simulation of fluid flow phenomena in three-dimensional vessel-like shape meshworks [12]. Each method (i.e. experimental measurements or computer simulations) has pros and cons and the best use is to combine them, using the results from one to validate the other and vice versa. We recently used CFD to perform numerical calculations of blood flow distribution inside an end-to-end, 25-month-old AVF [12]. Computations were based on real geometry meshwork of the AVF, reconstructed from orthogonal digital subtraction angiographies, and using blood properties (viscosity and density) that were measured in blood samples of that specific patient. The numerical run was transient using as input the blood flow wave form measured at the level of the radial artery using echo-color-Doppler US. Time average flow rate in the radial artery was 714 ml/min and pulse frequency was 68 beats/min. Using CFD analysis we were able to visualize velocity profiles and calculate WSS along the AVF wall. Shear stress at the level of the radial artery was low and within the physiological range [11] and fairly uniform along the vessel perimeter. Very high WSS (~350 dyn/cm^2), associated with high shear stress spatial gradients (more than 2,000 dyn/cm^3), developed in the bending zone, far exceeding the physiological range. Near the anastomosis an irregular geometry of the vein was present, probably due to old vein valves and increased hyperplasia within the suture zone. In this region recirculation flow occurred leading to positive and negative values of WSS, and thus to high shear stress gradients. More distally, on the cephalic vein, the flow disturbances were attenuated and WSS decreased returning to within the physiological range, without flow recirculation. In our AVF simulation study the flow pulsatility was limited, with the flow rate remaining sustained for the entire cardiac cycle. This condition resulted in almost null OSI along the entire vessel wall surface. It is interesting to note that the main flow characteristics we found in an end-to-end AVF by using CFD are quite similar to those obtained experimentally by Sivanesan et al. [10] in a side-to-end model of AVF.

These results indicate that oscillations in WSS may not be relevant for vascular wall changes in these types of AV shunts. The high shear stress gradients that develop near the bending and near the anastomotic zone may alter the functional state of the endothelial layer and probably of the underlying SMC.

Conclusions

Intensive investigations into VA for hemodialysis are still necessary to understand the reasons for primary and long-term failure of the shunt. New noninvasive investigation tools, such as US, and a detailed analysis of blood flow conditions may help elucidate the mechanisms for AVF failure and improve clinical outcomes of this crucial step in uremic patient management.

References

1 Feldman HI, Kobrin S, Wasserstein A: Hemodialysis vascular access morbidity. J Am Soc Nephrol 1996;7:523–535.
2 NKF-DOQI Clinical Practice Guidelines for Vascular Access. National Kidney Foundation-Dialysis Outcomes Quality Initiative. Am J Kidney Dis 1997;30:S150–S191.
3 Dhingra RK, Young EW, Hulbert-Shearon TE, Leavey SF, Port FK: Type of vascular access and mortality in US hemodialysis patients. Kidney Int 2001;60:1443–1451.

4 Kanterman RY, Vesely TM, Pilgram TK, Guy BW, Windus DW, Picus D: Dialysis access grafts: Anatomic location of venous stenosis and results of angioplasty. Radiology 1995;195:135–139.
5 Ku DN, Giddens DP, Zarins CK, Glagov S: Pulsatile flow and atherosclerosis in the human carotid bifurcation. Arteriosclerosis 1985;5/3:293–302.
6 DePaola N, Gimbrone MA Jr, Davies PF, Dewey CF Jr: Vascular endothelium responds to fluid shear stress gradients. Arterioscler Thromb 1992;12:1254–1257.
7 Robbin ML, Gallichio MH, Deierhoi MH, Young CJ, Weber TM, Allon M: US vascular mapping before hemodialysis access placement. Radiology 2000;217:83–88.
8 Allon M, Lockhart ME, Lilly RZ, Gallichio MH, Young CJ, Barker J, Deierhoi MH, Robbin ML: Effect of preoperative sonographic mapping on vascular access outcomes in hemodialysis patients. Kidney Int 2001;60:2013–2020.
9 Brimble KS, Rabbat CG, Schiff D, Ingram AJ: The clinical utility of Doppler ultrasound prior to arteriovenous fistula creation. Semin Dial 2001;14:314–317.
10 Sivanesan S, How TV, Black RA, Bakran A: Flow patterns in the radiocephalic arteriovenous fistula: An in vitro study. J Biomech 1999;32:915–925.
11 Giddens DP, Zarins CK, Glagov S: The role of fluid mechanics in the localization and detection of atherosclerosis. J Biomech Eng 1993;115:588–594.
12 Ene-Iordache B, Mosconi L, Remuzzi G, Remuzzi A: Computational fluid dynamics of a vascular access case for hemodialysis. J Biomech Eng 2001;123:284–292.

Giuseppe Remuzzi, MD, Research Coordinator, Clinical Research Center for Rare Diseases,
Aldo e Cele Daccò, Villa Camozzi, I–24020 Ranica (Italy)
Tel. +39 035 511111, Fax +39 035 514503, E-Mail gremuzzi@marionegri.it

Ronco C, La Greca G (eds): Hemodialysis Technology.
Contrib Nephrol. Basel, Karger, 2002, vol 137, pp 60–69

Quality Assurance and Continuous Quality Improvement in the Management of Vascular Access

Juan P. Bosch, Brian A.J. Walters

Gambro Healthcare, Scientific Affairs and Clinical Research,
Fort Lauderdale, Fla., USA

The quality of life and survival of patients on hemodialysis is, without question, directly linked to the establishment of a functioning vascular access. Following the introduction in 1997 of the Clinical Practice Guidelines for Vascular Access by the National Kidney Foundation in the United States [1] and an update in 2001 [2] there have been best practice guidelines published for vascular access management from peer review organizations in other countries [3]. While the importance of maintaining effective access to the patient's blood circulatory system to ensure proficient blood flow to the dialysis machine remains a primary goal in managing patients with end-stage renal disease (ESRD), it is surprising that vascular access outcome benchmarks remain suboptimal or have continued to deteriorate while other dialysis quality benchmarks have undergone significant improvement [4, 5]. Medical complications arising from the vascular access have been extensively documented in the medical literature and such evidence clearly indicates that the preferred method of vascular access is an arteriovenous fistulae (AVF), followed by an arteriovenous graft and least preferable is a permanent catheter. Our own studies and those of others continue to identify the use of catheters, either temporary or permanent, as a major cause of hospitalization, anemia and bacteremia within the hemodialysis population [6–8]. This has resulted in an escalation in the cost of providing care for these patients. In the United States, the movement towards increasing the accountability of providers of healthcare services to patients whose healthcare is covered by federal agencies such as Medicare has resulted in the introduction of vascular access Clinical Performance Measures by the Centers for Medicare and Medicaid Services

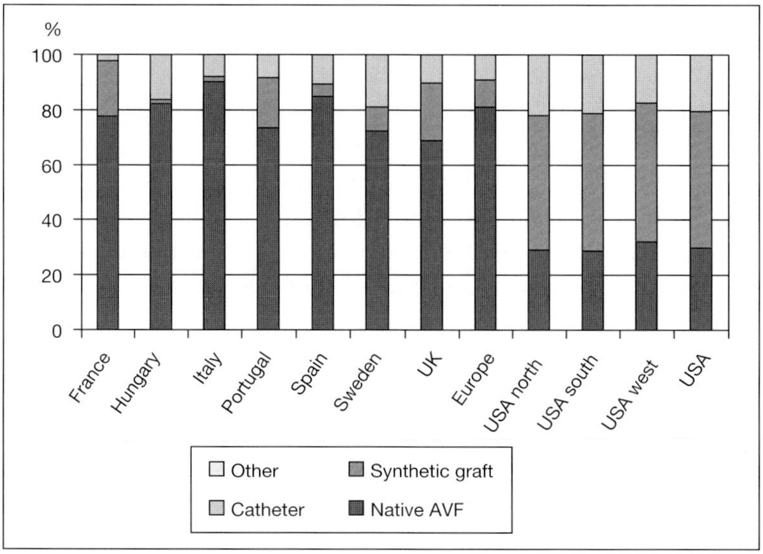

Fig. 1. Differences in vascular access among prevalent hemodialysis patients in Gambro Healthcare globally.

(CMS) – the regulatory body that finances the care for the majority of hemodialysis patients. The data on vascular access is collected through 18 regional networks and pressure is exerted upon the providers by the CMS to institute quality programs that will result in 50% of incident patients and 40% of prevalent patients having an AVF. In addition, the CMS has indicated that the use of catheters for primary vascular access be reduced to 10% in the prevalent dialysis population and a proactive surveillance system be developed to detect and correct problems before accesses thrombose or fail. The CMS used benchmarks published as an 'opinion' and a potential quality of care standard in the K/DOQI guidelines [2]. The magnitude of the challenge becomes clear when one considers that the most current data from the 18 dialysis networks in the United States indicates that only 28% of incident patients and 27% (range 15–40%) of prevalent patients are dialyzed with an AVF [4] and studies continue to demonstrate the care provided to predialysis patients is not optimal nor satisfactorily addresses access planning [9–11]. In addition, 14% (range 15–30%) of prevalent patients were dialyzed with a catheter. Data from Gambro Healthcare reflect the same trends in the United States as that reported from the ESRD Networks while confirming the differences between the United States and Europe (fig. 1).

The Facility Quality Control Team

The success of any program designed to survey and improve vascular access quality is determined by the level of participatory leadership from the upper management of the facility, in particular the physician/nephrologist. While ensuring that quality improvement is important it is essential that the physician participate as a team member allowing for a multidisciplinary approach to solving the problems by functioning as a leader and facilitator. The vascular access quality assurance (QA) program should become an integral component of the dialysis facility quality control team. The team should understand the structure-process-outcome framework used in quality measurement. In the vascular access program, 'structure' refers to the understanding by the team members of the surgical program within which the facility vascular access program operates. Who are the surgeons who are responsible for access placement and what data exists for surgeon-specific outcomes? What are the restraints under which the access placement program operates? These include access to operating room time and access to patients with chronic renal insufficiency within the immediate geographic location of the dialysis facility so that access placement can be coordinated prior to dialysis initiation. Studies within Gambro Healthcare suggest that the great variation in AVF placement in incident patients between facilities and within facilities is dependent on the medical community involvement of the nephrologist with his surgical and medical colleagues. In the United States, the nephrologist depends upon the primary care physician to refer the patient with ESRD with sufficient time before dialysis initiation to coordinate the surgical placement of the access. The reality is that this does not occur and more often catastrophic initiation of dialysis with a catheter is the norm.

The 'process' refers to the facility healthcare personnel, facility procedures and equipment available to monitor and ensure the success of the vascular access program. These include protocols, flow charts, access surveillance protocols such as venous pressure monitoring and routine measurement of blood flow rate through the access for the early detection of vascular accesses at risk for thrombosis. It also includes procedures that include medications such as tissue plasminogen activator and urokinase that are used to prevent catheter blockage prophylactically or to clear a blockage following a reduction in blood flow rates. The 'outcome' is then measured at an optimal frequency and reported back to the quality control team. The components and definitions used in the outcome measurement will be discussed in detail below. What is important from the perspective of the quality control team is that there is a regular feedback of outcomes and trends to document the value of interventions supported by the team. Quality does have a time component in that once the quality benchmark has been reached it should be maintained with as small a variation as possible. The standard deviation (SD) of the mean provides a measure of the variability and facilities with lower SD while maintaining the specified benchmark are considered to have a higher quality than facilities maintaining the benchmark with higher SD.

The Science of Quality: Medical Quality, QA and Continuous Quality Improvement

We are proposing that to orchestrate a change that will not only succeed in moving the current vascular access outcomes towards the benchmarks recommended, but also reverse the current trends that are going in the opposite direction will require invoking all of the basic tenets of QA and continuous quality improvement (CQI). Both QA and CQI are components of the science of quality. Medical quality is the adherence to recognized appropriate standards of peer-reviewed practices that have consistently been associated with the best patient outcomes. This definition has within its framework the innate ability to change and respond to change. As the program of quality proceeds benchmarks are raised, medical appropriateness, medical standards, the peer review process and what is considered to be the best patient outcomes will all undergo a redefining or upward trend. QA is essentially quality surveillance while CQI provides a methodology to improve outcomes through improving quality. The component steps of QA include (1) defining the quality standard (K/DOQI standard and/or facility-specific vascular access standard); (2) defining the rationale (understanding the impact on patient outcomes of not meeting the standard); (3) setting the quality threshold (AVF 40% prevalent patients; catheters <10%, access-related hospitalizations, thromboses requiring intervention, frequency of recirculation measurement or other access surveillance tool); (4) determining the survey frequency (monthly, quarterly or preferably rolling quarterly data collection), and (5) providing corrective action strategies if the standard cannot be attained. If improvements are not forthcoming then the process should be extended through a focused QA study to determine why the standard was unattainable. Often this leads to the formal institution of a CQI program.

CQI is more complex and requires a team, which, while committed to a common purpose, consists of individual members with different skill sets. The common purpose is also referred to as the vision of the team of which the most important component is 'beginning with the end in mind'. This is more than just defining clearly the objectives of the CQI team but defining the parameters to be measured, the outcome to be aimed for and providing an effective methodology

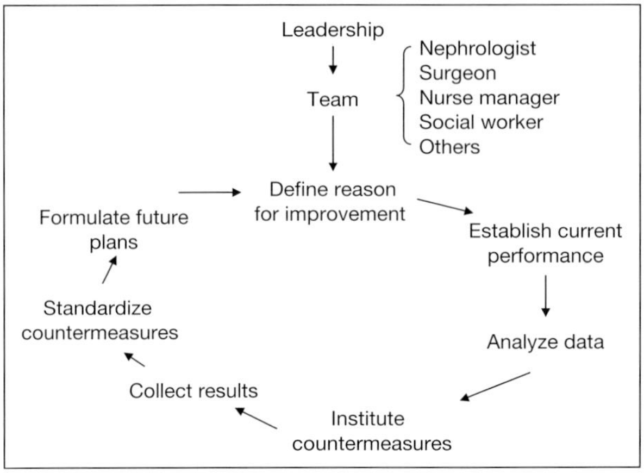

Fig. 2. Steps in the vascular access CQI program.

to achieve them. The link between proactivity and vision through methods based on a value system that includes the patient often involves rescripting which replaces ineffective patterns of medical practice and organizational processes with effective ones. Such a process involves defining all of the steps involved in the vascular access process and measuring the impact and importance of each step on the final outcome. Such rescripting may be essential for improving outcomes in vascular access through effectively utilizing improvements in technology and science at the level of the dialysis facility. The formation of the CQI team to address vascular access should include at a minimum the nephrologist medical director, the vascular surgeon, the nurse manager, a staff nurse, the patient care technician, and the social worker. The component steps utilized by the team in CQI are shown in figure 2 and are described in detail below.

Step 1: Defining the Reason for Improvement

The tools and techniques include a project planning sheet, trending graphs that monitor trends retrospectively and prospectively, control charts that compare the facility vascular access outcomes with their peers in the immediate geographic region standardized for age, ethnicity, gender and comorbidity and process flow charts that detail the steps involved in the process of vascular access management. Poor outcomes that are linked to vascular access problems are numerous but the most easily identifiable and the most important are increased hospitalization and infections. These outcomes have consistently been linked to the vascular access as the primary cause. Vascular access problems include cannulation technique, anticoagulant policies and procedures, increased frequency of venous stenosis due to subclavian catheter use, hypotension and different skill levels of the vascular surgeons. These can only be recognized if the dialysis facility has in operation a structured QA surveillance program with defined benchmarks. These document the acceptable frequency of complications and provide objective evidence that the acceptable frequency has been exceeded. The objective benchmarks define for the team the criteria used to identify that a vascular access problem exists and the impact on the patient. During the dialogue that develops within the team it will become clear that the commitment to improvement is patient-orientated and that the indicators used to monitor the problem correctly represent the problem to be addressed. This process of dialogue and commitment forms the basis of the CQI initiation process and assists in bonding within the team, which will solidify future commitment. It is important, during this time to revisit the data collected through the QA process to ensure that the need for the vascular access CQI program is justified. Finally, a schedule for completing the CQI program should be developed.

Step 2: State the Current Situation

The objective here is to select a problem(s) that has contributed to suboptimal vascular access outcomes within the facility and set a target for improvement. The target needs to be realistic and achievable. The tools and techniques here include control charts, histograms, Pareto charts and a check sheet. The responsibility of the team is to select a problem and set a target for improvement.

In most cases where vascular access is the major cause of increased hospitalization or infection rates the causes are multiple and the separate recognition of them demands a detailed surveillance program. In every dialysis facility in the United States the majority of patients begin dialysis with a catheter, so late referral to a nephrologist will always play a role. In addition, unless there has been a significant commitment by the dialysis quality control committee to providing surgeon-specific feedback of access survival data there will always be a spectrum of outcomes that are attributable to differences in the skill level of the vascular surgeons. The pervasive use of subclavian catheters add to the quality surveillance complexity by providing a background risk for venous stenosis that can mask other causes of venous stenosis that go undetected and untreated. The challenge is to stratify the data to a component level specific enough to analyze. Finally a problem statement is arrived at through an analysis of the data. The problem statement should address the gap between the current situation and the target set by the CQI team. The methodology in establishing the goals and target outcomes should be identified and finally the current situation analysis should ensure that the patient requirements were identified and were valid. This continual returning to the patient during the process maintains and strengthens the mission of the team, reestablishes commitment and prepares the team for constructive differences that may emerge during the analysis and interpretation steps to follow.

Step 3: Analysis

The objective is to identify and verify the root causes of poor vascular access outcomes within the facility being analyzed. The tools and techniques include cause and affect analysis, histograms, graphs, Pareto charts, scatter diagrams and use of a check sheet that lists all variables known to impact vascular access outcomes. Cause and effect diagrams sometimes called fishbone diagrams subdivide the program into the major responsible areas and then classify all of the causes within the responsible area that can affect the vascular access outcome. The primary causes of the problem often referred to as the root causes can then be identified through Pareto charts that classify causes and identify those that are significant from those that are not. Often these obey the 80:20 rule in that 80% of the poor outcomes results from only 20% of causes identified. It is important that the root causes of problems are not only identified but also taken to actionable levels and that the root causes with the probable greatest impact be selected for resolution. In all instances, access surveillance data are used to verify the root causes. The access surveillance program monitors hemodynamic changes within the access and is designed to detect vascular accesses at risk for thrombosis. The methods used depend on visual inspection, pressure measurements or access flow measurements. Whatever method is used, all are aimed at the early detection of stenotic lesions that can be corrected by angioplasty or surgical revision before there is thrombosis that occludes blood flow. While it is not the purpose of this review to discuss the relative merits of each surveillance program, it is important to mention that a detailed access inspection program that recognizes the value of collecting and trending changes in pressure or flow remains the foundation for initiating proactive interventions [12, 13].

Step 4: Institution of Countermeasures

The objective is to plan and implement countermeasures that will correct the root causes of the problem. Often this step might be field tested in a few patients or, in the case of a corporation or network, in a few facilities to confirm its effectiveness. In any case, a cost estimation must be performed to ensure that the cost is commensurate with the impact that the problem is having on the healthcare cost and patient outcomes. In the case of vascular access outcome improvement, it is a win-win for both the healthcare program and the patient because of the overwhelming volume of studies linking suboptimal vascular access outcomes with increases in hospital expenditure to the detriment of the healthcare program balance sheet. For a dialysis healthcare program that is outpatient driven, since the patient is not being treated by the facility while in hospital, there is a loss in productivity superimposed on increased personnel cost. Facilities that have acute contracts with the hospital and often benefit financially from performing the dialysis treatment in the hospital may consider the impact of vascular access improvement on reducing infections, the third major cause of mortality for hemodialysis patients [2]. Tools commonly used include a countermeasure matrix with a chart listing barriers and aids to the countermeasures. When the team has finally approved the countermeasures to be instituted an action plan is developed. The action plan attempts to answer the questions of who, what, where and how. It must reflect the barriers and aids necessary for successful implementation. The countermeasures are analyzed themselves to ensure that they attack the root causes in step 3 and that the countermeasures were consistent with patients' needs that were identified in step 1.

Step 5: Results

The objective here is to confirm that the problems and root causes impacting on suboptimal vascular access outcomes have been decreased and the target for improvement has been met. It is important that the tracking indicator or QA marker used to demonstrate the improvement is the same one that was used to identify the problem in the first place. If the results did not meet or exceed the target then the cause of the failure needs to be addressed.

Step 6: Standardization

The objective is to standardize the countermeasures by reporting them to the upper management and the medical leadership of the network or corporation so that policies may be written or revised to incorporate the countermeasures. They should become an integral part of the standard operating procedures in the network or the dialysis facility. This will prevent the problem and its root causes from recurring. To achieve this goal there must be developed a method to assure that the countermeasures become part of the daily work. Most often this involves developing an educational training program to ensure that the countermeasures are adopted by the current staff and that the countermeasures are included in the training of new staff. A program of periodic checks must be put in place with assigned responsibility to monitor the countermeasures. The QA checks should be reported to the facility Quality Control Committee for a defined period of time to ensure that there is no deterioration in their value and that the root causes of the problems identified do not reemerge.

Step 7: Future Plans

Often the process of CQI identifies problems that were not immediately obvious when the process began and these need to be addressed. In our own experience, the CQI vascular access program identified a group of patients with reduced responsiveness to erythropoietin [7]. It is not surprising that the presence of a catheter may lead to a heightened state of inflammation which has been linked to erythropoietin resistance. Other instances of opportunities for improvement resulting for the CQI vascular access program include the recognition of occult infections in nonfunctioning grafts responsible for inflammation and this has led to programs that monitor the origin of primary bacteremias within the facility. The remaining non-root cause problems identified need to be resolved and the process of plan-do-check-act should be applied to the lessons learned.

Conclusions

We have outlined a process of CQI from a generic perspective that we have found to be successful in improving vascular access outcomes within our own experience [14]. The process requires dedication and leadership from the nephrologist but depends upon the presence of an already established quality surveillance program that contains accurate, valid retrospective data on vascular access outcomes. The process establishes the link between improvement in vascular access outcomes and cost-effective healthcare delivery that always places the patient at the center of the circle of concern. The process recognizes that excellence in providing quality in vascular access management begins before the patient initiates dialysis and we challenge the CQI team to design plausible proactive opportunities to reach into the domain of chronic renal insufficiency and catalyze change. The great successes of CQI often are realized in the step labeled 'future plans' and the great challenge is to expand the circle of influence created during the CQI process to ensure that every opportunity to improve quality of life and life expectancy for the patient is exhausted.

References

1 National Kidney Foundation-Dialysis Outcomes Quality Initiative Clinical Practice Guidelines for Vascular Access. Am J Kidney Dis 1997;30(suppl 3):S150–S189.
2 National Kidney Foundation. K/DOQI Clinical Practice Guidelines for Vascular Access 2000. Am J Kidney Dis 2001;37(suppl 1):S137–S181.
3 Jindal KK, Ethier JH, Lindsay RM, Barre PE, Kappal JE, Carlisle EJF, Common A: Clinical practice guidelines for vascular access. J Am Soc Nephrol 1999;10:S287–S321.
4 HealthCare Financing Administration: 2000 Annual Report: ESRD Clinical Performance Measures Project. Am J Kidney Dis 2001;37(suppl 3):S1–S74.
5 Excerpts from the United States Renal Data System's 2001 Annual Data Report: Atlas of end stage renal disease in the United States. Am J Kidney Dis 2001;38(suppl 3):S79–S90.

6 Bleyer AJ, Rocco MV, Burkart JM: The costs of hospitalizations due to hemodialysis access management. Nephrol News Issues 1995;9:19–22.
7 Walters BAJ, Carter WB, Augustine BA, Bander SJ: Central venous catheters contribute to low blood hemoglobin in hemodialysis patients (abstract). J Am Soc Nephrol 2000;11:295A.
8 Walters BAJ, Molina M, Rosenthal RF, DiDominic V, Bander SJ: Incidence of bacteremia in hemodialysis patients 1993–1994 (abstract). J Am Soc Nephrol 1995;6:567.
9 Beserab A: Vascular access in Europe and the United States: Striking contrasts. Contemp Dial Nephrol 1999;20:22–28.
10 Astor BC, Eustace MB, Powe NR, Klag MJ, Sadler JJH, Fink NE, Coresh J: Timing of nephrologist referral and arteriovenous fistulae use: The CHOICE study. Am J Kidney Dis 2001;38: 494–501.
11 Allon M, Ornt DB, Schwab SJ, Rasmussen C, Delmez JA, Greene T, Kusek JW, Martin AA, Minda S, for the Hemodialysis (HEMO) Study Group: Factors associated with the prevalence of arteriovenous fistulas in hemodialysis patients in the HEMO study. Kidney Int 2000;58:2178–2185.
12 Leypoldt KJ: Standards for reproducible access flow measurements. Blood Purif 2002;20:20–26.
13 Beserab A: Preventing vascular access dysfunction: Which policy to follow. Blood Purif 2002;20: 26–35.
14 Duda CR, Spergel LM, Holland J, Tucker T, Bander SJ, Bosch JP: How a multidisciplinary vascular access care program enables implementation of the DOQI guidelines. Nephrol News Issues 2000;14/5:13.

Dr. Juan P. Bosch, Director Renal Division,
George Washington University, The H.B. Burns Memorial Building,
2150 Pennsylvania Ave., N.W. No. 505, Washington, DC 20037 (USA)

Ronco C, La Greca G (eds): Hemodialysis Technology.
Contrib Nephrol. Basel, Karger, 2002, vol 137, pp 70–77

Membranes for Dialysis

Composition, Structure and Function

William R. Clark[a,b], *Dayong Gao*[c], *Claudio Ronco*[d]

[a]Renal Division, Baxter Healthcare Corp., McGaw Park, Ill.; [b]Nephrology Division, Indiana University School of Medicine, Indianapolis, Ind., and [c]Center for Biomedical Engineering, University of Kentucky, Lexington, Ky., USA; [d]Nephrology Department, St. Bortolo Hospital, Vicenza, Italy

In the first clinical hemodialysis performed in 1923 by Haas et al. [1], collodion tubes served as the semipermeable membrane. Since that time, a variety of different hemodialyzer configurations and membranes have been used. The current HD membrane market is based almost exclusively on hollow fiber technology, which provides the foundation for the annual production of approximately 90 million dialyzers now. The purpose of this article is severalfold. First, a brief historical review of the different membrane and dialyzer configurations used for HD therapy is provided, with emphasis placed on the factors that have led to the present situation of hollow fiber predominance. Second, the general characteristics of hollow fiber membranes used for HD are discussed. Third, an overview of the factors primarily determining a membrane's characteristics that are most relevant clinically is provided. These characteristics are small solute removal capabilities, middle and large molecule removal attributes, and the 'inflammatory' nature of a membrane, including its complement activation potential and its ability to prevent cytokine-inducing substance (CIS) transfer from dialysate to blood.

Hemodialyzer Configurations: Historical Perspective

The first HD apparatus considered suitable for widespread human use was the rotating drum kidney [2]. This device consisted of a 30-meter cellophane tube with an inner diameter of 35 mm that was spirally wrapped around a cylinder which rotated in a stationary dialysate bath. The device was characterized by a very low blood compartment resistance, a desirable feature in that dialysis could be achieved without a blood pump. However, this was an undesirable feature from the perspective of ultrafiltration, which was limited by the very low transmembrane pressures generated. To address this problem, Alwall [3] developed a modified version in which the cellophane tubing was placed between two cylinders rather than only being wrapped around one. This resulted in a restricted blood pathway and higher blood compartment pressures, which in combination with the generation of negative pressure in the dialysate compartment, permitted significant plasma water ultrafiltration to occur. A general limitation of this type of device was the large extracorporeal blood volume requirement (500–700 ml).

The next major development was the coil dialyzer in which [4] cellophane tubing surrounded by a fiberglass screen were wound together in a single coil which in turn was situated circumferentially in a cylinder. Dialysate was recirculated from a large tank at 30 liters/min. Because the blood compartment inner diameter was controlled by specific spacing of the screens, relatively high blood compartment resistance (i.e. pressure) was generated. Unfortunately, a mandatory net ultrafiltration volume of approximately 700 ml during a typical 5-hour treatment was created as a result of the high blood path resistance. This type of dialyzer was commercialized as the 'twin-coil' [5] which had two coils providing a total surface area of 1.8 m^2.

In the late 1940s [6, 7], multiple-use parallel-flow dialyzers in which the blood pathway was created by stacking cellophane tubes or flat sheets were first described. This configuration created a relatively narrow blood channel (short mass transfer length) and with acceptable blood compartment high resistance. A specific dialyzer of this type, described by Kiil [8], consisted of four parallel cellophane channels (formed by eight flat sheet membranes) which in turn were supported by plastic boards. Diffusive mass transfer in this dialyzer was relatively favorable due to the relatively narrow blood channels (created by the compression effect of the boards) and the use of a new thin-walled membrane, Cuprophan. (Dialyzer designs previously had employed relatively thick cellophane membranes (30–40 μm in thickness) whereas Cuprophan's thickness in this dialyzer was 15 μm.) A modified version of the multiple-use Kiil dialyzer became commercially available and was widely used in the 1960s [9]. Subsequently, disposable single-use parallel flow dialyzers were developed, including the Rhone-Poulenc (RP) dialyzer [10].

The deficiencies of the above configurations, especially those related to high blood compartment resistance and inefficient mass transfer, led to the development of the hollow fiber artificial kidney (HFAK) [11]. The HFAK had several advantages, including decreased blood compartment channel distance, improved blood rheology, and the decreased boundary layer effects due to the attainment of relatively high shear rates with modest axial pressure drops. These favorable mass transfer and hydrodynamic characteristics of the HFAK led to a rapid increase in the use of this type of dialyzer, which is essentially the only kind used in contemporary HD.

Hollow Fiber Membrane Characteristics

Hollow Fiber Dimensions

An individual hollow fiber is a cylinder with an inner annular region serving as the blood compartment. The relatively standard dimensions of hollow fibers used for HD (blood compartment inner diameter, 180–220 μm; length, 20–24 cm) represent a compromise between opposing forces that exist during a typical treatment. Decreasing hollow fiber inner diameter improves diffusive mass transfer by shortening path length and attenuating boundary layer effects through higher shear rates [12]. However, the factors constraining decreases in hollow fiber inner diameter become evident with knowledge that axial (i.e. from arterial to venous end) flow in the lumen of a hollow fiber is governed by the Hagen-Poiseuille equation [13]:

$$Q_B = \Delta P/R \quad (1)$$

In this equation, Q_B is blood flow rate, ΔP is axial pressure drop, and R is the resistance to flow. (Note that resistance to flow differs from diffusive mass transfer resistance discussed previously.) Resistance is directly proportional to blood viscosity and fiber length and indirectly proportional to the fourth power of the hollow fiber inner diameter. As such, a small decrease in hollow fiber inner diameter induces a large increase in flow resistance, which in turn results in a proportional increase in axial pressure drop (at constant blood flow rate). Therefore, hollow fiber lumen dimensions represent a compromise that reflects both mass transfer and hydrodynamic considerations.

For a particular hollow fiber, the inner annular surface represents the nominal blood compartment surface area and is the theoretically maximal area available for blood contact. For the entire group of fibers comprising a dialyzer, total nominal surface area then depends on fiber length, inner diameter, and overall number, the latter of which varies generally from approximately 7,000 to 14,000.

Water Permeability (Flux)

Several approaches have been used to characterize and quantify the flux properties of HD membranes. One approach assumes that all of a membrane's pores have the same radius (r_p), and the directional orientation of the cylinders is assumed to be perpendicular to the flow of blood and dialysate. Because the Hagen-Poisseuile equation can also be used here to characterize fluid flow through the pores, ultrafiltrate flux is also directly proportional to r_p. As described by Handley et al. [14] recently, a more sophisticated approach accounts for tortuosity of pores in a membrane:

$$K_f = n\pi r^4/\tau\mu\Delta x \qquad (2)$$

In this equation, K_f is the hydraulic permeability of the membrane, n is the number of pores per unit area (i.e. pore density), r is the pore radius, τ is a factor accounting for pore tortuosity, μ is the viscosity of the ultrafiltrate, and Δx is the membrane wall thickness. Since the rate of ultrafiltrate flow is directly related to the fourth-power of the pore radius in both of these approaches, the membrane characteristic that most directly influences water permeability is mean pore size.

Depuration Properties

On the other hand, the diffusive properties of a dialysis membrane are determined mainly by the porosity (pore density) and, to some extent, the pore size [15]. Diffusion during HD can be characterized by solute flux (φ: mass removal rate per unit surface area of membrane). Based on the (straight) cylindrical pore model, diffusive solute flux can be expressed as:

$$\varphi = \lambda D\rho\Delta C/\Delta x \qquad (3)$$

where λ is the solute partition coefficient, D is solute diffusivity, ρ is membrane porosity, and ΔC is the transmembrane concentration gradient. The partition coefficient is inversely proportional to the degree to which a solute is excluded from entering a pore while membrane porosity ($\rho = n\pi r^2$) is a function of both pore size and number. Thus the membrane-related factors providing relatively high diffusive permeability are high porosity and low wall thickness. Of note, high porosity does not necessarily imply large mean pore size, as porosity can be manipulated by changes in both pore size and pore density.

The removal of relatively large compounds, such as peptides and proteins, during HD occurs primarily by nondiffusive mechanisms, namely convection and adsorption. For a specific solute, its sieving coefficient is typically used to characterize the convective removal capabilities of a membrane. Although the cylindrical pore model described previously is a good first-order approximation, actual membranes used for clinical HD actually have a distribution of pore sizes. As described recently by Ronco et al. [16], the nature of this pore size distribution may significantly influence a membrane's sieving properties. Desirable features for a high-flux membrane include a large number of relatively large pores (as large as 45 Å) having a narrow distribution of sizes. This type of distribution leads ideally to a solute sieving coefficient vs molecular weight profile with a sharp cut-off at a molecular weight just below that of albumin, similar to that of the native kidney. In actual practice, all highly permeable membranes have measurable albumin sieving coefficient values, such that the design of this type of membrane involves striking a balance between optimized large molecular weight toxin removal and minimal albumin losses.

Another convection-related mechanism by which large uremic toxins can be removed relates to fluid flow within the filter. Under normal operating conditions of high-flux dialysis, the large axial pressure drop that occurs in such highly permeable membranes typically results in pressures in a certain portion of the distal (venous) end of the fiber that are less than the corresponding dialysate compartment pressure. This results in the routine occurrence of backfiltration of dialysate during high-flux HD. Although the combination of significant backfiltration and contaminated dialysate raises many concerns (see below), this internal filtration ('Starling's flow') mechanism can significantly augment larger molecule removal. In fact, attempts at accentuating this internal filtration mechanism, either through a decrease in hollow fiber inner diameter or manipulations in dialysate compartment pressure, have been described recently [17].

Adsorption (membrane binding) is another mechanism by which hydrophobic compounds like peptides and proteins may be removed during HD. Although adsorption during HD is a relatively poorly understood phenomenon, certain membrane characteristics play an important role. First, adsorption primarily occurs within the pore structure of the membrane rather than at the nominal surface contacting the blood only [18]. Therefore, the open pore structure of high-flux membranes affords more adsorptive potential than do low-flux counterparts. Second, synthetic membranes, many of which are fundamentally hydrophobic, generally are much more adsorptive than hydrophilic cellulosic membranes [19].

The adsorptivity of a membrane also appears to influence the 'inflammatory' potential of a dialysis treatment. Dialysate may contain both endotoxin-related and exotoxin-derived compounds, which have collectively been called cytokine-inducing substances (CIS) due to their ability to stimulate cytokine production by mononuclear cells in vitro. CIS transfer may play a causative role in the occurrence of both acute and chronic adverse effects in ESRD patients treated with HD. The size range of these CIS is such that the majority of them have the potential to be 'backtransported' by either diffusion or convection from dialysate to blood during HD. The potential for convective CIS transport from contaminated dialysate in association with backfiltration across a highly permeable dialyzer membrane has received the most attention. However, several groups have demonstrated in vitro CIS transfer from highly contaminated dialysate is abrogated either significantly or totally by certain high-flux synthetic HD membranes [20, 21]. This attenuation has been attributed to adsorptive removal of CIS by the membrane via nonspecific hydrophobic interactions. CIS backtransport from contaminated dialysate can occur across dialyzer membranes of relatively low water permeability, for which the only relevant mechanism is diffusion. Thus, mean pore size alone does not determine the extent of CIS transfer and other membrane-related factors, such as hydrophobicity and diffusive characteristics, also play important roles.

Membrane Composition and Structure

Unmodified Cellulosic Membranes

The constituent component of cellulosic membranes is cellobiose and a characteristic feature of unmodified versions of this type is a high density of hydroxyl groups. Although this feature largely accounts for the exuberant complement activation that characteristically occurs with clinical use of these membranes, they have a number of features which render them very useful for diffusive HD. Specifically, these fibers can be manufactured to have low wall thickness (see below) and high porosity, both of which provide excellent diffusive transport properties. However, these membranes generally have low mean pore size and pronounced hydrophilicity, such that neither transmembrane nor adsorptive removal of middle and larger sized uremic toxins is significant typically [22].

Modified Cellulosic Dialyzers

These membranes retain the desirable diffusive properties of regenerated cellulose membranes but are associated with less-pronounced complement activation and generally have larger mean pore size [23]. The attenuation of complement activation is achieved either by substituting a high percentage of hydroxyl groups with a relatively small chemical compound (e.g. cellulose diacetate, cellulose triacetate) or by substituting a relatively small percentage of hydroxyl groups (less than 5%) with a bulky chemical compound (e.g. Hemophan, synthetically modified cellulose). Thus, either by a direct effect or a steric mechanism, both of the approaches result in diminished ability of complement proteins to interact with the membrane surface and thus initiate the complement activation process [24].

Synthetic Membranes

Although synthetic membranes were initially manufactured exclusively with high water permeability [25] to allow use in hemofiltration, this class displays varying water permeability now. As opposed to the relatively thin-walled, symmetric structure of cellulosic membranes, synthetic membranes are thicker (>20 μm) and may be either symmetric or asymmetric. An asymmetric structure implies a blood-contacting 'skin' layer (approximately 1 μm) and a support layer which comprises the remaining wall thickness. The pore structure of this support layer, which varies considerably among the various synthetic membranes [17, 26–28] is much more open than the skin layer and has little influence on the transmembrane solute removal capabilities of a membrane, although it may be an important determinant of adsorptivity. In addition, for a given asymmetric membrane, the mean pore size in the support layer may vary considerably depending on radial location. In general, the average pore size of the inner skin layer of a high-flux synthetic membrane falls in the 30–50 Å, range, while pore sizes in the support layer may be greater than 100 Å. On the other hand, a typical low-flux synthetic membrane has a skin layer mean pore size of approximately 10 Å.

References

1 Haas G: Dialysis of flowing blood in the patient. Klin Wochenschr 1923;70:1888.
2 Kolff W, Berk H: The artificial kidney: A dialyzer with a great area. Acta Med Scand 1944;117:121–134.
3 Alwall N: On the artificial kidney. I. Apparatus for dialysis of blood in vivo. Acta Med Scand 1947; 128:317–325.
4 Kolff W, Watschinger B, Vertes B: Results in patients treated with the coil kidney. JAMA 1956; 161:1433–1437.
5 Vertes V, Aoyama S, Kolff W: The twin-coil disposable artificial kidney. Trans Am Soc Artif Intern Organs 1958;3:119–121.
6 MacNeill A, Doyle J, Anthone R, Anthone S: Technique with parallel flow, straight tube blood dialyzer. NY State J Med 1959;59:4137–4149.
7 Skeggs L, Leonards J: Studies on the artificial kidney. I. Preliminary results with a new type of continuous dialyzer. Science 1948;108:212–213.
8 Kiil F: Development of a parallel-flow artificial kidney in plastics. Acta Chir Scand Suppl 1960; 253:142–150.
9 Cole J, Pollard T, Murray J: Studies on the modified polypropylene Kiil dialyzer. Trans Am Soc Artif Intern Organs 1963;9:67–70.
10 Funck-Brentano J, Sausse A, Vantelon J, Granger A, Zingraff J, Man NK: A new disposable plate-kidney. Trans Am Soc Artif Intern Organs 1969;15:127–130.
11 Lipps B, Stewart R, Perkins H, Holmes G, McLain E, Rolfs M, Oja P: The hollow fiber artificial kidney. Trans Am Soc Artif Intern Organs 1967;13:200–207.
12 Clark WR, Gao D: Properties of membranes used for hemodialysis therapy. Semin Dial 2002; 15:1–5.
13 Bird RB, Stewart WE, Lightfoot EN: Velocity distributions in laminar flow; in Bird RB, Stewart WE, Lightfoot EN (eds): Transport Phenomena, ed 1. New York, Wiley, 1960, pp 34–70.
14 Handley HH, Gorsuch R, Levin NW, Ronco C: Intravenous catheter for intracorporeal plasma filtration. Blood Purif 2002;20:61–69
15 Clark WR, Hamburger RJ, Lysaght MJ: Effect of membrane composition and structure on performance and biocompatibility in hemodialysis. Kidney Int 1999;56:2005–2015.
16 Ronco C, Bowry S: Nanoscale modulation of the pore dimensions, size distribution, and structure of a new polysulfone-based high-flux dialysis membrane. Int J Artif Organs 2001; 24:726–735.

change of its state from liquid to gas. For this reason the inactivation of the spores can be obtained at a lower temperature and shorter duration with moist heat than with dry heat.

Standard cycles are known (i.e. 121°C for 15 min at a pressure of 1 atm or 134°C for 4 min at a pressure of 2 atm) for the inactivation of the spores of the pathogenic bacilli (i.e. tetanus bacillus, gas gangrene Clostridium) and of environmental mesophile bacilli with moist heat. These cycles are obtained with boiling water in an autoclave, that is an hermetically sealed boiler where steam and pressure increase proportionally. For the sterilization effect it is necessary that steam is saturated; in fact, the killing time of the micro-organisms gets longer proportionally to the content of air in steam. It is, therefore, necessary that the air inside the autoclave is eliminated through a dedicated exit site and replaced with steam originating in the boiler. Only when the air has been completely removed (a thick jet of steam comes from the exit site) does the valve close automatically; a certain time is necessary until the manometer and the thermometer show the validated parameters (i.e. 1 atm and 121°C). The duration of the sterilization step may vary considerably (i.e. from 15 to 30 min or more) according to the quantity and quality of the load to be sterilized; this is in relation to the difficulties which the steam may encounter in penetrating materials such as gauze or linen and to the time needed for the temperature to become uniform (from the periphery to the centre of the load) in autoclaves of big dimensions.

Dry and wet steam sterilisations are possible only in thermostable materials. Steam sterilisation avoids many of the problems occurring with other sterilisation methods, but it retains the capacity to modify the physical characteristics of the materials. It may cause an enlargement of pores in some PS membranes (low flux PS) resulting in an increase in Ko and Kuff compared with the same product treated with EO. In some other membranes, such as the high-flux polysulphone, these phenomena seem to be minimised or absent suggesting that the methods of manufacturing or the polymer brands may play a role in such phenomena. As in gamma radiation, steam sterilisation can cause cracking of the macromolecule of the potting resin producing MDA and, therefore, it is advisable to additionally rinse the product before use to eliminate any microparticles or breakdown products.

EO Sterilisation

Applicable official standards are:

(1) EN 550: 1994: sterilisation of medical devices – validation and routine control of EO sterilisation,

(2) ISO 11135: 1994: medical devices – validation and routine control of EO sterilisation, and

(3) EN ISO 30993-7: 1993: biological evaluation of medical devices – part 7: EO sterilization residuals.

The EO sterilization has been used by the medical device companies for 40 years as the most common sterilization process. Generally, disposable medical devices are made from plastic materials that change their characteristics when exposed to the temperatures necessary in autoclaves for the heat and radiation sterilisation. The EO sterilisation is, therefore, recommended since it represents a reliable sterilisation process, which ensures that the necessary sterility assurance level (SAL) is reached at a temperature compatible with most of the plastic materials.

The European norm EN 550 (1994) is responsible for the design, the routine validation, the process control and the monitoring of the EO sterilisation of medical devices. The formula of EO is C_2H_4O, which assumes the gas state at 10.73°C and 760 mbar; it is supplied as liquid in stainless steel cylinders. EO is effective against all micro-organisms and bacterial spores. Its microbicidal activity comes from the lability of oxygen bound, which allows the radical CH_2-CH_2 to fix on the active groups COOH, NH_2, SH_2, OH; in this way the ionisation processes of the proteins are denaturated and the enzymatic activities are blocked. The sterilising effect depends on the gas concentration, the exposure time, the pressure, the temperature and the humidity. Such parameters are related to the characteristics of the load to be sterilised and are to be defined during the process validation. The remarkable penetration capacity of EO makes the EO sterilisation highly effective, but there is also a high EO adsorption by the material in relation to the initial EO concentration, the load configuration and the composition of the material (latex rubber and PVC have a maximum adsorbance).

Both EO and its derivatives have a remarkable irritating effect on mucous membranes and skin; additionally they can cause acute or delayed allergic reactions, hemolysis and alterations in coagulation. Residual quantities remaining in the dialyser, particularly in the polyurethane headers following de-aeration, have been implicated in the aetiology of the 'first use syndrome'. Between 15 and 17% of patients receiving regular dialysis treatments are known to have anti-EO IgE antibodies.

Validation of the Process

The sterilisation process has to be validated according to official standards. The main content of the validation process is the verification through a worst condition procedure that the product is sterile with the standard process in all cases. In fact the sterilisation process is defined as a special production process which needs validation since it is not possible to verify the sterility of all products after the sterilisation process. The concept of validation also includes the verification that the sterilisation process does not interfere with the product performance and safety.

Verification of the Influence of the Sterilization Process

The verification of the effects of the sterilisation process has to take into consideration the 'state of the art', based on the scientific literature, and the manufacturer's experience. Through the sterilisation validation process and the verification of the effects on the product, it is possible to define the process parameters and the control activities to be performed in the routine process. There is no specific norm for the performance verification, so the manufacturer has to use his own experience and the available official relevant tests listed in the pharmacopoeias or internal standards. For these reasons an internal experiment is presented. Anyway, the performance verification should include the following: physical inspection, functional inspection (verification of the integrity of the membranes, mechanical strength, in vitro verification of the performances), chemical verification (qualitative and quantitative investigation, EO residual content, in case of EO sterilisation, visible and not visible particle counts, heavy metals).

Most of the tests are aimed to verify the possible toxicity; biological tests are performed according to EN 30993, and also include the pyrogen test, LAL test and bioburden.

Ageing tests are usually carried out to verify the stability of the product with time and define its shelf life.

All above tests are also considered relevant for the definition of the standard sterilisation procedure.

Conclusion

The sterilisation method alone does not identify a product as 'good' or 'not good' in the same way as no sterilisation method is better than another. Each one offers advantages and disadvantages in relation to the different aspects of the device to be sterilised. The sterilisation method most suitable for a certain device is chosen after a careful short- and long-term evaluation, sterilisation validation, of the interaction of the characteristics of the device in question with the sterilisation method itself.

References

1 Frankenberger H: Sterile Medizinprodukte – Forderungen an Hersteller, Konsequenzen für Betreiber? Medizinproduktejournal 1994;1:12–19.
2 Europäische Norm 550 (Stand 1994): Sterilisation von Medizinprodukten: Validierung und Routineüberwachung für die Sterilisation mit Ethylenoxid.
3 Europäische Norm 552 (Stand 1994): Sterilisation von Medizinprodukten: Validierung und Routineüberwachung für die Sterilisation mit Strahlen.
4 Europäische Norm 554 (Stand 1994): Sterilisation von Medizinprodukten: Validierung und Routineüberwachung für die Sterilisation mit feuchter Hitze.
5 Europäische Norm 556 (Stand 1994): Sterilisation von Medizinprodukten: Anforderungen an Medizinprodukte, die als 'STERIL' gekennzeichnet werden.
6 Association of International Industrial Irradiation: Newsletter, April 1997, No 31.
7 Williams D: The 'sterile' debate: The effects of radiation sterilisation on polymers. Med Device Technol 1997;7/8:6–9.
8 Brinston RM: Gaining the competitive edge with gamma sterilization. Med Device Technol 1991;2/5:28–33.
9 Buchalla R, Schüttler C, Bögl KW: Die Strahlensterilisation von Medikalprodukten aus Kunststoffen – eine übersicht. Teil I. Bundesgesundheitsblatt 1994;6:261–268.
10 Van Doorne H, Bosch EH, Zwaving JJ, Elema ET: Gamma irradiation of *Sennae folium*, microbiological and phytochemical studies. Pharm Weekbl 1988;10:217–220.
11 Stock A, Gebhardt G, Helle N, Schüttler C, Bögl KW: Strahlenbehandlung von Arzneidrogen. Bundesgesundheitsblatt 1992;9:458–463.
12 Danielsson M: Hypersensivität und Sterilisationsmethoden in der Hämodialyse. EDTA-ERCA J 1993;19/3:12–22.
13 Sakai K: Structure and permeability of dialysis membranes sterilized by various methods. J Biomater Appl 1989;4:71–101.
14 Sakai K, Takesawa S, Mimura R, Ohashi H: Structural-analysis of hollow fiber dialysis membranes for clinical use. J Chem Eng Jpn 1987;20:351.

G. Gavioli, B. Braun Carex S.p.A.,
Via XXV Luglio, 11, I–41037 Mirandola (Italy)
Tel. +39 0535 616711, Fax +39 0535 23137, E-Mail giuliana.gavioli@bbraun.com

Ronco C, La Greca G (eds): Hemodialysis Technology.
Contrib Nephrol. Basel, Karger, 2002, vol 137, pp 85–94

Nano-Controlled Membrane Spinning Technology: Regulation of Pore Size, Distribution and Morphology of a New Polysulfone Dialysis Membrane

Sudhir K. Bowry

Fresenius Medical Care, Bad Homburg, Germany

Haemodialytic modalities that enhance the removal of large-molecular weight solutes are today established therapy modes for chronic haemodialysis patients [1]. The advantages of convective therapies such as haemodiafiltration and haemofiltration have been reported and discussed extensively in the literature in recent years [2–4]. A number of approaches can be taken to increase convective transport, e.g. increased ultrafiltration, internal filtration and high substitution rates [1, 3, 4], but the fundamental component that determines the convective characteristics of filters is the membrane: the membrane fine structure should be such that it provides increased permeability to solutes as well as to fluid [1].

This paper presents the application of advanced membrane fabrication techniques, based upon nanotechnology principles, towards the development of a new high-flux polysulfone membrane (Helixone®) having a refined, inner separating-surface features that permit the controlled elimination of large-molecular weight toxins in an extremely narrow size-range [5, 6]. The result of this development is, firstly, a membrane that has an elevated high sieving coefficient for β_2-microglobulin but without causing leakage of useful proteins such as albumin. Secondly, the surface membrane nano-structure is such that an enhanced clearance of small-molecular-weight substances is achieved per unit membrane surface area. Thus, the development strategy of Helixone® resulted in a membrane structure that provides advantages in terms of a more effective elimination of a broad spectrum of substances (both high and low molecular weight) that are considered as uremic toxins [7, 8].

Essential Solute-Removal Requirements of High-Flux Membranes

Even before high-flux dialysis and haemodiafiltration became established routine therapies for chronically ill renal patients, Lindsay and Henderson [9] had proposed that the adequacy of dialysis therapy should be evaluated using both small- and middle-molecule clearance. Thus, in considering high-flux membranes or dialysers, discussions should not be restricted only to the benefits of removal of large uraemic toxins, but also simultaneously include small uraemic toxin removal [7, 8].

The total flux of solute through a given dialyser is the sum of the diffusive and the convective flux: both diffusive and convective transport of high flux membranes are influenced by the structure and characteristics of the membrane [10]. The diffusive transport is predominantly a function of membrane thickness and membrane porosity; the latter, in turn, is a function of both the pore size and number [11]. Diffusive transport is thus favourable for low-molecular-weight solutes not only because of the inverse relationship between molecular weight and diffusivity, but also because of the greater accessibility of small solutes to the membrane pore structure.

In convective transport, an augmentation of solute transport across the membrane occurs if a high rate of fluid transport across the membrane is facilitated, i.e. solutes are dragged along by fluid movements [1]. Again, the permeability characteristics of the membrane determine the quality and quantity of the convective flux [11]. The membrane property having the largest impact on water permeability is also pore size; the solute concentration in the ultrafiltrate depends on the membrane porosity and is expressed by the sieving coefficient (SC). If the membrane pore size is sufficiently large enough to allow a given molecule to pass totally unimpeded, the SC is 1 (as is the case of most small solutes), and zero if the molecule is so large that it is completely impeded by the pores [10, 11].

Development Approach of the New High-Flux Polysulfone Membrane, Helixone

The aforementioned theoretical considerations constituted the fundamental developmental basis for Helixone, a membrane that has been designed specifically to achieve high sieving coefficients for β_2-microglobulin (β_2-m 11,800 daltons). As removal of β_2-m (identified as a precursor of amyloid deposits in long-term dialysis patients) is considered to be beneficial [12, 13], it is generally acknowledged to represent the target size-range (>10 kD) of large molecules or uremic toxins whose elimination is desirable [14].

However, the separation characteristics of virtually all dialysis membranes are still essentially based upon size-exclusion principles, i.e. centred around pore dimensions. In making a membrane more permeable to larger substances in the size range of β_2-m, an inevitability of membrane fabrication procedures to date has been the inability to restrict the number of larger pores that may allow the passage of useful plasma proteins into the dialysate. Hence, a focus point of the developmental strategy of Helixone was to achieve significant removal of β_2-m without compromising the albumin retention characteristics of the membrane – achieved through the application of a new, advanced membrane spinning technology [15].

Helixone: The Application of Nanotechnology Principles to the Production of Dialysis Membranes

Nanotechnology has been defined, in general terms, as any technology related to features of nanometer scale: thin films, fine particles, chemical synthesis, advanced microlithography, and so forth [16]. The term *nanotechnology* was first widely used to what is today defined as molecular nanotechnology, which resembles and overlaps with other fields. Drexler [16] compares and describes the essentials of several nanotechnology-based fabrication procedures, including their applicability to solution-phase chemistry, akin to the process principles involved in the manufacture of solution-spun dialysis membranes such as Helixone.

Most membranes used for haemodialysis are prepared by phase inversion processes all of which are based upon the same thermodynamic principles [17]. The main stages and critical steps of the hollow-fibre membrane fabrication process are the composition of the polymer dope (i.e. the polymer spinning solution involving the solvent and the various polymers in the blend) and the core fluid, the coagulation bath where the precipitation occurs and the extraction bath [18]. Other preparation procedures include polymer concentration, humidity temperature, composition of the casting solution and the spinning rate [17]. All these stages and parameters determine the ultimate membrane morphology, performance, and hence its exact application, in terms of flux and selectivity of removal of solutes of varying size.

To attain the unique membrane fine structure of Helixone (described below), a number of crucial refinements were made to various parameters in the membrane fabrication process that resulted in an increase of the local membrane porosity (to increase the hydraulic permeability and diffusive transport). The increase of the mean pore size at the innermost separating 'skin' region together with the narrow pore size distribution (sharp molecular weight cut-off) results in elevated sieving coefficients for larger solutes. Finally, an optimisation of the surface distribution of the pores (pore area-to-polymer ratio) has a direct bearing on the clearance of small solutes in particular by providing a more effective surface area for separation.

Refinements to the precipitation step, together with the application of a thorough, more homogeneous polymer mixing mode, were decisive towards determining the controlled nanoscale morphology of the inner surface of Helixone. By controlling the exchange of solvent and nonsolvent, together with the thermodynamics of the initial stage of phase transition (the process of 'solidification' whereby the polymer solution is transformed from liquid to solid state upon immersion into the coagulation bath containing nonsolvent), an inner region with high local porosity was defined for Helixone according to the desired properties that had been laid down at the outset of the membrane development programme.

Characterisation of the Membrane Structure of Helixone

The detailed structure and characteristics of the new membrane were evaluated by a number of techniques:

(1) *The sieving coefficient* profile of a membrane provides important information about the probability of a specific molecule (of a given size) traversing the membrane upon reaching the membrane surface. A number of methods are available for the measurement of the sieving coefficients of dialysis membranes. For Helixone, the sieving coefficients for, β_2-microglobulin and albumin were measured under the most realistic and application-relevant conditions as described previously [5].

(2) *Pore size and distribution*: Although, for all practical purposes, the sieving coefficient profiles enable an assessment of the extent to which a molecule passes a given membrane, information about the mean pore size as well as the pore size distribution is often additionally sought or required. There are several methods to determine mean pore sizes, and for Helixone a method based upon the application of the aforementioned experimentally-derived sieving coefficients was used [5, 19]. The dimensions of the porous structures of a given membrane essentially define the separation characteristics of a given membrane. However, although characterisation of the size of the pores of membranes is important, it is often not a clearly defined entity. Significantly, the pore size dimensions that determine which substances cross the membrane and which are retained, are only important for the more dense 'innermost' porous part of the lumen side of a hollow fibre membrane. 'Pore size' dimensions, therefore, essentially refer to pore diameter, or more arbitrarily, pore width.

(3) *Scanning and transmission electron microscopy (SEM and TEM)*: The visualisation and assessment of the detailed structures of Helixone were determined, firstly, using a high resolution field-emission SEM microscope. Secondly, transmission electron micrographs were obtained using a state-of-the-art transmission electron microscope (TEM) to show more the details of the membrane porosity at the inner (lumen) region of the membrane [5].

(4) *Computer image analysis to determine local membrane porosity*: TEM images of thin (200 nm) cross-sections were analysed using a computer-enhanced image analysis (CEIA) technique to ascertain the intensity profiles that provide a relative measure of the degree of porosity of the thin, innermost, separating region of the membrane as well as providing an indication of the structure and geometry of the pores in that region. This approach was undertaken to eliminate the bias that is normally associated with the subjective evaluation of SEM and TEM micrographs [5].

Essentially, the technique determines the dark (black) intensity levels (i.e. indicating the presence of the polymer within the membrane structure) as well as the 'white level' of the brighter areas of the image where no membrane material (i.e. 'porous' spaces only) was present. By assessing the degree of 'darkness' (polymer) and 'whiteness' (porosity) along the entire section of the membrane, an accurate intensity profile of the membrane wall can be plotted as a curve that is characteristic for a given membrane type. The local intensity level was thus determined by an integration of adjoining vertical lines, having a width of one pixel only, parallel to the membrane surface. For each of these lines, the mean value was determined and plotted versus the distance in nanometers of the particular line from the membrane inner surface.

As in TEM-based computer image analysis a number of factors may influence the evaluation of the intensity distribution of an image to introduce potential arbitrariness of the quantitative measurements, a number of criteria were applied to minimise the risk of misinterpretation of the data; these have already been described in [5].

(5) *Atomic force microscopy* (AFM) enables the characterisation of the surface of materials, providing 3-dimensional topographic or surface roughness information of the material down to the nanometer scale [6]. On appropriate samples resolution even at a molecular level may also be obtained. A sharp cantilever tip (silicone nitride) with a diameter of smaller than 10 nm scans across the test surface and London-van der Waals interactions occur between the atoms in the tip and the surface of the membrane and these forces are amplified and detected [6]. This will result in a line scan or profile of the surface.

Surface Elemental Composition of Helixone

Electron spectroscopy for chemical analysis (ESCA) enables the determination of the elemental chemical composition and the chemical binding of the membrane surface at a depth of between 1 and 5 nm. The general principle of the method is that the surface is excited by means of radiation bombardment and the emission products, which provide information about the presence of specific chemical groups, atoms, or bonds, are detected.

The relative surface elemental composition of the membranes was obtained in terms of the percentage of the constituent elements present. Based upon the chemical structure of the polymer (polysulfone, from which both Helixone and Fresenius Polysulfone membranes are manufactured), carbon (C), oxygen (O), and sulphur (S) were measured. However, in addition, N was found to be present which is derived from the presence of PVP (polyvinylpyrrolidone) that is used in the fabrication of the dialysis membranes.

Consequences of the Helixone Nanostructure on Dialyser Performance

As already described, the diffusive transport as well as the convective transport (i.e. hydraulic permeability and sieving coefficient) properties of a membrane are defined by the morphology of the membrane wall. As a result of the mean pore size (i.e. diameter) of 3.3 nm and an extremely narrow pore size distribution, Helixone acquires a sieving coefficient for β_2-m of as high as 0.8 while that for albumin is <0.001 which is critical in that the membrane does not permit any leakage of essential proteins.

Further evidence of the unique inner membrane structure of Helixone is provided by the computer image analysis data derived from TEM microscopy (fig. 1). Unlike all contemporary dialysis membranes, Helixone not only has a high local porosity (less polymer, more porous spaces) at the innermost membrane region, but the degree of porosity increases steadily into the membrane interior, especially within the first 500 nm from the interface, permitting a more free initial access and penetration of solutes into the membrane interior. Other synthetic dialysis membranes have a much denser inner region up to 1,000–2,000 nm, whereby the increased resistance to solute transfer is less favourable to efficient mass transfer. The advantages of the reduced initial resistance to solute transport together with the increased pore size at the blood-contacting surface are reflected in the classical performance properties of the Helixone: improved clearance of both low and high MW substances.

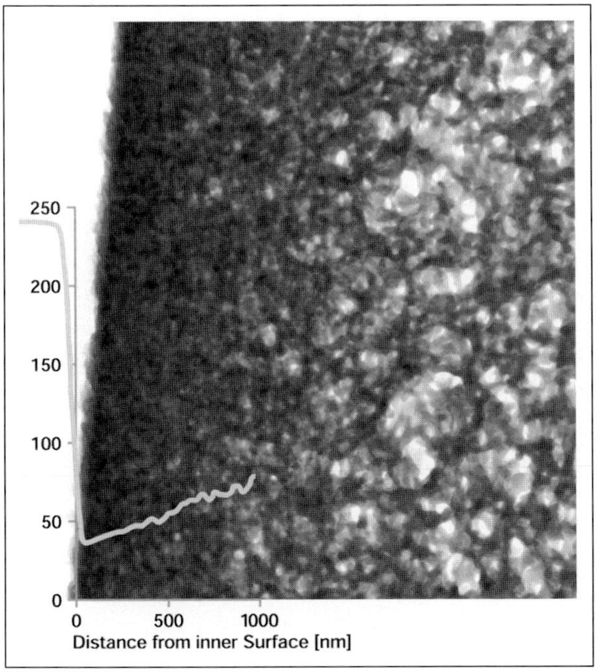

Fig. 1. Computer image analysis of the degree of porosity of separating region of Helixone transmission electron micrograph. The intensity profile shows a high and gradually increasing local porosity within the innermost 'skin' region of the membrane.

A further outcome of the nano-controlled spinning technology employed for Helixone is the unprecedented *surface distribution* of the (large) pores at the blood-contacting surface. Helixone possesses a significantly larger proportion of pores per unit area than membranes prepared by conventional technologies. In other words, the pore-area to polymer-surface area ratio is higher for Helixone than for all other synthetic dialysis membranes. The availability of more pores per unit surface area, increases the probability of a solute molecule encountering and traversing the pores, resulting in a higher effective clearance efficiency at a smaller unit surface area, especially for smaller solutes.

To illustrate the example further, figure 2 considers the clearance properties of dialysers made from two different technologies: the F60S dialyser containing the Fresenius Polysulfone is compared with the FX50 dialyser having the Helixone membrane. The clearance profiles for low-molecular-weight solutes are highly comparable for the two dialyser types – despite the fact that the specified surface area for the two dialysers (calculated conventionally on

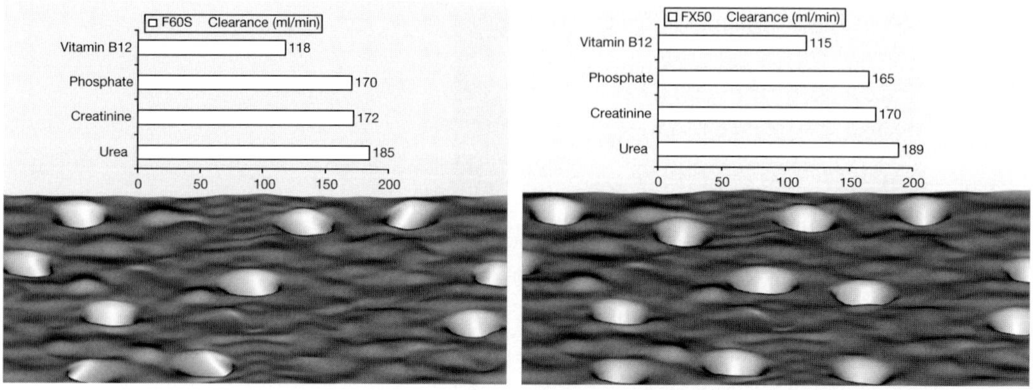

Fig. 2. Comparison of the surface distribution of pores of the Helixone membrane prepared by nano-controlled spinning (NCS) technology and membranes prepared by conventional membrane spinning processes. The availability of more pores per unit surface area for Helixone enables the FX50 dialyser (1.0 m^2) to have an equivalent low-molecular-weight solute clearance as the F60S dialyser (1.3 m^2). Additionally, Helixone has an elevated β_2-m sieving coefficient (0.8), facilitating the elimination of larger uraemic toxins.

the basis of the inner diameter, length of each cylindrical fibre and the total number of fibres within the housing) being vastly different (the FX50 dialyser type has a 'conventional' surface area of 1.0 m^2 while that of the F60S dialyser type is 1.3 m^2).

Hence, a direct consequence of the novel nano-controlled membrane spinning technology (porosity, pore size and pore distribution) is the increased clearance efficiency of the new dialyser range: smaller dialysers containing the Helixone membrane provide equivalent treatment efficiency to the larger-sized dialysers containing membranes with conventional pore size/distribution. It must be added, however, that the increased performance efficiency of the FX class of dialysers (which contain the Helixone membrane) is attributed to additional factors related to the design features of this dialyser series. Furthermore, usage of dialysers of reduced size (without compromising performance), provides advantages in terms of environmental issues during production as well as with the dispensing of the used dialysers.

In achieving the unique structural refinements of Helixone via diverse alterations and refinements of the membrane spinning process, there was the possibility that the procedures could inadvertently lead to changes of the membrane surface chemistry which could negatively influence the properties of the membrane during blood-material interaction. To investigate this eventuality, surface elemental composition of Helixone was compared with that of

Table 1. Relative surface elemental composition of Helixone and Fresenius Polysulfone as measured by ESCA

Material	C %	O %	N %	S %
Helixone				
Mean	81.2	12.7	4.2	1.9
SD	0.4	0.5	0.4	0.4
Fresenius Polysulfone				
Mean	81.3	12.6	4.0	2.2
SD	0.4	0.3	0.2	0.1

The mean values represent measurements from four different points on the membrane surface. The maintenance of the exact chemical composition of the inner blood-contacting surfaces of the two membranes ensures that Helixone retains the recognised biocompatibility features of Fresenius Polysulfone.

Fresenius Polysulfone which is commonly regarded as a standard in terms of its highly favourable biocompatibility profile. The results in table 1 show a remarkable consistency of the elemental composition of the two membranes despite significant structural differences that were derived for the new Helixone membrane relative to the original polysulfone membrane. The maintenance of the exact chemical composition of Helixone similar to that of the Fresenius Polysulfone was crucial towards retaining the recognised biocompatibility profile of the Fresenius Polysulfone that has contributed to its extensive clinical application.

Conclusions

Major advances have been made in recent years towards the improvement of the efficiency of modern haemodialytic therapies involving convective mechanisms of solute removal [1, 20]. These improvements rely, to a significant extent, upon the structural features and composition of the membrane. The modulation of the fine structure of the inner separating region of Helixone at the nano-scale level has resulted in a membrane that is specifically suited to high-flux treatment modalities. Despite the morphological alterations, Helixone (a polysulfone-based membrane) maintains the essential, established characteristics of the Fresenius Polysulfone membrane, namely inline-steam sterilisation, endotoxin retention properties and biocompatibility.

References

1 Ledebo I: Principles and practice of hemofiltration and hemodiafiltration. Artif Organs 1998; 22:20–25.

2 de Francisco ALM, Ghezzi PM, Brendolan A, Fiorini F, La Greca G, Ronco C, Arias M, Gervasio R, Tetta C: Hemodiafiltration with on-line regeneration of the ultrafiltrate. Kidney Int 2000;58 (suppl 76):66–71.

3 Ronco C, Brendolan A, Lupi A, Metry G, Levin NW: Effects of reduced inner diameter of hollow fibres in hemodialyzers. Kidney Int 2000;58:809–817.

4 Leypoldt JK, Cheung AK, Carroll CE, Stannard C, Pereira BJG, Agodoa LY, Port FK: Effect of dialysis membranes and middle molecule removal on chronic hemodialysis patients survival. Am J Kidney Dis 1999;33:349–355.

5 Ronco C, Bowry S: Nanoscale modulation of the pore dimensions, size distribution and structure of a new polysulfone-based high-flux dialysis membrane. Int J Artif Organs 2001;24:726–735.

6 Bowry SK, Ronco C: Surface topography and surface elemental composition analysis of Helixone®, a new high-flux polysulfone dialysis membrane. Int J Artif Organs 2001;24:757–764.

7 Vanholder R, De Smet R: Pathophysiologic effects of uremic retention solutes. J Am Soc Nephrol 1999;10:1815–1823.

8 Horl WH: Uremic toxins: New aspects. J Nephrol 2000;13(suppl 3):S83–88.

9 Lindsay RM, Henderson LW: Adequacy of dialysis. Kidney Int 1988;33(suppl 24):S92–S99.

10 Berland Y, Brunet P, Dussol B: Ultrafiltration and depurative parameters; in Bonomini V, Berland Y (eds): Dialysis Membranes: Structure and Predictions. Contrib Nephrol. Basel, Karger, 1995; vol 113, pp 45–49.

11 Clark WR, Hamburger RJ, Lysaght MJ: Effect of membrane composition and structure on solute removal and biocompatibility in hemodialysis. Kidney Int 1999;56:2005–2015.

12 Gejyo F, Yamada T, Odani S, Nakagawa Y, Arakawa M, Kunitomo T, Kataoka H, Suzuki M, Hirasawa Y, Shirahama T, Cohen AS, Schmid K: A new form of amyloid protein associated with hemodialysis was identified as beta-2 microglobulin. Biochem Biophys Res Commun 1985; 129:701–706.

13 Schiffl H, Fischer R, Lang SM, Mangel E: Clinical manifestations of AB-amyloidosis: Effects of biocompatibility and flux. Nephrol Dial Transplant 2000;15:840–845.

14 Vanholder R, De Smet R, Lameire NH: Redesigning the map of uremic toxins. Contrib Nephrol. Basel Karger, 2001, vol 133, pp 42–70.

15 Ronco C, Nissenson AR: Does nanotechnology apply to dialysis? Blood Purif 2001;19:347–352.

16 Drexler KE: Nanosystems Molecular Machinery, Manufacturing and Computation. Chichester, Wiley, 1992.

17 Mulder M: Characterisation of membranes; in: Basic Principles of Membrane Technology. Dordrecht, Kluwer Academic, 1998, pp 157–209.

18 Lysaght MJ: Evolution of hemodialysis membranes; in Bonimini V, Berland Y (eds): Dialysis Membranes: Structure and Predictions. Contrib Nephrol. Basel, Karger, 1995, vol 113, pp 1–10.

19 Nakao S: Determination of pore size and pore size distribution. 3. Filtration membranes. J Membr Sci 1994;131–165.

20 Ronco C, Ballestri M, Cappelli G: Dialysis membranes in convective treatments. Nephrol Dial Transplant 2000;15(suppl 2):31–36.

Dr. S.K. Bowry, Fresenius Medical Care, Else-Kröner-Strasse 1
D–61352 Bad Homburg (Germany)
Tel. +49 6172 609 2128, E-Mail sudhir.bowry@fmc-ag.com

Ronco C, La Greca G (eds): Hemodialysis Technology.
Contrib Nephrol. Basel, Karger, 2002, vol 137, pp 95–105

Vitamin E-Modified Dialyzers

Francesco Galli

Department of Internal Medicine, Section of Applied and Clinical Biochemistry, University of Perugia, Italy

In chronic hemodialysis (HD), oxidant stress is believed to be the result of combined effects of two factors [reviewed in 1–3]. The first is the repeated contact of blood components with nonself materials of the extracorporeal circulation. The second is the effect of the abnormal chemistry of the uremic environment that can impair antioxidant defenses and exacerbate the reactivity of some pro-oxidants.

Therefore, the relative risk of oxidant stress in dialysis patients is assumed to depend mainly on the so-called 'biocompatibility' of the materials in the extracorporeal circulation and on the quality of dialysis treatments. Actually, fewer biocompatible membranes lead to a chronic activation of leukocytes, overproduction of proinflammatory cytokines and pro-oxidant toxins. These factors can trigger tissue-oxidant stress through a sustained production of reactive oxygen/nitrogen species (ROS/RNS) and consumption of antioxidant defenses [3].

New generations of synthetic membranes have overwhelmingly – but not completely – reduced this drawback of the HD treatments [4, 5]. At the same time, as in the overall healthy population, antioxidant supplements are increasingly adopted in an attempt to prevent oxidant stress-related comorbidity in maintenance HD patients, and particularly atherosclerotic cardiovascular disease (ACVD) [3]. In this context, vitamin E appears to be one of the most promising antioxidant drugs. Indeed, the controlled trial SPACE [6] has recently suggested a role of the vitamin E in lowering the incidence of some major cardiovascular endpoints associated with chronic HD, and particularly myocardial infarction.

In the last decade, in searching for the solutions that could lower oxidant stress some original strategies have been proposed [1–3, 7]. A promising approach to the antioxidant therapy in HD consisted of the infusion of ascorbic acid (vitamin C) with the dialysate, and the recirculation of the dialysate through cartridges filled with vitamin E-enriched liposomes. The combination of these strategies has been proposed in the so-called hemolipodialysis [7]. This technique is addressed on one hand to compensate the intradialytic loss of vitamin C and on the other hand to neutralize activated lipids and other reactive substances by the scavenging function of vitamin E. Conceptually, other antioxidants and supplements could be used in this HD procedure and its versatility could make it possible to combine antioxidants with different types of dialyzers and dialysis modalities. These aspects let us envision a wide space to further advancements in developing this technique, but so far its real impact on oxidant stress remains to be confirmed by a suitable clinical experience.

The concept of a proper antioxidant intervention in HD patients should go hand in hand with that of a high standard of biocompatibility and removal of proinflammatory/pro-oxidant toxins. These aspects have been approached through the development of high-efficacy dialysis techniques, in which synthetic materials have been used to produce membranes with a high permeability in order to remove toxins with a broad range of molecular weights [8]. Sorbents could be also used in this context to prevent dialysate contamination by endotoxins, another possible source of leukocyte activation and oxidant stress during HD. They can also remove oxidant stress-sustaining uremic toxins, among which there are reactive carbonyls, homocysteine and phagocyte-stimulating high-molecular-weight toxins such as advanced glycation and oxidation protein products [9]. However, conclusive evidence of the expected beneficial role of the approach to these new uremic toxins by convective techniques and sorbents still has to be put forward.

So far, among the strategies expected to help lowering the incidence of oxidant stress in HD the most frequently investigated one is that of vitamin E-modified dialyzers (CLE; commercial name Excebrane). The original concept adopted with this type of membrane is that of giving a specific and timely protection against the ROS/RNS on the membrane surface, the main site of their production [10, 11]. Actually, CLE are cellulose-based hollow-fiber dialyzers coated on the blood surface with a two-layer synthetic copolymer that binds a film of oleic alcohol, to which α-tocopherol is bound by hydrophobic interaction.

This membrane has been widely tested during an approximately 6-year clinical experience, with more than 15,000 patients treated in Japan and approximately 3,000 in Europe since 1996, and has now also been introduced in the USA market (information provided by Terumo Co., Rome Branch). As a consequence of this experience 23 clinical and basic studies have been published in peer-reviewed journals. Furthermore, a previous number of this book series was entirely dedicated to CLE [reviewed in 1] and collected studies on (1) membrane manufacturing and technical tips, (2) overall biological role of the vitamin E, and (3) early investigation featuring bioactivity and biocompatibility properties of this membrane.

This paper provides an up-to-date review of this literature on CLE grouped into four main areas of interest: (1) antioxidant properties, (2) endothelial protection and antiatherogenic effects, (3) leukocyte function and activation, and (4) anticoagulant and antianemic effects.

Antioxidant Properties

Once we assume that a defective antioxidant protection plays a role in the causes of oxidant stress in HD [2, 3], efforts to protect or strengthen the antioxidant network in blood and tissues become a main goal in fighting this HD-related drawback. In more detail, the impaired antioxidant defense in HD patients is believed to follow as a consequence of these events [reviewed in 3, 12]:

(1) increased consumption by chronic leukocyte activation with increased generation of ROS, and abnormal accumulation and/or insufficient removal of pro-oxidant toxins (such as reactive carbonyls, protein and lipid oxidation byproducts),

(2) intra-HD leakage of dialyzable nonenzymatic antioxidants such as vitamin C and thiol-containing amino acids and proteins, and

(3) inactivation of individual enzymes and pathways with antioxidant function such as the extracellular glutathione peroxidase, LDL-associated paraoxonase, and the hexose monophosphate shunt that provides reducing equivalents to different antioxidant systems including that of the glutathione.

The cross talk between different antioxidant compartments together with their ubiquity results in an overlapping and usually redundant defense against a given pro-oxidant insult [13]. These key features of the whole antioxidant system in our body demonstrate the importance of providing timely and sufficient protection against oxygen and other pro-oxidants. However, specific defects in some antioxidants could be responsible for the damage on a particular class of biomolecules. As an example, cell membrane and lipoprotein polyunsaturated lipids in HD patients have been demonstrated to be particularly susceptible to oxidative damage [reviewed in 3].

Almost surprisingly, total blood levels of vitamin E – the most abundant and biologically active nonenzymatic liposoluble antioxidants – have been observed to be normal or only slightly decreased in HD patients [14, 15]. However, a defective concentration in some lipoprotein subclasses [16, 17] as well as blood cell membranes [reviewed in 18] together with the challenge of the uremic environment and HD on proinflammatory cells [19] and/or the administration of pro-oxidant drugs [20, 21] have suggested the possibility that target elements in

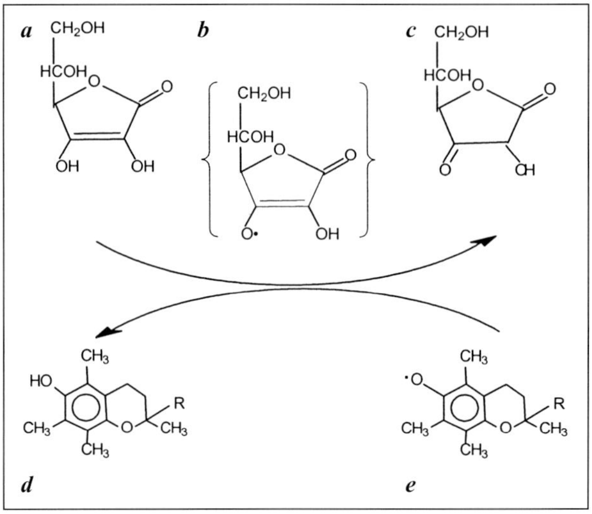

Fig. 1. Redox coupling of the vitamin C (ascorbic acid, ***a***) and vitamin E (α-tocopherol, ***e***). The one-electron reaction of the ascorbate (***a***) to semidehydroascorbate (***c***) is shown. The two-electron process gives origin to the product dehydroascorbate (not shown). During its oxidation the vitamin C gives origin to an ascorbyl radical intermediate (***b***). Other antioxidants such as the same vitamin E and/or the cysteine-containing tripeptide glutathione are able to restore the ascorbic acid from its oxidation products ascorbyl radical and dehydroascorbic acid. In this reaction the tocopherol (***d***) also generates a radical intermediate or tocopheryl radical (***e***). This reactive intermediate shows a good level of stability when compared to hydroperoxyl and alkoxyl radicals formed during the lipid oxidation reactions in cell membranes and lipoproteins, and then it can act as an effective antioxidant for polyunsaturated lipids [3].

body fluids and tissues could face a condition of relative deficiency of this antioxidant vitamin, and ultimately an increased risk of oxidant stress.

In the meanwhile, a clear-cut trend toward an antioxidant imbalance in these patients is due to the chronic loss during HD of vitamin C, uric acid and to some extent of thiol containing amino acids and proteins [12]. These hydrosoluble molecules other than to be main contributors to the total antioxidant capacity in plasma are the most important coantioxidants of the vitamin E [3, 13]. Interestingly, in a recent study by Clermont et al. [22] it was demonstrated that HD leads to an accumulation of the ascorbil radical, i.e. the radical produced through the one-electron oxidation of the vitamin C (fig. 1). Therefore, this important antioxidant vitamin not only undergoes a massive depletion, but its redox appears to be disrupted as a result of the HD. In this study the ratio ascorbil radical/ascorbic acid was improved by CLE compared to standard dialyzers.

Based on the data of this study and accordingly to the data provided by Eiselt et al. [23] it could be suggested that CLE sustains the levels of ascorbic acid both in the intra- and inter-HD intervals. This appears to be a direct demonstration of a vitamin E-dependent restoration of the ascorbic acid redox during HD.

A similar effect could be observed for other vitamin E coantioxidants. In fact, we preliminarily observed that the use of CLE may sustain the levels of GSH in red blood cells [24], while others have described that CLE can increase the content of vitamin E and β-carotene in lipoprotein subfractions [17].

These findings are in agreement with our early in vitro studies, in which the vitamin E bound to the blood surface of the dialyzers was demonstrated to be redox-active with respect to classical coantioxidants such as vitamin C and glutathione [10]. Therefore, the cross talk between the vitamin E and its coantioxidant could be important for both its antiperoxidative activity and for the overall regulation of nonenzymatic antioxidants and the glutathione-dependent enzymatic defense. This effect of support of different antioxidant systems could also depend on a 'supplementation-like' function [10] that this membrane has been proposed to exert with respect to blood vitamin E levels. Actually, increased levels of this antioxidant vitamin have been observed in four separate studies on CLE [10, 17, 25, 26], while Mune et al. failed to confirm this result [27]. The increased bioavailability of vitamin E in the blood of patients treated with CLE can also be deduced from the effective protection against lipid peroxidation [10, 14, 26] and cell damage [25].

Endothelial Protection and Antiatherogenic Function

Endothelial dysfunction and damage are commonly observed in populations at risk of ACVD including chronic HD patients [27–29]. An increased chemical injury on circulating lipoproteins is thought to play a key pathogenic role in HD-related ACVD [16, 27, 29]. Several lines of research have supported the use of vitamin E in preventing atherosclerotic lesions, but conclusive clinical evidence of its antiatherogenic effect has not yet been reached [reviewed in 30]. Early small-population intervention studies performed in patients on regular HD seem to encourage the use of vitamin E supplements as positive results in the prevention of lipoprotein and endothelial damage were observed [reviewed in 3]. This assumption has found an important confirmation in the first large-population controlled study – i.e. the SPACE study [6] – that has demonstrated the role of vitamin E in preventing some major cardiovascular endpoints and particularly myocardial infarction.

Two independent studies have demonstrated that the use of CLE can prevent the acute impairment of the endothelial elasticity due to HD [29] and the accumulation of advanced lesions, as measured by the aortic calcification index [27]. In both these studies the protective effect of CLE on the endothelium was related to a lowering of the indices of LDL oxidation. Bonnefont-Russelot et al. [17] observed that CLE can decrease the in vitro oxidizability of HDL and markers of lipid peroxidation in plasma. These findings are correlated with the increased content of vitamin E and carotenoids in the lipoprotein subfractions collected after the treatment with CLE.

Recently, these findings of a lower degree of endothelial activation and LDL injury by CLE compared to cellulosic dialyzers found a confirmation in a controlled A-B-A prospective study, in which the release of the endothelial protein von Willebrand factor and the titer of autoantibodies against oxidized LDL was measured [31]. These are recognized markers of the HD-related endothelial activation and damage [32]. It is suggested that the data observed in this study show a possible cause-effect relationship between the increased titer of oxidized LDL autoantibodies and that of von Willebrand factor. This study also gave some insight into the critical role of patient selection as an important prerequisite to a proper investigation of the effect of CLE – and/or vitamin E per se – on the HD-associated ACVD. In fact, dialysis age and preexisting severe ACVD could be important confounding factors in this context.

Unfortunately, the largest part of the available studies on the effect of CLE on the indices of ACVD has been carried out only comparing this type of membrane with cellulosic ones. However, more recent studies have demonstrated that CLE shows a performance as regards leukocyte activation and some indices of oxidant stress comparable with the last generation of synthetic membranes including polysulfone (PS), AN69, polymethylmethacrylate (PMMA) and polyamide (PA; see the next section on Leukocyte Function and Activation).

Moreover, so far these studies on CLE as well as the intervention studies on vitamin E that appeared in the literature in uremic and nonuremic subjects have been affected by a common bias, that is the absence of a detailed investigation of vitamin E metabolism and bioavailability. This makes the information coming from this research work incomplete regarding the mechanism through which vitamin E supplements – or the coating of vitamin E on the CLE membrane – can exert their antiatherogenic function. These aspects strongly suggest the need for other studies aimed to further elucidate the antiatherogenic mechanism of the vitamin E and its role when used as a modifier of the HD membrane.

Leukocyte Function and Activation

The key role of the chronic leukocyte activation as pathogenic contributor to the whole HD-associated comorbidity is now universally accepted. This unwanted consequence of the blood-membrane interaction exerts its noxious effects through the release of cytokines, chemotactic factors, pro-oxidant enzymes, complexes of transition metals with proteins, and ROS [2, 33, 34]. Polymorphonuclear cells (PMN or neutrophils) and monocyte-macrophages are the two populations of leukocytes mainly involved in these processes.

CLE membranes have been evaluated for their effect on the activation of these cell populations. Girndt et al. [35] first investigated in a crossover study design CLE in comparison with hemophan (HP) as a low-biocompatibility membrane and PA as a biocompatible membrane. In this study it was demonstrated how CLE in comparison to PA was able to preserve the in vitro proliferation capability of monocytes that was significantly reduced by HP. In the same way CLE and PA maintained an optimal inter-HD ratio between IL-10 – a key subject in the negative feedback of proinflammatory cells – and the proinflammatory cytokine IL-6. Importantly, the intra-HD production of IL-6 was described to be lower with CLE in comparison with PA.

In a prospective study still in progress in Italy the intra-HD generation of IL-6 over 6 months of treatment with CLE was demonstrated to remain steady compared to the levels observed during the basal step, in which the patients were treated with PS [pers. commun.]. Other studies have demonstrated that CLE can restore the depressed function of PMN and mononuclear phagocytes [36, 37], and at the same time it can lower the amount of reactive oxygen species produced upon their activation [10, 34, 38], the expression of surface molecules involved in leukocyte activation and cell adhesion [39]. Some of these effects can be ascribed to the in vivo antioxidant function of CLE as shown in the EPR study of Shimazu et al. [37].

In contrast, in a study contributed by Dhondt et al. [40], CLE has been proposed to activate during HD both PMN and monocytes more than low-flux PS-based membranes as assessed by surface molecule expression. Even though this remains an isolate finding, it should be considered for its possible clinical relevance after appropriate revision of the methods used and the study design.

Oxidant stress is known to sustain cell death pathways that can be among the underlying factors for leukopenia and increased susceptibility to infectious diseases in HD patients [reviewed in 41, 42]. The vitamin E has been proved to regulate the apoptotic signaling and CLE can play a role in decreasing the proapoptotic effect of the uremic environment [41]. Recently in a study by Tarng et al. [25] CLE was shown to antagonize the leukocyte DNA damage induced by HD. This latter effect was demonstrated to be comparable to that of biocompatible membranes such as PS, AN69 and PMMA membranes. Accordingly, in another study the levels of 8-OH-dG in plasma of diabetic uremic patients were observed to decrease after 6 months of treatment with CLE [43].

Pertosa et al. [44] showed that CLE compared to cellulosic dialyzers modified with the same synthetic layer present on the CLE – but without the presence of oleic alcohol and vitamin E – can decrease the expression of the inducible form of the pro-oxidant enzyme nitric oxide synthase in mononuclear leukocytes. The same comparison carried out in a recent study contributed by Tsuruoka et al. [36] demonstrated that the lipid coating (oleic alcohol plus vitamin E) is responsible for a specific control of PMN function.

Anticoagulation and Antianemic Function

In a study by Huraib et al. [45] CLE was observed to reduce dialyzer clotting, as well as heparin and erythropoietin requirement in comparison with PS membranes. Other studies by the Usberti group [46] have also suggested that CLE by itself or in combination with supplemental glutathione can improve the number of RBC through a better survival of them. These recent findings, if confirmed by further studies, could be of impressive clinical and economic relevance in HD.

Concluding Remarks

In the last few years, efforts in improving materials and dialysis methods have led to an increasing interest in the antioxidant therapy to fight the HD-associated oxidant stress and its different pathogenic effects [47]. Vitamin E could be considered as one of the most promising antioxidants for this type of use in HD [3]. In particular, the study of CLE dialyzers has provided biological and clinical evidence that supports a role of this membrane in regulating the antioxidant network of plasma and blood cells [10, 17, 22–24], leukocyte activation and viability [10, 35–39, 41], lipoprotein injury [17], and endothelial dysfunction and damage [27, 29, 31].

In the light of these studies, the early use of CLE appears to be a possible specific strategy for slackening the chronic-degenerative processes that contribute to the pathogenesis of one of the most severe comorbidity of the HD, i.e. the ACVD. The possible lag in the onset and progression of proatherogenic events in patients treated with CLE could be due to a lower generation of pro-oxidant and proinflammatory mediators by (1) lower leukocyte activation, (2) ROS scavenging, and (3) increased bioavailability of the vitamin E. A 'supplementation-like' effect of CLE on the pool of vitamin E of tissues and body fluids has been demonstrated in 4 out of 5 studies in which vitamin E levels were investigated (see above). All these aspects can be taken into account to explain the function of CLE – and vitamin E supplements overall – as a possible antiatherogenic tool that can act through both antioxidant and nonantioxidant mechanisms [48]. However, the way in which the effects of the points 1 and 2 can be attained appears an exquisite peculiarity of the CLE membrane. In fact, contrary to oral supplements of vitamin E, CLE can selectively exert these functions both at the site in which these events take place, i.e. the membrane surface, and at the systemic level.

During the intensive investigation carried out over the last years on this membrane some interesting aspects of the oxidant stress and antioxidant therapy in HD have been further elucidated and others demonstrated for the first time. Anyway, it seems important to proceed with further studies that could better describe the clinical relevance of this type of dialyzers and of the overall antioxidant therapy in HD.

References

1 Galli F, Ronco C: Oxidant stress in hemodialysis. Nephron 2000;84:1–5.

2 Wratten ML, Tetta C, Ursini F, Sevanian A: Oxidant stress in hemodialysis: Prevention and treatment strategies. Kidney Int 2001;59(suppl 78):S32–S36.

3 Galli F, Canestrari F, Bellomo G: Physiopathology of the oxidative stress and its implication in uremia and dialysis. Contrib Nephrol. Basel, Karger, 1999, vol 127, pp 1–31.

4 Cristol JP, Canaud B, Rabesandratana H, Gaillard I, Serre A, Mion C: Enhancement of reactive oxygen species production and cell surface marker expression due to haemodialysis. Nephrol Dial Transplant 1994;9:389–394.

5 Markert M, Wauters JP: New aspects on oxidative metabolism of neutrophils during hemodialysis on different dialyzer membranes. Adv Exp Med Biol 1991;297:207–213.

6 Boaz M, Smetana S, Green MS: Secondary prevention with antioxidants of cardiovascular disease in end-stage renal disease (SPACE): Randomised placebo-controlled. Lancet 2000;356:1213–1218.

7 Wratten ML, Navino C, Tetta C, Verzetti G: Haemolipodialysis. Blood Purif 1999;17/2–3: 127–133.

8 Buocristiani U, Galli F, Benedetti S, Errico R, Beninati S, Ghibelli L, Rovidati S, Floridi A, Canestrari F: Quantitative and qualitative assessment and clinical meaning of molecules removed with BK membranes. Contrib Nephrol. Basel, Karger, 1998, vol 125, pp 133–158.

9 Galli F, Buoncristiani U, Floridi A, Ronco C: In vitro removal of oxidation and glycation-related toxins from uremic plasma by a new sorbent cartridge (abstract). 38th ERA-EDTA Congress, Vienna, 2001, p 217.

10 Galli F, Rovidati S, Chiarantini L, Kulurianu H, Canestrari F, Buoncristiani U: Bioreactivity and biocompatibility of a vitamin E-modified multi-layer hemodialysis filter. Kidney Int 1998;54: 580–589.

11 Sasaki M, Hosoya N, Saruhashi M: Vitamin E modified cellulose membrane. Artif Organs 2000; 24:779–789.

12 Galli F, Floridi A, Buoncristiani U: Oxidant stress in hemodialysis patients. Contrib Nephrol. Basel, Karger, 2002, vol 137, pp 371–378.

13 Diplock AT, Chaleux J-L, Crozier-Willi G, Kok FS, Rice-Evans C, Roberfroid M, Stahl W, Wiña-Ribes J: Functional food sciences and defenses against reactive oxygen species. Br J Nutr 1998;80:S77–S112.

14 Galli F, Varga Z, Balla J, Ferraro B, Canestrari F, Floridi A, Kakuk G, Buoncristiani U: Vitamin E, lipid profile, and peroxidation in hemodialysis patients. Kidney Int 2001(suppl 78):S148–S154.

15 Weiss MF: Vitamin E for dialysis patients. Semin Dial 2001;14:71–72.
16 Hasselwander O, Young IS: Oxidative stress in chronic renal failure. Free Radic Res 1998;29:1–11.
17 Bonnefont-Rousselot D, Lehmann E, Jaudon MC, Delattre J, Perrone B, Rechke JP: Blood oxidative stress and lipoprotein oxidizability in haemodialysis patients: Effect of the use of a vitamin E-coated dialysis membrane. Nephrol Dial Transplant 2000;15:2020–2028.
18 Usberti M, Bufano G, Lima G, Gazzotti RM, Tira P, Gerardi G, Di Lorenzo D: Increased red blood cell survival reduces the need of erythropoietin in hemodialyzed patients treated with exogenous glutathione and vitamin E-modified membrane. Contrib Nephrol. Basel, Karger, 1999, vol 127, pp 208–214.
19 Maccarrone M, Meloni C, Manca-di-Villahermosa S, Cococcetta N, Casciani CU, Finazzi-Agro A, Taccone-Gallucci M: Vitamin E suppresses 5-lipoxygenase-mediated oxidative stress in peripheral blood mononuclear cells of hemodialysis patients regardless of administration route. Am J Kidney Dis 2001;37:964–969.
20 Roob JM, Khoschsorur G, Tiran A, Horina JH, Holzer H, Winklhofer-Roob BM: Vitamin E attenuates oxidative stress induced by intravenous iron in patients on hemodialysis. J Am Soc Nephrol 2000;11:539–549.
21 Nemeth I, Turi S, Haszon I, Bereczki C: Vitamin E alleviates the oxidative stress of erythropoietin in uremic children on hemodialysis. Pediatr Nephrol 2000;14:13–17.
22 Clermont G, Lecour S, Cabanne J, Motte G, Guilland J, Chevet D, Rochette L: Vitamin E-coated dialyzer reduces oxidative stress in hemodialysis patients. Free Radic Biol Med 2001;31:233–241.
23 Eiselt J, Racek J, Trefil L, Opatrny K Jr: Effects of a vitamin E-modified dialysis membrane and vitamin C infusion on oxidative stress in hemodialysis patients. Artif Organs 2001;25:430–436.
24 Buoncristiani U, Galli F, Rovidati S, Albertini MC, Covarelli C, Canestrari F: Oxidative damage during hemodialysis using a vitamin E-modified dialysis membrane: A preliminary characterization. Nephron 1997;77:57–61.
25 Tarng DC, Huang TP, Liu TY, Chen HW, Sung YJ, Wei YH: Effect of vitamin E-bonded membrane on the 8-hydroxy 2′-deoxyguanosine level in leukocyte DNA of hemodialysis patients. Kidney Int 2000;58:790–799.
26 Mydlik M, Derzsiova K, Racz O, Sipulova A, Lovasova E, Petrovicova J: A modified dialyzer with vitamin E and antioxidant defense parameters. Kidney Int 2001(suppl 78):S144–S147.
27 Mune M, Yukawa S, Kishino M, Otani H, Kimura K, Nishikawa O, Takahashi T, Kodama N, Saika Y, Yamada Y: Effect of vitamin E on lipid metabolism and atherosclerosis in ESRD patients. Kidney Int 1999(suppl 71):S126–S129.
28 Gris J-C, Branger B, Vécina F, Al Sabadani B, Fourcade J, Schved J-F: Increased cardiovascular risk factors and features of endothelial activation and dysfunction in dialyzed uremic patients. Kidney Int 1994;46:807–813.
29 Miyazaki H, Matsuoka H, Itabe H, Usui M, Ueda S, Okuda S, Imaizumi T: Hemodialysis impairs endothelial function via oxidative stress: Effects of vitamin E-coated dialyzer. Circulation 2000;101:1002–1006.
30 Keaney JF, Simon DI, Freedman JE: Vitamin E and vascular homeostasis: Implications for atherosclerosis. FASEB J 1999;13:965–976.
31 Bufano G, Usberti M, Mandolfo S, Testa S, Ferraro B, Galli F: Von Willebrand factor and autoantibodies against oxidized LDL in hemodialysis patients treated with vitamin E-modified dialysers. J Am Soc Nephrol 2001;12:355A.
32 Holvoet P, Donck J, Landeloos M, Brouwers E, Luijtens K, Arnout J, Lesaffre E, Vanrenterghem Y, Collen D: Correlation between oxidized low density lipoproteins and von Willebrand factor in chronic renal failure. Thromb Haemost 1996;76:663–669.
33 Pertosa G, Grandaliano G, Gesualdo L, Ranieri E, Monno R, Schena FP: Interleukin-6, interleukin-8 and monocyte chemotactic peptide-1 gene expression and protein synthesis are independently modulated by hemodialysis membranes. Kidney Int 1998;54:570–579.
34 Galli F, Rovidati S, Benedetti S, Canestrari F, Ferraro B, Floridi A, Buoncristiani U: Lipid peroxidation, leukocyte function and apoptosis in hemodialysis patients treated with vitamin E-modified filters. Contrib Nephrol. Basel, Karger, 1999, vol 127, pp 156–171.

35 Girndt M, Lengler S, Kaul H, Sester U, Sester M, Kohler H: Prospective crossover trial of the influence of vitamin E-coated dialyzer membranes on T-cell activation and cytokine induction. Am J Kidney Dis 2000;35:95–104.

36 Tsuruoka S, Kawaguchi A, Nishiki K, Hayasaka T, Fukushima C, Sugimoto K, Saito T, Fujimura A: Vitamin E-bonded hemodialyzer improves neutrophil function and oxidative stress in patients with end-stage renal failure. Am J Kidney Dis 2002;39:127–133.

37 Shimazu T, Ominato M, Yasuda T, Sato T, Maeba T, Owada S, Ishida M: Effect of a vitamin E bonded dialysis membrane on neutrophil superoxide anion radical production. Kidney Int 2001; 59(suppl 78):137–143.

38 Omata M, Higuchi C, Demura R, Sanaka T, Nihei H: Reduction of neutrophil activation by vitamin E-modified dialyzer membranes. Nephron 2000;85:221–231.

39 Zaluska WT, Ksiazek A, Roliski J: Effect of vitamin E modified cellulose membrane on human lymphocyte, monocyte, and granulocyte CD11b/CD18 adhesion molecule expression during hemodialysis. ASAIO J 2001;47:619–622.

40 Dhondt A, Vanholder R, Glorieux G, Waterloos MA, De Smet R, Lesaffer G, Lameire N: Vitamin E-bonded cellulose membrane and hemodialysis bioincompatibility: Absence of an acute benefit on expression of leukocyte surface molecules. Am J Kidney Dis 2000;36:1140–1146.

41 Galli F, Canestrari F, Buoncristiani U: Biological effects of oxidative stress in hemodialysis: The possible roles of the vitamin E. Blood Purif 1999;17:79–94.

42 Jaber BL, Cendoroglo M, Balakrishnan VS, Perianayagam MC, King AJ, Pereira B: J. Apoptosis of leukocytes: Basic concepts and implications in uremia. Kidney Int 2001(suppl 78):S197–S205.

43 Satoh M, Yamasaki Y, Nagake Y, Kasahara J, Hashimoto M, Nakanishi N, Makino H: Oxidative stress is reduced by the long-term use of vitamin E-coated dialysis filters. Kidney Int 2001; 59:1943–1950.

44 Pertosa G, Grandaliano G, Valente M, Montinaro V, Soccio M, Gesualdo L, Schena FP: In vivo evaluation of biocompatibility of a new dialyzer employing the vitamin E-modified cellulose membrane 'Excebrane E': Study of mechanisms involved in mononuclear cell activation. Contrib Nephrol. Basel, Karger, 1999, vol 127, pp 200–207.

45 Huraib S, Tanimu D, Shaheen F, Hejaili F, Giles C, Pagayon V: Effect of vitamin-E-modified dialysers on dialyser clotting, erythropoietin and heparin dosage: A comparative crossover study. Am J Nephrol 2000;20:364–368.

46 Usberti M, Bufano G, Lima G, Gazzotti RM, Tira P, Gerardi G, Di Lorenzo D: Increased red blood cell survival reduces the need of erythropoietin in hemodialyzed patients treated with exogenous glutathione and vitamin E-modified membrane. Contrib Nephrol. Basel, Karger, 1999, vol 127, pp 208–214.

47 Senior K: Antioxidants improve brain function in advanced renal failure. Lancet 2001;358:1075.

48 Ricciarelli R, Zingg JM, Azzi A: Vitamin E: Protective role of a Janus molecule. FASEB J 2001;15:2314–2325.

Francesco Galli, PhD, Department of Internal Medicine,
Section of Applied and Clinical Biochemistry, University of Perugia,
Via del Giochetto, I–06100 Perugia (Italy)
Tel. +39 075 5857445, Fax +39 075 5857441, E-Mail f.galli@unipg.it, fragalli@libero.it

Ronco C, La Greca G (eds): Hemodialysis Technology.
Contrib Nephrol. Basel, Karger, 2002, vol 137, pp 106–110

Modified Cellulose Triacetate Membranes

Toshiaki Masuda

Nipro Corporation, Dialysis-Related Products, Osaka, Japan

Cellulose triacetate (CTA) is cellulose, three hydroxyl radicals of which are all replaced with acetyl radicals. This is classified as cellulose acetate and defined as a synthetic fiber in the field of fiber industries. In the meantime, regenerated cellulose is classified as a regenerated fiber, which belongs to the category of chemical fibers [1].

In 1927, cellulose acetate in rod and sheet forms and in 1929, cellulose acetate pellets for molding products became widely available on the market. Such cellulose acetate is thermoplastic and can be easily used to mold products of various designs for use in many fields, the same as conventional plastics.

Reverse osmosis modules, ultrafiltration modules, dialyzers, hemofilters, plasma separators and microfilters are examples of currently used devices receiving mass separation CTA membranes.

Methods of Spinning CTA Hollow Fiber

The CTA hollow fiber is spun based on dry and wet processes. After the addition of solvent and nonsolvent (swelling agent), necessary to form pores in the wall of CTA hollow fibers, these are mixed, heated, and then the mixture is extruded through an orifice of a double nozzle structure to spin the fiber. During the extrusion, core gas or liquid such as nitrogen or nontoxic isopropyl myristate is put into the fiber lumen to maintain its circularity and properly control the fiber wall thickness. In the next step, during the free running of the fiber in atmospheric air and dipping in the coagulation bath, the solvent or nonsolvent (swelling agent) is released by diffusion so that pores are formed in the fiber wall. After rinsing the fiber with hot water, the water contained in the pores is replaced with glycerin because of its high boiling temperature (290°C)

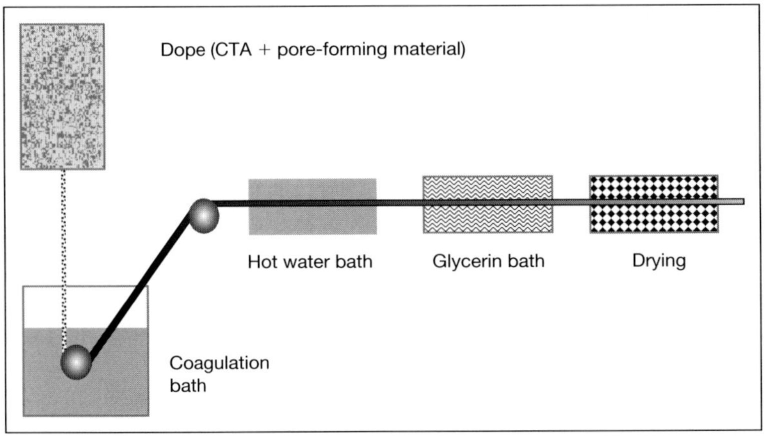

Fig. 1. Spinning process.

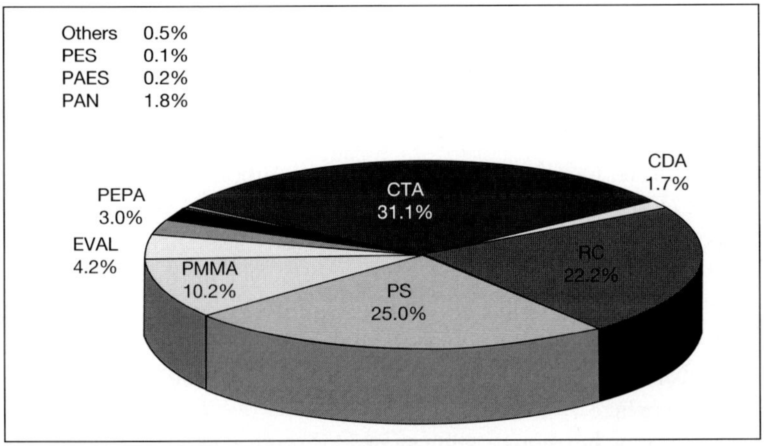

Fig. 2. The market share of each dialyzer membrane in Japan (2000; JSDT December 31, 2000).

and nontoxicity suitable for avoiding pore deformation by drying and membrane deterioration during storage. Finally, the CTA hollow fiber for dialysis is obtained by drying. A flow chart of the manufacturing process of the CTA hollow fiber is shown in figure 1.

Furthermore, the pore size of CTA hollow fibers can be controlled by the selection of an appropriate combination of solvents and nonsolvents and their contents in CTA hollow fibers, which means that it is possible to obtain a membrane with specific characteristics. CTA hollow fiber dialyzers are widely used in Japan, as shown in figure 2 [2].

Features of CTA Membrane

Characteristics

CTA has a relatively hydrophobic property, as all hydrophilic hydroxyl radicals are replaced with acetyl radicals. In contrast to regenerated cellulose which swells in water, no swelling is caused when CTA is dipped into water, resulting in no changes in the fiber wall thickness and internal diameter. CTA has characteristics which can resist the exposure to gamma irradiation under certain conditions; this means that the application of gamma sterilization is possible [3].

Mass Transfer Properties

CTA dialyzers perform better in removing β_2-microglobulin, small molecular weight solutes such as urea and creatinine, and inorganic phosphate than conventional cellulose diacetate dialyzers. About half the CTA membrane area is sufficient to obtain the same clearance of small molecular weight solutes as with the conventional ones. And a significant increase in removal rates of middle molecular weight solutes and low molecular weight proteins is recognized with CTA dialyzers.

β_2-Microglobulin is not absorbed by the CTA membrane surface, and the sieving coefficient is unchanged during dialysis [4]. Mass removal of this substance by diffusion is, therefore, realized.

Additionally, the formation of an albumin monolayer on the CTA membrane surface by contact with blood leads to a negligible albumin loss during dialysis and gives a very sharp molecular weight cutoff property. This characteristic is derived from the low-charged membrane surface specific to CTA and the smooth internal surface finish of the fiber.

Furthermore, various hormones, such as erythropoietin and insulin, are not adsorbed on the surface of the CTA membrane, and almost all the mass removals are caused by diffusion.

Clearance of negatively charged inorganic phosphate depending on zeta potential is well known. CTA membrane is also considered suitable for effective removal of inorganic phosphate, since removal is not adversely affected by the charge distribution due to low zeta potential and high porosity of the membrane.

Transfer of endotoxins into the blood from dialysate had been suspected in the use of high-flux dialyzers due to their relatively high ultrafiltration rate. However, according to the study conducted to examine endotoxin permeation through the membrane by the determination of levels of cytokines produced by monocytes, it was reported that the transfer through the CTA membrane was smaller than through the polysulfone membrane [5].

Furthermore, the transfer of *Escherichia coli*-derived pyrogen from dialysate to blood was not detected by the evaluation conducted by adding the pyrogen to dialysate.

It can be noted, however, that the control of dialysate to reduce contamination as much as possible is very important in order to perform the dialysis treatment more safely.

Blood-Membrane Interaction

When the CTA membrane is used, complement activation and changes of the WBC count and granulocyte elastase level are low during dialysis [6]. This fact proves that interaction between blood and the membrane is very small.

This is considered to be the result of appropriate hydrophobicity of the CTA membrane caused by the replacement of hydroxyl radicals of cellulose with acetyl radicals.

It was also reported that blood coagulation by contact with the CTA membrane was very low [7].

Safety

The safety of dialyzers is very important in addition to a high performance. The CTA membrane satisfies all the requirements for extraction and biological tests necessary to assure its safety as specified by various standards. Maintaining safe and stable characteristics of the CTA dialyzers for at least 3 years has already been confirmed by long-term storage tests to determine changes in the characteristics.

Conclusion

Features of the CTA membrane are safety, excellent biocompatibility and performance that fully comply with the requirements of every type of dialyzer.

References

1 Kroschwitz JT: Cellulose Esters. Organic Encyclopedia of Polymer Science and Engineering. New York, Wiley-Interscience,1987, vol 3, p 166.

2 Numerical Statement of the Japanese Society for Dialysis Therapy. Tokyo, JSDT, 2000.

3 Masuda T, Ohmiya H, Ono Y: Japan Patent Publication Number 50946/1993 (radiation sterilization for hollow fiber blood treatment device). Tokyo, Japanese Patent Office.

4 Mineshima M, Hosono T, Era K, Sasaki Y, Agishi T, Ota K: Diffuse and convective mass transport characteristics in beta2-microglobulin removal. Trans Am Soc Artif Organs 1987;33:103–106.

5 Lonnemann G, Schindler R, Lufft V, Mahiout A, Shaldon S, Koch K: The role of plasma coating on the permeation of cytokine-inducing substances through dialyzer membranes. Nephrol Dial Transplant 1995;10:207–211.
6 Nishibori H, Itoh K, Ohdan T, et al: Clinical evaluation of a new porous membrane dialyzer composed of cellulose triacetate. Jpn Artif Organs 1993;22/1:43–46.
7 Fukui H: Dialysis with nonanticoagulant. Toseki Front 1997;7/2:19–23.

Toshiaki Masuda, MD, Nipro Corporation, 3-9-3, Kitaku, Osaka 531–8510 (Japan)
Tel. +81 6 6373 0092, Fax +81 6 6373 8978, E-Mail masuda-toshiaki@nipro.co.jp

Ronco C, La Greca G (eds): Hemodialysis Technology.
Contrib Nephrol. Basel, Karger, 2002, vol 137, pp 111–119

The AN69ST Dialysis Membrane

A New Approach for Reducing Systemic Heparinization

Jean-Louis Renaux, Mauro Atti

Hospal International Marketing, Lyon, France

Interactions between blood components (cells and proteins) and the extracorporeal circuit induce the activation of several biological systems such as platelets, leukocytes, complement and coagulation cascades. The coagulation system generates a key enzyme, factor IIa or thrombin, responsible for blood clotting in the dialysis circuit (blood lines, dialyzer, needles). For routine delivery of hemodialysis (HD), the blood's tendency to clot must be stopped by using anticoagulation procedures. Clotting in the circuit may reduce dialysis efficiency and, if persistent, will increase transfusion requirements by reducing hematocrit. Conversely, excessive anticoagulation can induce a significant increase in the risk of bleeding. Practically every dialysis session needs to achieve a balance between circuit anticoagulation and the patient's bleeding risk. Clearly, this balance is influenced by the immediate side effects of the anticoagulants while the consequences of long-term anticoagulation have yet to be assessed. New dialysis membranes are continuously being developed, but none of them are able to dispense anticoagulants for routine HD. This paper presents (1) a brief review of routine anticoagulation in HD and (2) an original way of modulating the anticoagulation-bleeding balance in dialyzed patients: the preheparinized AN69ST membrane.

Anticoagulation in HD

Unfractionated Heparin

Systemic heparinization is the most common anticoagulation procedure routinely adopted in HD. Heparin is an anionic sulfated mucopolysaccharide extracted from bovine or pig tissue. Unfractionated heparin (UFH or standard heparin) is a heterogeneous mixture of glycosaminoglycans varying in size from 5 to 50 kD. Its anticoagulant effect primarily depends on its ability to bind the plasma protein antithrombin III (ATIII). The UFH-ATIII complex inactivates several coagulation factors such as thrombin, factor IXa, Xa and XIa. More recently, chemical or enzymatic depolymerization of UFH has resulted in several heparin preparations called 'low molecular weight heparins' because the mean molecular size is around 3.5 kD (2–8 kD). For routine HD, only some features are clinically relevant: (1) binding to ATIII to inhibit factor Xa but not thrombin; (2) as a consequence, clotting times such as activated partial thromboplastin time (aPTT) cannot be used and should be replaced by anti-Xa heparin activity, and (3) the pharmacological property allows for a single predialysis dose even for a 5-hour dialysis session. The other beneficial effects compared to UFH (lipid metabolism, bleeding complications, osteoporosis) remain unclear, perhaps due to heterogeneity among the different LMWH preparations (enoxaparin, dalteparin, nadroparin…).

What is Adequate Heparinization Strategy for HD?

No consensus exists for the heparinization procedures. The anticoagulation level is monitored by the visual inspection of the extracorporeal circuit, the routine practices of the center and sometimes by the heparin activity (anti-Xa activity) or coagulation time (aPTT) assessments. As the thrombin generation is a rapid and autoamplified phenomenon, the heparin dose (necessary to inhibit thrombin induced by blood-material contact) should be significant compared to the 'steady-state' dose (e.g. for patients with no known bleeding problems, loading dose ≥65% of total dose).

Two basic techniques are routinely used for UFH administration.

(1) A heparin loading dose (1,000–5,000 IU) is followed by a continuous heparin infusion (500–1,000 IU/h) discontinued 30 or 60 min before the end of the session.

(2) Repeated heparin bolus, e.g. for a 4-hour session, a heparin loading dose (1,500–5,000 IU) is followed by a second midsession bolus (1,000–2,500 IU).

For LMWH, the most rational strategy is a single bolus (4,000–6,000 IU) per 4- to 5-hour session. However, pharmacological clinical studies including chronic hemodialyzed patients have to be performed so as to better define the optimal anticoagulant strategy for each LMWH commercial preparation.

Independently of the blood-material interactions, many parameters affect heparinization, such as the blood flow rate, hematocrit, fistula quality, air-blood contact, dialysis time, bleeding from needle sites postdialysis or drugs interfering with the hemostasis system, such as oral anticoagulant, nonsteroidal anti-inflammatory agents or antiplatelet agents.

Complications Associated with Heparin Therapy

Apart from bleeding, the administration of UFH has also been associated with dyslipidemia, hypoaldosteronism and hyperkalemia, thrombopenia, osteoporosis, pruritus, itching and hypersensitivity reactions [see review in 1].

Alternatives to Standard Heparinization

To limit and prevent the drawbacks of UFH, several anticoagulation strategies have been developed based on regional heparinization with protamine, low-dose heparin, no anticoagulation or other drugs such as citrate or hirudin. Nowadays the main clinical factor for these alternatives is still the acute side effect of bleeding. Several authors have suggested a system for classifying the bleeding risk in HD patients [2, 3]. Various techniques have been described to reduce bleeding complications. Regional heparinization consists of heparin neutralization (continuously infused into the arterial line) by protamine infusion into the venous line. Due to a possible complex dissociation and technical difficulties, this procedure has been abandoned in favor of low heparinization or heparin-free dialysis. Low-dose heparinization is carried out in the centers using coagulation time to adjust the doses but for practical reasons high-bleeding-risk patients are mostly treated by heparin-free dialysis. Heparin-free dialysis is performed with periodic saline flushes through the dialyzer (100–200 ml, every 30 or 60 min). Some studies have shown clotting events located in the dialyzer or in the venous drip chamber [4, 5], leading to low dialysis efficiencies.

Two strategies directly affecting the coagulation cascade have been described. Using a calcium-free dialysate, citrate continuously infused into the arterial line is able to decrease the calcium in the dialyzer and thus to locally inhibit thrombin generation. For obvious safety reasons, calcium chloride 5% is infused into the venous line. A potential risk of alkalosis associated with the complexity of the technique has limited citrate anticoagulation. Hirudin reacts with thrombin to form an inhibitory thrombin complex. Nevertheless, its pharmacological properties (long half-life) and the absence of long-term studies limit the spread of hirudin.

The last technique for reducing heparinization is based on dialysis membranes preprimed with heparinized saline, as described hereafter.

AN69ST Dialysis Membrane

The dream of every medical equipment company is to identify and develop the most biocompatible environment applicable to the patients. The thromboresistance of the vascular wall requires the endothelium lining to be compatible with the cells (platelets) and plasma coagulation proteins. Unlike artificial materials, the endothelium does not induce coagulation. This is partially due to the glycoaminoglycans layer present on the endothelial cell surface.

For more than 12 years, Hospal's Research Division has been studying the development of a new high-flux dialysis membrane based on the significant reduction of coagulation system activation. Two different approaches have been conducted in parallel (1) reduction of coagulation contact phase activation by the dialysis membrane and (2) limitation of thrombin generation due to 'extramembrane' stimuli (vascular access, needles, blood lines) by heparin adsorption on the membrane. In order to process the original AN69 membrane with a polycationic polymer a spraying method is used for the flat sheet membrane and a washing method for hollow fiber AN69ST dialyzers. The gamma sterilization step reinforces the polyethylenimine (PEI) coating network at the surface and results in a homogeneous treatment with a reduction of AN69ST roughness compared with the AN69 membrane (mean roughness = 18 ± 2 vs. 30 ± 7 nm; unpubl. data). The physical and core electrical properties of the original AN69 membrane are preserved as demonstrated by Randoux et al. [6]. They showed that native β_2-microglobulin mass transfer was similar through the AN69 and AN69ST membranes, as was the fraction of native β_2-microglobulin binding to the membrane. The PEI surface effect does not alter the bulk adsorption properties of AN69 [6], while clinical trials of AN69ST have shown that the 'standard' biocompatibility (C3a generation, leukocytes and platelet counts) of AN69ST is similar to that of the well-known AN69 (unpubl. data: clinical study report Nephral 400ST Hospal internal data).

Reduction of Contact Phase Activation

Like almost every commercial dialysis membrane, polyacrylonitrile membranes have an electronegative surface. The AN69 membrane is electronegative as measured by zeta potential (−70 mV). Partial neutralization (by chemical grafting) of the AN69 surface-electronegative charges with a high molecular weight cationic polymer called PEI results in a significant increase in zeta potential as compared with AN69 (−15 ± 5 vs. −70 ± 10 mV) [7]. This surface treatment prevents contact phase system activation and bradykinin generation measured in the acidic medium [7].

Heparin Adsorption on the AN69ST Membrane

The AN69ST dialysis membrane is able to adsorb heparin through its polycationic polymer-coated surface (fig. 1). In vitro experiments [8] have shown that during routine priming with heparinized saline (5,000 IU/l), heparin kinetic adsorption is a very rapid phenomenon, saturable after 3–5 min for a 100 ml/min flow rate. Around 800–1,000 IU/m^2 of standard heparin is adsorbed on AN69ST membrane, slightly more than dalteparin (500–700 IU/m^2) and significantly more than enoxaparin or nadroparin (100–200 IU/m^2). Using healthy human citrated plasma, 100% of adsorbed enoxaparin and nadroparin are desorbed,

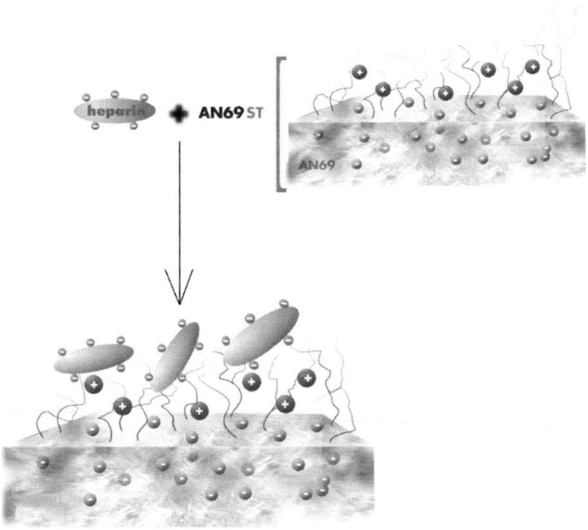

Fig. 1. AN69ST 'heparinization process'. Heparinized saline priming of AN69ST leads to heparin binding to the cationic polymer present on the membrane surface.

50% of dalteparin and only 15% of UFH. The discrepancies in these data can be accounted for by the size variability of the different heparin preparations. Following these in vitro data, we suggest (1) using standard heparin (5,000 or 10,000 IU/l) in saline solution at 100 ml/min during the priming procedure of the AN69ST membrane and (2) avoiding saline heparinization with LMWH (the dalteparin case requires clinical confirmation).

An experimental protocol testing the AN69ST membrane without systemic heparinization was performed in sheep. The extracorporeal circuit was primed with 2 liters of saline containing 5,000 IU/l of UFH. The dialysis sessions were delivered for more than 6 h without massive clotting. In comparison massive clotting of the extracorporeal circuit occurred within 30–40 min of AN69 dialysis.

First Clinical Experiences of Low Systemic Heparinization with AN69ST

UFH Dose Finding. Lavaud et al. [9] reported a prospective monocentric study focused on the systemic heparin dose reduction in AN69ST dialyzers. Thirteen stable chronic hemodialyzed patients were followed up over a 7-week period in order to define the appropriate UFH dose. The patients received bicarbonate HD with AN69ST dialyzers (1.25 m^2), thrice weekly for 4 h per session at blood flow rates of 300–350 ml/min. Subjects receiving oral anticoagulants, antiplatelet or nonsteroidal anti-inflammatory agents were excluded.

Table 1. Heparin dose

	Week						
	0	1	2	3	4	5	6
Loading dose, IU	4,000	4,000	4,000	3,000	2,000	1,000	0
Bolus, IU	2,000	1,000	0	0	0	0	0

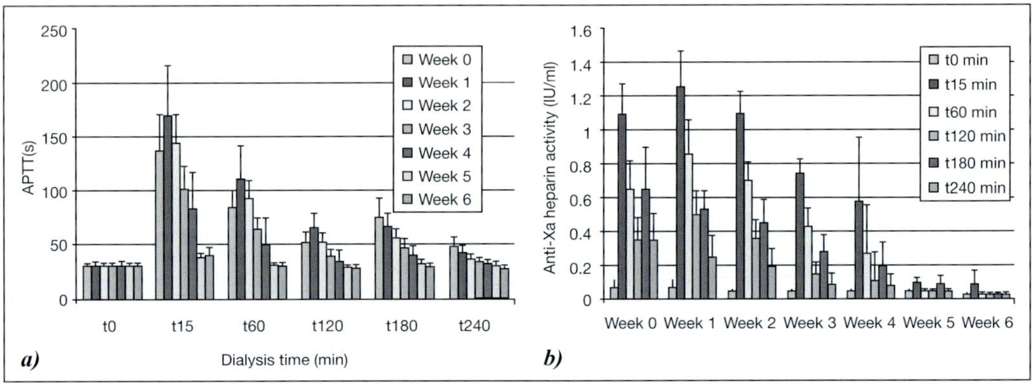

Fig. 2. Changes in aPTT (***a***) and heparin anti-Xa activity (***b***) in the heparin dose found with AN69ST dialyzers. The heparinization strategies are shown in table 1.

The AN69ST dialyzers were primed with 2 liters of heparinized saline (5,000 IU/l). The evaluation of the range of the heparin dose started with 4,000 IU of UFH (loading dose) and 2,000 IU bolus at midsession. The heparin dose decreased by 1,000 IU per week as shown in table 1.

Three massive circuit thromboses and fifteen partial thromboses occurred in the 256 dialysis sessions. From week 3, venous drip chamber clotting (variable intensity) was seen in two thirds of dialysis sessions. Nevertheless, the dialysis efficiency, measured by ionic dialysance with Diascan module, was not modified throughout the study. After loading doses, anti-Xa and aPTT increased markedly and moved closely with the heparin injections (fig. 2a, b, table 1). From week 2, none of the end-session values showed heparin activity and anticoagulation process. At week 6 we observed a slight increase in anti-Xa (0.2 IU/ml) and aPTT (49 s) after 15 min of dialysis (fig. 2a, b). This observation results from two phenomena: (1) heparinized saline priming solution is partly infused into the patient at the onset of dialysis, and (2) a low heparin

Table 2. Systemic heparin-free HD: comparison between preheparinized AN69ST and saline flush technique with polysulfone membrane (PS)

	AN69ST	PS
Sessions, n	67	67
Saline flushes, l	0	1.1 ± 0.2*
Ultrafiltration, l/session	2.9 ± 0.8	3.8 ± 1.3*
BW deviation, kg	0.4 ± 0.4	0.8 ± 0.6*
Kt l/session	50 ± 3	48 ± 3*
Hb g/l	105 ± 6	95 ± 9*
Weekly EPO, IU	15,000	15,000
Circuit aspect	57A/7B/3C	19A/7B/41C*

Circuit aspect notation: A = Good, B = partial thrombosis, C = massive thrombosis and dialyzer replacement. Student's *t* test was used for paired comparisons:* $p < 0.001$.

desorption occurred as shown by our in vitro experiments [8] and confirmed by Tielemans et al. [10], who measured thrombin time elevation within the first 30 min of dialysis. However, it should be pointed out that after 1 h of dialysis no blood heparin activity was detected; thus the 'preheparinized' AN69ST maintains the heparin activity at its surface. Lastly, changing the heparin strategy to 1,000 IU (loading dose) and 1,000 IU (bolus at midsession) has allowed us to limit venous drip chamber clotting.

Heparin-Free Dialysis with AN69ST. HD without systemic anticoagulation is frequently required in chronic renal disease. To take advantage of the AN69ST properties (heparin adsorption and active heparinized surface), Arkouche et al. [11] have compared two clinical heparin-free dialysis modalities. In 2 patients at risk of hemorrhage, they compared frequent saline flush HD with the polysulfone membrane (n = 67 sessions) with 'preheparinized' AN69ST dialysis without flushes (n = 67). Both dialyzers were primed with 2 liters of heparinized saline (5,000 IU/l). Table 2 showed that AN69ST heparin-free dialysis results in an improved dry weight achievement, higher hemoglobin levels (for identical EPO therapy) and significantly lower extracorporeal circuit clotting. Due to less clotted circuit changes, the AN69ST technique is more comfortable for the patients and involves a lower workload for the staff.

Clinical Perspectives

Due to the ionic nature of UFH and the AN69ST membrane, heparin binding during the priming phase allows for a significant reduction in the systemic heparin dose. This membrane specificity paves the way for new therapeutic perspectives. In HD patients serious bleeding complications are currently described and so HD techniques which can avoid systemic heparinization are required (hemorrhagic pericarditis, gastrointestinal bleeding, pre-post surgery). It has been assumed that heparinization would encourage retinal bleeding in diabetic patients and cholesterol embolus mobilization. For these clinical indications, minimal heparinization or heparin-free HD with AN69ST can be guaranteed. The last potential AN69ST indication in HD is the reduction of blood triglycerides. In the short term, the heparin effect on endothelial lipoprotein lipase release leads to triglycerides catabolism and free fatty acid generation. In the long term, repeated heparin infusions induce lipoprotein lipase depletion and could increase the amount of triglycerides.

Conclusions

Systemic exposure to approximately 600,000–1,200,000 IU of UFH per year is unique in chronic HD patients. The side effects of heparinization are well-known but their influence on HD patients' complications are not currently being studied. Hospal has conducted original research into reduced contact phase activation together with the heparinized-like dialysis membrane. Even though further multicenter clinical studies will still have to be launched in order to confirm its clinical benefits, AN69ST can help us to understand the consequences of long-term heparinization and can also reduce heparin side effects in chronic HD patients.

References

1 Lane DA, Lindahl U: Heparin. Chemical and Biological Properties, Clinical Applications. London, Arnold, 1989.
2 Lohr JW, Schwab SJ: Minimizing hemorrhagic complications in dialysis patients. J Am Soc Nephrol 1991;2:961–975.
3 Ward DM: The approach to anticoagulation in patients treated with extracorporeal therapy in the intensive care unit. Adv Ren Replace Ther 1997;4:160–173.
4 Keller F, Seemann J, Preuschof L, Offermann G: Risk factors of system clotting in heparin-free haemodialysis. Nephrol Dial Transplant 1990;5:802–807.
5 Sanders PW, Taylor H, Curtis JJ: Hemodialysis without anticoagulation. Am J Kidney Dis 1985;5:32–35.
6 Randoux C, Gillery P, Georges N, Lavaud S, Chanard J: Filtration of native and glycated beta2-microglobulin by charged and neutral dialysis membranes. Kidney Int 2001;60:1571–1577.
7 Renaux JL, Thomas M, Crost T, Loughraieb N, Vantard G: Activation of the kallikrein-kinin system in hemodialysis: Role of membrane electronegativity, blood dilution and pH. Kidney Int 1999;55:1097–1103.
8 Renaux JL, Thomas M, Crost T, Paris JM: Heparin adsorption on Nephral ST: In vitro/ex vivo results. Nephrol Dial Transplant 2001;16:A165.

9 Lavaud S, Canivet E, Mohajer M, Crost T, Wuillai A, Renaux JL, Chanard J: Change in membrane electronegativity induces heparin sparing for hemodialysis. J Am Soc Nephrol 2000;11:281A.
10 Tielemans C, Neyens C, Warnimont M, Husson C, Muniz MC, Pradier O, Nortier J: Hémodialyse sans anticoagulation systémique grâce à la membrane AN69ST. Néphrologie 2001;22:263.
11 Arkouche W, Delawari E, Renaux JL, Sibaï-Galland R, Pachot M, Traeger J: Benefits of AN69ST membrane on heparin free dialysis. J Am Soc Nephrol 2001;12:261A.

J.-L. Renaux, PhD, Hospal International Marketing,
61, avenue Tony Garnier, F–69007 Lyon (France)
Tel. +33 4 37 28 10 25, Fax +33 4 37 28 11 01, E-Mail jean-louis.renaux@hospal.com

Ronco C, La Greca G (eds): Hemodialysis Technology.
Contrib Nephrol. Basel, Karger, 2002, vol 137, pp 120–128

Flow Distribution and Cross Filtration in Hollow Fiber Hemodialyzers

Claudio Ronco[a], *Alessandra Brendolan*[a], *Carlo Crepaldi*[a], *Fiorella Gastaldon*[a], *Nathan W. Levin*[b]

[a] Department of Nephrology, St. Bortolo Hospital, Vicenza, Italy;
[b] Renal Research Institute, New York, N.Y., USA

Since the beginning of dialytic therapy, diffusion and convection have been combined in an attempt to replace renal function [1]. The knowledge of diffusion came from the industrial chemistry and dialyzers were designed to be ideal countercurrent exchangers. Only later, convection was used in clinical practice showing potential advantages. Although ultrafiltration (UF) was employed first to treat overhydrated patients, convective solute removal was subsequently employed to enhance solute removal. Blood flow greatly affects the clearance of small solutes like urea while UF rate primarily affects the removal of larger solutes like inulin. Increases in dialysate flow rate become important only with large surface area dialyzers and mostly affect the clearance of small solutes. All these aspects must also consider the type of membrane utilized and the hydraulic conditions within the hemodialyzer.

Diffusion and Convection

Diffusion is a process in which molecules randomly move in all directions. Statistically this movement results in a passage of solutes from a more concentrated area to a less concentrated one. Besides the concentration gradient (dc), the solute diffusive flux (Jd) through a semipermeable membrane depends on the temperature (T), the surface area and the diffusivity (D) of the solute, while it is inversely proportional to the membrane thickness (dx):

$$Jd = D \cdot A \cdot T\ (dc/dx)$$

The convective process requires a fluid movement caused by a transmembrane pressure (TMP) gradient. Therefore, the convective flux of a solute (Jc) will depend on the UF rate (Qf), the solute concentration in plasma water (Cb) and the solute sieving coefficient (S):

$$Jc = Qf \cdot Cb \cdot S$$

being in ideal conditions: $S = 1 - \sigma$, where σ is the reflection coefficient of the membrane. These definitions present convection and diffusion as two separate phenomena. However, it is impossible to precisely define the contribution of each single process to the removal of solutes because of their continuous interactions.

Membranes, Diffusivity and Sieving

Different membranes are utilized in extracorporeal therapy. Cellulosic membranes are considerably hydrophilic, with wall thickness values in the 5- to 15-μm range. Such membranes offer remarkable diffusive performances with limited solute sieving properties. Original synthetic high-flux membranes had an internal skin layer surrounded by a microporous structure with a total thickness up to 100 μm. The polymer was hydrophobic and its efficiency in diffusion was poor. Only recently, partially hydrophilic synthetic membranes with a reduced wall thickness have been developed making the combination of diffusion and convection possible, as in the case of high-flux dialysis or hemodiafiltration.

As solute molecular weight increases the diffusivity coefficient tends to decrease. Thus, the characteristics of the solute are extremely important and diffusion of solutes in the range of 5,000–20,000 daltons may be poor even in the presence of a very permeable membrane. In this case, transport is mainly limited by the low diffusivity of the molecule rather than by the sieving characteristics of the membrane. In addition to the hydrophobic nature of the membrane, the membrane wall thickness and considerable amount of unstirred fluid inside the support structure remarkably slow down the solute transport. The structure of the recent synthetic high-flux membranes partially avoids the above-mentioned problems combining a relatively less hydrophobic nature with a reduced wall thickness and a more homogeneous structure.

Solute diffusivity also plays an important role in blood and dialysate. The resistances generated by blood, dialysis fluid and membrane can be reported as a percent of the overall resistance to solute transport (total resistance = R blood + R membrane + R dialysate). At the cutoff value, the resistance of the membrane represents 100% of the total resistance. This resistance progressively decreases for smaller solutes while the resistances in the blood and dialysate compartments become increasingly important.

The resistance to the transport of larger solutes due to their poor diffusion coefficients can be overcome by the use of convection. The convective flux is influenced by the permeability of the membrane, which is characterized by the observed sieving coefficient. The sieving coefficient is the ratio between the solute concentration in the filtrate and the solute concentration in plasma water in the absence of a gradient for diffusion. However, solute distribution in the blood compartment is not homogeneous depending on polarization and other phenomena. As UF increases, part of the solute tends to accumulate at the blood/membrane interface, thus creating gradients for diffusion both towards the bulk region inside the hollow fiber and towards the dialysate compartment across the membrane. As a consequence diffusion is continuously interfering with convection and the sieving coefficient can be overestimated. In fact, the concentration in the bulk region (which is the value measured empirically) is generally lower than that at the blood/membrane interface. Therefore, the difference between the observed sieving coefficient (So) and the true sieving coefficient (St) can be significantly affected by the amount of convection used. With low UF values, So and St tend to be equal while large differences can be observed at high UF rates [2].

The Membrane and the Blood Compartment

For all membranes to some extent but particularly in the case of synthetic membranes, a protein layer is deposited on the internal surface of the fiber. This slightly reduces the membrane sieving coefficient with a rather constant trend. However, in case of high UF rates or high filtration fractions, a thick protein deposit on the membrane is induced by the additional phenomenon of polarization. This progressively reduces the membrane permeability and So becomes proportional to a new reflection coefficient (σ_1) of the membrane. This layer is a function of several variables, and above all the value of the 'shear rate' at the wall. As the blood enters the hollow fiber, the shear stress generates different layers of blood from the bulk phase to the membrane interface flowing at different velocities. The ratio between the differential velocity of the fluid threads in the fiber and the differential distance from the center of the fiber (shear rate expressed in s^{-1}) is a function of blood viscosity and shear stress. The shear rate is also proportional to the blood flow per single fiber. The thickness of the protein layer at the blood membrane interface depends on the wall shear rate value, and is extremely important for the membrane performance. The shear rate value linearly correlates with the shear stress in case of Newtonian fluids and the velocity profile is regularly parabolic. Blood approaches Newtonian behavior only at shear rates higher than 200 s^{-1} [3].

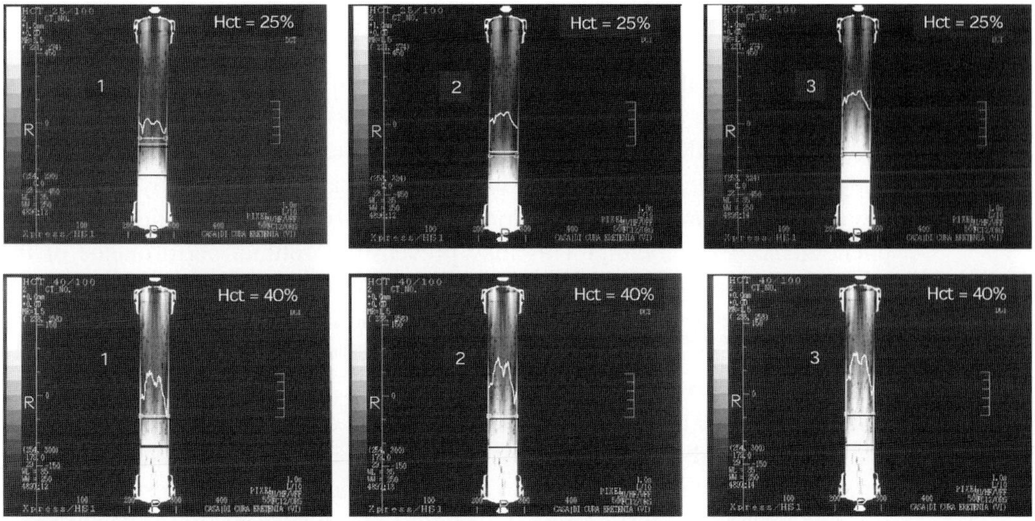

Fig. 1. Typical parabolic distribution of blood flow in the fiber bundle documented by dye injection in the blood compartment and image reconstruction by a helical scanner. The increase in hematocrit further enhances the discrepancy between central and peripheral fibers in terms of relative flow velocity.

UF and solute sieving coefficients are considerably influenced by the wall shear rate because it contributes to keeping the polarization layer very thin. This is particularly important for solutes in the middle-high range. Diffusion is also affected by the value of the shear rate since high shear rates contribute to maintaining the diffusion distance from blood to dialysate within minimal values. This is because concentration polarization and the secondary layer of proteins lead to the formation of a pseudomembrane whose thickness is added to that of the original membrane. In clinical practice, high wall shear rates are obtained with high blood flows and appropriate device geometry with relative preservation of UF rates and solute clearances. In a recent study carried out with dye injection in the blood compartment of different hollow fiber dialyzers, we could demonstrate that in peripheral fibers, blood flows and shear rates much lower than those observed in the central fibers of the bundle are observed [4]. This is even more evident when hematocrit rises above 35% (fig. 1). Based on the above-mentioned issues we could speculate that blood flows higher than 350–400 ml/min must always be utilized in the presence of a 1.8- to 2.0-m^2 dialyzer, if an optimal performance of all the fibers is to be achieved.

The Dialysate Compartment

While several attempts have been made to optimize the blood compartment, by creating adequate blood ports and flow distributors at the inlet of the dialyzer, very little attention has been paid to the dialysate compartment. The dialysate distribution may in fact be asymmetrical inside the dialyzer, presenting a nonhomogeneous distribution within the fiber's bundle and consequent phenomena of channeling. This may prevent the optimal performance of the dialyzer and may affect the final performance of the treatment.

Some attempts to avoid dialysate channeling have been made by new filter design. For example, an increased length of the fibers reduces contact because of a waived configuration of the fiber. An external irregular surface makes it possible to avoid the perfect contact of adjacent fibers. Different systems of nonparallel orientation of the fibers or the use of tissue structures within the bundle may further help to maintain adequate distances between the external surface of adjacent fibers. The most recent approach is the use of spacing filaments ('spacer yarns') between the fibers or the creation of waved fibers (moiré structure). We carried out a complex evaluation using an helical CT scan to achieve a detailed imaging of the dialysate distribution pattern after dye injection. The modified dialysate compartment with the spacing filaments between the fibers and the moiré structure displayed a more homogeneous distribution of the dye, as compared to the standard dialyzers in which a typical channeling effect was displayed in the peripheral regions [5] (fig. 2).

Interference between Diffusion and Convection

Although convection and diffusion are described as two separate phenomena, in practice we cannot distinguish between the single contributions given by the two mechanisms separately. Moreover, especially in treatments that present a combined utilization of diffusion and convection, there is a continuous interference between the two transport mechanisms [6]. In such circumstances, enhancement of one type of transport can produce effects on the other mechanism of transport that may be beneficial or detrimental.

In hemodiafiltration, solutes are carried across the membrane at the same concentration as in plasma water because of the high UF rate. This phenomenon mostly takes place in the proximal side of the filter and reduces the driving force for diffusion. In this case convection negatively affects diffusion that becomes more important in the distal side of the filter where UF approaches zero. This emphasizes the importance of the surface area for the diffusive performance in hemodiafiltration. However, in hemodiafiltration the backdiffusion

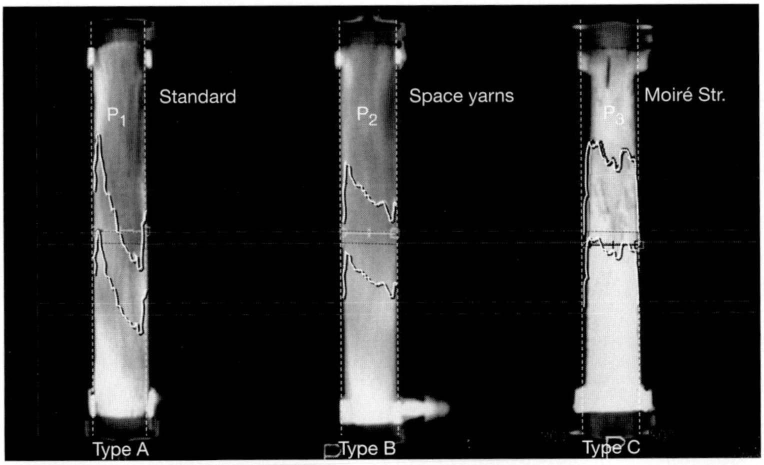

Fig. 2. Distribution of dialysate in three different hemodialyzers: standard configuration (type A), spacing filament configuration (type B) and moiré structure configuration (type C). It is evident that the most homogeneous distribution is obtained with the micro-ondulation design of the hollow fibers (type C).

of substances such as buffers from dialysate into the blood may also be negatively affected at least in the proximal side of the filter where UF is higher. In high flux dialysis a typical filtration-backfiltration profile occurs [7]. The minimal interference between convection and diffusion is achieved in the central part of the dialyzer at which the water flux in both directions is near zero. In the region near the blood ports, convection may interfere with diffusion both in the filtration and backfiltration modes.

Internal Filtration and Backfiltration

Hemodiafiltration enhances middle molecule clearances; however, the need to replace the ultrafiltrate with sterile solutions makes this modality complex and costly. Volumetrically controlled hemodialysis with high-flux membranes (high-flux dialysis) also improves middle molecule clearances as compared to standard hemodialysis without the need for substitution fluid. In this modality, however, the convective removal of middle molecules is limited by the rate of internal filtration.

Internal filtration is governed by the hydraulic and oncotic forces acting along the length of the dialyzer on each side of the membrane. In each point of the dialyzer, the local pressure differential is termed TMP. When the TMP is positive, the water flux is from the blood compartment to the dialysate compartment. When the TMP is negative, backfiltration occurs. Thus, removal of middle molecules can be enhanced by increasing the positive pressure differential in the proximal part of the dialyzer, thus increasing internal filtration. Adequate net filtration is maintained by the UF control system by a parallel increase of the negative pressure differential in the distal part of the dialyzer. This results in increased proximal filtration and distal backfiltration without affecting the 'net' filtration rate.

When high rates of backfiltration are utilized, a high quality of dialysate is needed to prevent any inconvenience or side effect related to pyrogen transfer into the patient's circulation. For this treatment, the use of the last-generation hemodialysis machines is strongly suggested. New machines are equipped with a built-in pyrogen filter to prepare ultrapure dialysate. The reinfusion via backfiltration provides an extra step of safety since the fluid is filtered again across the hemodialysis membrane prior to reaching the blood compartment.

Several experimental approaches have been tried out to increase the rate of internal filtration including modifications of the geometry of the dialyzer and the application of an o-ring in the middle portion of the hemodialyzer [8, 9]. The most practical modification has been shown to be a reduction of the inner diameter of the hollow fiber. This is an interesting approach to increasing the positive pressure differential across the membrane in the proximal and distal regions of the hemodialyzer without introducing major changes in the dialyzer design. In recent observations [6], this approach resulted in a definite increase of internal filtration.

The difference in pressure drop between the two filters is significant as it is predicted by the Hagen-Poiseuille formula:

$$\Delta P = Qb \times (8\eta\, l/\pi r^4)$$

where ΔP = end-to-end pressure drop, Qb = blood flow, η = blood viscosity.

Since the pressure drop in a fiber correlates with the internal radius of the fiber to the fourth power, it seems logical to attempt solutions that involve modifications of the fiber geometry. In this circumstance even small changes of the inner diameter of the fiber may result in dramatic changes in its performance. In our study, a reduction of the inner diameter of the fiber resulted in an improved filtration rate in the proximal half of the dialyzer with a complementary increase in backfiltration in the distal part of the dialyzer (fig. 3). With net filtration rates near zero, the increases in filtration and backfiltration were doubled compared to the standard high-flux dialyzer with a similar length and surface area.

One may speculate that a reduction of the inner diameter of the hollow fiber will also result in an increase of the average blood flow velocity per fiber and a

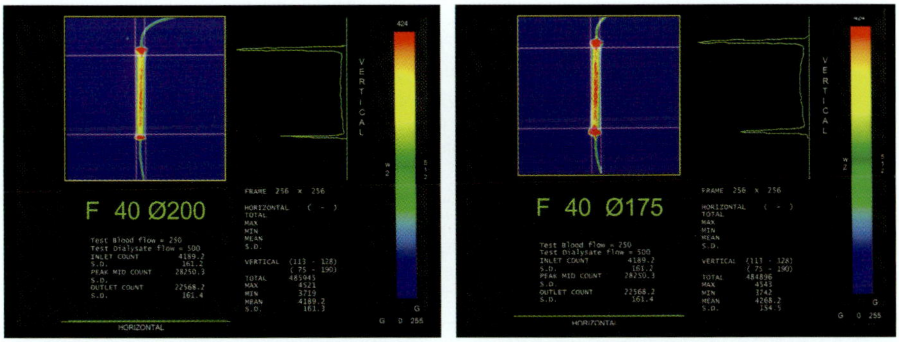

a *b*

Fig. 3. ***a***, ***b*** Images of two filters analyzed with the gamma camera. The increased concentration of the labeled nondiffusable marker molecule in the central portion of the modified hemodialyzer (***b***, reduced inner diameter of the fibers) can be visually captured from the change in color. The curve of the radioactive count is displayed on the right side of the filter image. The relative changes in concentration of the marker molecule are displayed for the two filters along the length of the fibers. It is evident that no net filtration occurred since the concentration of the molecule is equal at the inlet and at the outlet of the filters. The peak values are obtained at 4/10 of the filter length and are significantly different for the two filters. The peak change in concentration, as compared to the inlet value, for the modified dialyzer is 22.94% implying filtration-backfiltration rates of 48.2 ml/min. The peak concentration change for the standard dialyzer is only 10.06% implying a 23.1 ml/min UF-backfiltration.

consequent increase in wall shear rates. This additional factor may in fact result in a 'cleaning' effect at the blood/membrane interface. Higher shear rates lead to a reduction of the thickness of the protein boundary layer and improve membrane permeability counterbalancing the concentration polarization phenomenon. This will certainly help not only to obtain a better performance of the membrane in terms of filtration rates at a given local TMP gradient, but also an optimal utilization of the sieving capacities of the membrane.

An in vivo analysis of middle molecule removal demonstrated the benefits of increased internal filtration resulting from the change in hollow fiber geometry. Although urea, creatinine and phosphorus clearances were not changed as expected by their high-diffusion coefficients (poorly affected by changes in convection), the clearance of vitamin B_{12} and inulin were improved by more than 30% using the modified dialyzer.

In conclusion, modifications in the design of hollow fibers may lead to new interesting performances of hemodialyzers. Newly conceived dialyzers may, therefore, appear in the future with an enhanced capability of convective transport, leading to simplified hemodiafiltration techniques without the need for replacement solutions, but simply utilizing internal filtration as a main way to increase convective transport.

References

1 Hoenich N, Ronco C: Dialyzer evaluation; in Winchester J, Koch K, Jacobs C, Kjiellestrand C (eds): Replacement of Renal Function by Dialysis. Dordrecht, Kluwer Academic Publishers, 1996, pp 256–270.

2 Ronco C, Clark W: Factors affecting hemodialysis and peritoneal dialysis efficiency. Semin Dial 2001;4:257–262.

3 Ronco C: Extracorporeal therapies: Should we use plasma instead of blood? Int J Artif Organs 1999;5:342–346.

4 Ronco C, Ghezzi PM, Metry G, Spittle M, Brendolan A, Rodighiero M, Milan M, Zanella M, La Greca G, Levin N: Effects of hematocrit and blood flow distribution on solute clearance in hollow fiber hemodialyzers. Nephron 2001;89:243–250.

5 Ronco C, Brendolan A, Crepaldi C, Rodighiero MP, Everard P, Ballestri M, Cappelli G, Spittle M, La Greca G: Dialysate flow distribution in hollow fiber hemodialyzers with different dialysate pathway configuration. Int J Artif Organs 2000;9:601–609.

6 Ronco C, Brendolan A, Lupi A, Metry G, Levin N: Effects of a reduced inner diameter of hollow fibers in hemodialyzers. Kidney Int 2000;58:809–817.

7 Ronco C: Backfiltration: A controversial issue in modern dialysis. Int J Artif Organs 1988;11: 69–74.

8 Ronco C, Brendolan A, Feriani M, Milan M, Conz P, Lupi A, Berto P, Bettini MC, La Greca G: A new scintigraphic method to characterize ultrafiltration in hollow fiber dialyzers. Kidney Int 1992;41:1383–1393.

9 Ronco C, Brendolan A, Lupi A, Bettini MC, La Greca G: Enhancement of convective transport by internal filtration in a modified experimental hemodialyzer. Kidney Int 1998;54:979–985.

Claudio Ronco, MD, Department of Nephrology,
St. Bortolo Hospital, Viale Rodolfi, I–36100 Vicenza (Italy)
Tel. +39 0444993869, Fax +39 0444993949, E-Mail cronco@goldnet.it

Ronco C, La Greca G (eds): Hemodialysis Technology.
Contrib Nephrol. Basel, Karger, 2002, vol 137, pp 129–137

Optimal Use of Hemodialyzers

John K. Leypoldt[a,c,d], *Alfred K. Cheung*[b,c]

[a]Research and [b]Medical Services, VA Salt Lake City Health Care System and Departments of [c]Internal Medicine and [d]Bioengineering, University of Utah, Salt Lake City, Utah, USA

An adequate dose of hemodialysis depends on achieving adequate clearances of small solutes, expressed either as a minimum urea reduction ratio of 65% or a minimum single pool urea Kt/V of 1.2 [1]. Solute clearance from the hemodialyzer depends fundamentally on three parameters: the blood flow rate through the hemodialyzer, the dialysate flow rate and the mass transfer-area coefficient for the solute of interest. Each of these parameters has units of volume per unit time (e.g., ml/min) and can be viewed as a potential clearance. The quantitative relationship among these parameters is governed by an equation described by Michaels [2]; however, this equation is not easily used during routine hemodialysis because it is complex and depends on transcendental mathematical functions. This paper describes an approximate equation for predicting hemodialyzer clearance of urea that provides a more simple interpretation of this relationship and can be readily applied during routine hemodialysis. Urea clearances are predicted using the Michaels equation to illustrate the effects of altering blood flow, dialysate flow and the mass transfer-area coefficient on hemodialyzer clearance of urea. Furthermore, guidelines based on these concepts are suggested for optimal use of hemodialyzers in routine hemodialysis.

Theory

The dependence of solute clearance (K) on hemodialyzer blood flow rate (Q_b), dialysate flow rate (Q_d) and the mass transfer-area coefficient (K_oA) is described by the following equation [2]:

$$K = Q_b \{\exp[K_oA/Q_b \times (1 - Q_b/Q_d)] - 1\}/\{\exp[K_oA/Q_b \times (1 - Q_b/Q_d)] - Q_b/Q_d\} \quad (1)$$

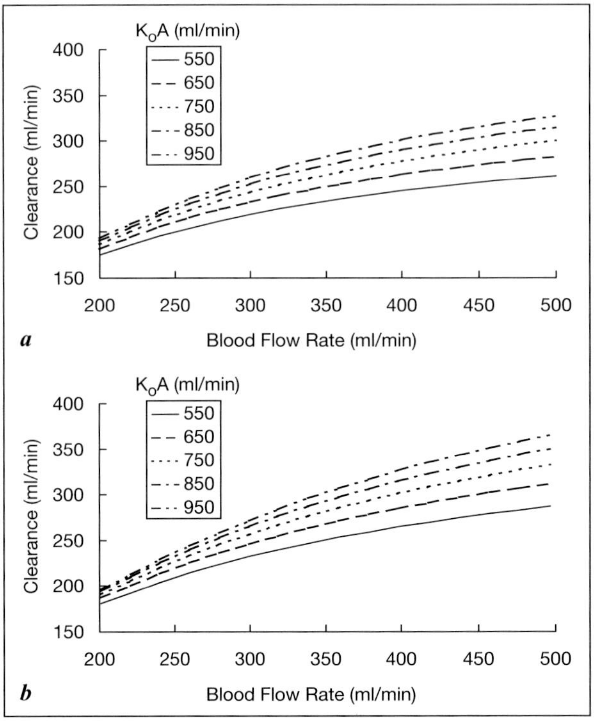

Fig. 1. Dependence of urea clearance on blood flow rate for 5 different hemodialyzers with urea mass transfer-area coefficients (K_oA) of 550, 650, 750, 850 and 950 ml/min at a dialysate flow rate of either 500 ml/min (***a***) or 800 ml/min (***b***). Results are based on equation (1) of the main text.

The dependence of K on Q_b in equation 1 for various hemodialyzers (i.e., K_oA values) is shown in figure 1a and b for dialysate flow rates of 500 and 800 ml/min, respectively. The K_oA values chosen are representative of those for urea in most current commercial hemodialyzers under in vivo conditions. For given Q_b and Q_d, K is larger for high values of K_oA. Comparison of figure 1a with b shows that dialyzer K is larger at high Q_d.

An approximation to equation (1) is the following:

$$0.664/K = 1/Q_b + 1/Q_d + 1/K_oA \quad (2)$$

The percent error in predicting K using equation (2) compared with equation (1) is a maximum of 10.5% over the range of Q_b from 200 to 500 ml/min, Q_d from 500 to 800 ml/min, and K_oA from 550 to 950 ml/min. This equation is plotted in figure 2a and b, corresponding to the predictions in figure 1a and b, respectively.

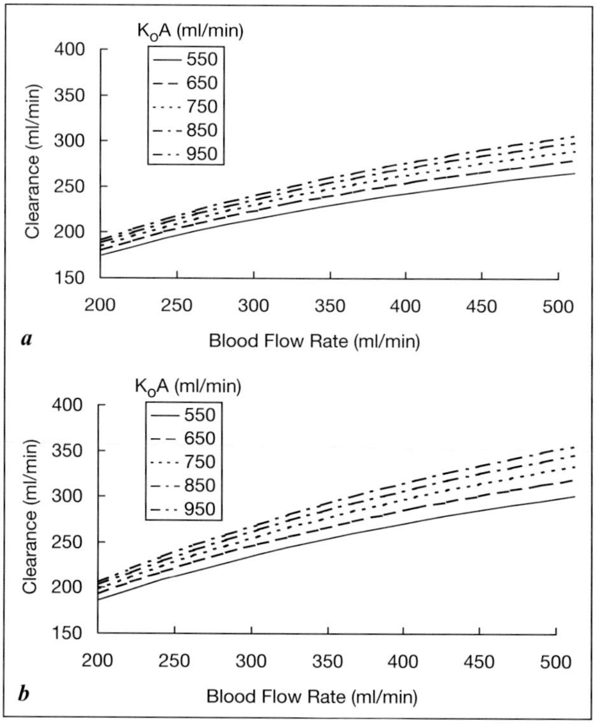

Fig. 2. Dependence of urea clearance on blood flow rate for 5 different hemodialyzers with urea mass transfer-area coefficients (K_oA) of 550, 650, 750, 850 and 950 ml/min at a dialysate flow rate of either 500 ml/min (***a***) or 800 ml/min (***b***). Results are based on equation (2) of the main text.

Unlike equation (1), equation (2) has a simple interpretation. Recall that the solute removal rate during hemodialysis (Q_s) can be calculated by the following equation:

$$Q_s = K\,C_b \qquad (3)$$

Relating Q_s with electrical current and C_b with the electrical potential, equation (3) indicates that the relationship between the solute removal rate and solute concentration has an analog in electrical circuits if the inverse of clearance (i.e., 1/K) is considered the electrical resistance. Consequently, equation (2) states that the overall resistance to solute removal (1/K) is proportional to the sum of three separate series resistances to solute removal: that due to slow blood flow ($1/Q_b$), that due to slow dialysate flow ($1/Q_d$) and that due to a low mass transfer-area coefficient of the dialysis membrane ($1/K_oA$).

The simplicity of equation (2) for conceptualizing hemodialyzer clearance of urea is apparent. The relative importance of the potential clearances (Q_b, Q_d and K_oA) in limiting urea removal during hemodialysis can be identified simply by comparing their absolute magnitudes. For example, the lowest value of Q_b, Q_d or K_oA identifies the limiting resistance to urea removal from the hemodialyzer. Further, equation (2) suggests that the essential relationships between Q_b, Q_d and hemodialyzer K_oA on K are all approximately similar.

In predicting urea clearances using the above equations, several caveats are important to note. First, in vivo values of hemodialyzer K_oA for urea are significantly lower than those determined in vitro [3, 4]. Recent work from the HEMO Study has shown that in vivo urea K_oA values were, on average, only 80% of those observed in vitro [3, 4]. These results further suggest that in vivo urea K_oA values are only approximately 70% of the in vitro values reported by the manufacturer. Second, hemodialyzer K_oA for urea is dependent on Q_d. An increase of Q_d from 500 to 800 ml/min has been shown to increase average in vitro urea K_oA by 14% [5]. Recent work suggests that the effect of Q_d on urea K_oA in vivo is more modest however [3, 4, 6]. The average increase in urea K_oA after increasing Q_d from 500 to 800 ml/min in vivo was only 6% in the HEMO Study [3, 4]. Third, the true blood water flow rate used in the above equations is not equal to the blood pump speed during routine hemodialysis. This discrepancy is caused both by a high negative prepump pressure in the dialysis arterial tubing that lowers the true blood flow rate for most hemodialysis delivery systems [7] and recognition that blood consists of only approximately 89.4% of water at a hematocrit of 30% [8]. The first concern can be modeled by assuming that the true blood flow rate is related to the blood pump speed (Q_{bps}) by the following equation [4]:

$$Q_b = Q_{bps} - 0.05 \times Q_{bps} \times (Q_{bps} - 200)/100 \qquad (4)$$

Equation (4) states that the blood flow rate is reduced by 5% for each 100 ml/min of nominal flow greater than 200 ml/min. The caveats mentioned in the above two paragraphs were included in the predictions described below.

Predictions for Hemodialyzer Clearance for Urea

The importance of the blood flow rate in determining urea clearance has been recently reviewed [9]. Typical blood flow rates are the lowest of the potential clearances, and therefore low blood flow substantially limits urea clearance. If the vascular access is adequate, increasing Q_{bps} (and therefore Q_b) will produce substantial increases in K (table 1). The effect of Q_{bps} is greater in the presence of large K_oA and large Q_d (data not shown), but the effect of increasing

Table 1. Increase in hemodialyzer urea clearance (K) when increasing blood pump speed (Q_{bps}) at a constant dialysate flow rate of 500 ml/min

Urea K_oA ml/min	Initial Q_{bps} ml/min	Initial K ml/min	Final Q_{bps} ml/min	Final K ml/min	Increase in K, %
650	200	168.8	300	216.4	28.2
850	200	174.2	300	230.6	32.3
650	300	216.4	400	245.4	13.4
850	300	230.6	400	266.4	15.5
650	400	245.4	500	263.8	7.5
850	400	266.4	500	289.4	8.6

Table 2. Increase in hemodialyzer urea clearance (K) when increasing dialysate flow rate (Q_d) at different mass transfer-area coefficients (K_oA) and blood pump speeds (Q_{bps})

Urea K_oA[a] ml/min	Q_{bps} ml/min	Initial Q_d ml/min	Initial K ml/min	Final Q_d ml/min	Final K ml/min	Increase in K, %
650	300	500	212.9	800	225.8	6.1
850	300	500	227.8	800	238.7	4.8
650	400	500	240.5	800	261.6	8.8
850	400	500	262.1	800	282.8	7.9
650	500	500	258.0	800	285.7	10.7
850	500	500	284.0	800	313.4	10.3

[a]Value at Q_d of 500 ml/min. The K_oA value at Q_d of 800 ml/min is assumed to be 6% higher.

Q_{bps} becomes less substantial at high Q_{bps} (i.e., there is diminishing return). To illustrate this point, over the range of hemodialyzer K_oA and Q_d values considered here, increasing Q_{bps} from 200 to 300 ml/min will produce approximately a 30% increase in K, from 300 to 400 ml/min will produce approximately a 15% increase in K, but from 400 to 500 ml/min will produce only approximately an 8% increase in K.

An optimum rate of dialysate flow has been suggested based on theoretical considerations by Sigdell and Tersteegen [10, 11]. These workers suggested that an upper limit for an optimal Q_d is twice the blood flow rate and a potentially feasible optimal value for Q_d in practice is equal to the blood flow rate. The effect of increasing Q_d on urea clearance is shown in table 2. In general, the effect of increasing Q_d is greater at higher Q_{bps}. At low Q_{bps} (200–300 ml/min),

Table 3. Increase in hemodialyzer urea clearance (K) when increasing mass transfer-area coefficient (K_oA) at different dialysate flow rates (Q_d) and blood pump speeds (Q_{bps})

Q_d ml/min	Q_{bps} ml/min	Initial K_oA ml/min	Initial K ml/min	Final K_oA ml/min	Final K ml/min	Increase in K, %
500	300	650	212.9	850	227.8	7.0
800	300	689	225.8	901	238.7	5.7
500	400	650	240.5	850	262.1	9.0
800	400	689	261.6	901	282.8	8.1
500	500	650	258.0	850	284.0	10.1
800	500	689	285.7	901	313.4	9.7

increasing Q_d has only a minimal impact on urea clearance. At high Q_{bps} (400–500 ml/min), the increase in urea clearance upon increasing Q_d from 500 to 800 ml/min is generally around 10%.

Table 3 shows the effect of increasing K_oA on urea clearance. The effect of increasing K_oA is greater at high Q_{bps} and at low Q_d.

Discussion

Traditional flow conditions during hemodialysis are a blood flow rate of 200 ml/min and a dialysate flow rate of 500 ml/min. The above analysis shows that a blood flow rate of 200 ml/min will not provide high clearances for small solutes such as urea. Increasing the blood flow rate from 200 to 300, 400 or 500 ml/min will produce substantial increases in hemodialyzer clearance of urea. These increases in clearance will, however, only be productive if the blood flow rate can be increased without causing access recirculation or high negative prepump pressures in the dialysis arterial tubing.

The optimal dialysate flow rate for a given hemodialyzer and blood flow rate remains unclear. The theoretical analysis of Sigdell and Tersteegen [10, 11] suggests that the dialysate flow rate should be between 1 and 2 times the blood flow rate. Others have suggested that the dialysate flow rate should be between 1.5 and 2 times the blood flow rate [9]. The current analysis shows that only relatively small increases in urea clearance are obtained by increasing the dialysate flow rate to 800 ml/min unless the blood pump speed is at least 400 ml/min or greater (i.e., 2 times the blood flow rate). The effect of increasing dialyzer mass transfer-area coefficient from 650 to 850 ml/min produces similar increases in urea clearance to increasing dialysate flow rate from 500 to

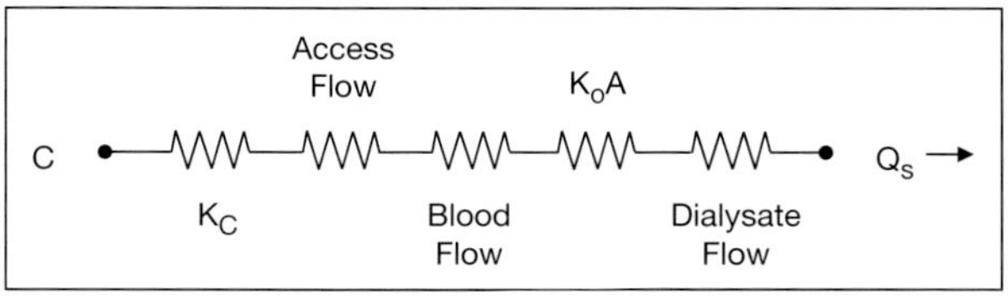

Fig. 3. Electrical circuit conceptual model describing the limitations to urea removal during hemodialysis (Q_s). Urea removal depends on its concentration in blood water (C) and several resistances to urea transport. The resistances include those in the hemodialyzer due to slow blood flow, slow dialysate flow and low mass transfer-area coefficients for urea (K_0A) and those in the patient due to low vascular access blood flow and low intercompartmental transfer of urea (K_c).

800 ml/min. If urea clearance needs to be increased for a given patient, the options of using a more efficient hemodialyzer or increasing dialysate flow rate will depend on the relative economics of these options.

The concept embodied in equation (2) for understanding factors that influence hemodialyzer clearance readily explain the examples described above. For example, increasing the blood flow rate has the most substantial impact on increasing urea clearance since its value is usually the lowest among the potential clearances. In addition, there is no obvious extra financial cost associated with increasing the blood flow rate. In general, increasing either the dialysate flow rate or the mass transfer-area coefficient when their values are already 2 or more times the blood flow rate produces little increase in urea clearance. The similar influence of dialysate flow rate and urea mass transfer-area coefficient on urea clearance is also predicted by equation (2).

The concept of series resistances to overall small solute removal can be further generalized to include two other potential clearances: the vascular access flow rate and the intercompartmental mass transfer coefficient for urea (fig. 3). The vascular access flow rate may limit blood flow through the hemodialyzer since a blood flow rate higher than the access flow rate primarily produces access recirculation [12]. Thus, the magnitude of these potential clearances can be compared among each other to identify the flow rates and membrane and physiological clearance parameters that are most influential in limiting urea clearance from the patient.

The above theoretical analyses apply primarily to urea but may apply similarly to other small solutes. The approach for optimizing hemodialyzer clearance of middle molecules is also of interest but simpler. For middle molecules, including low molecular weight proteins, hemodialyzer clearances are limited primarily by the value of the mass transfer-area coefficient of the dialysis membrane. Therefore, the most effective approach to increase hemodialyzer clearance of middle molecules would be to increase either K_0 and/or A. The use of high flux hemodialyzers provides substantial increases in dialyzer clearances for middle molecules because of the increase in K_0. Thus, the use of high flux hemodialyzers with large surface area will lead to substantial increases in hemodialyzer clearance for these molecules. As discussed elsewhere [13], the use of convective therapies, such as hemofiltration and hemodiafiltration, can be used to further augment clearance of middle molecules. Whether increases in hemodialyzer clearance of middle molecules will increase their overall removal from the patient depends to a large extent on the intercompartmental mass transfer coefficient for these solutes.

Acknowledgments

This material is based upon work supported by the office of Research and Development, Medical Research Service, Department of Veterans Affairs (USA) and the Dialysis Research Foundation (Ogden, Utah, USA).

References

1 National Kidney Foundation: K/DOQI clinical practice guidelines for hemodialysis adequacy, 2000. Am J Kidney Dis 2001;37(suppl 1):S7–S64.
2 Michaels AS: Operating parameters and performance criteria for hemodialyzers and other membrane-separation devices. Trans Am Soc Artif Intern Organs 1966;12:387–392.
3 Depner T, Greene T, Daugirdas J, Gotch F, Kusek J, Leypoldt J, McGillicuddy JR: Simultaneous estimation of delivered blood flow (Qb) and in-vivo urea mass transfer coefficient (KoA) from the cross-dialyzer extraction ratio (ER) (abstract). The HEMO Study Group. J Am Soc Nephrol 2000;11:317A–318A.
4 Depner TA, Greene T, Daugirdas JT, Cheung AK, Gotch FA, Leypoldt JK: Dialyzer performance in the HEMO Study: In vivo KoA and true blood flow determined from a model of cross-dialyzer urea extraction. The HEMO Study Group, in review.
5 Leypoldt JK, Cheung AK, Agodoa LY, Daugirdas JT, Greene T, Keshaviah PR: Hemodialyzer mass transfer-area coefficients for urea increase at high dialysate flow rates. The Hemodialysis (HEMO) Study Group. Kidney Int 1997;51:2013–2017.
6 Ouseph R, Ward RA: Increasing dialysate flow rate increases dialyzer urea mass transfer-area coefficients during clinical use. Am J Kidney Dis 2001;37:316–320.
7 Depner TA, Rizwan S, Stasi TA: Pressure effects on roller pump blood flow during hemodialysis. ASAIO Trans 1990;36:M456–M459.
8 Daugirdas JT, Van Stone JC: Physiologic principles and urea kinetic modeling; in Daugirdas JT, Blake PG, Ing TS (eds): Handbook of Dialysis, ed 3. Philadelphia, Lippincott Williams & Wilkins, 2001, pp 15–45.
9 Ward RA: Blood flow rate: An important determinant of urea clearance and delivered Kt/V. Adv Ren Replace Ther 1999;6:75–79.
10 Sigdell JE, Tersteegen B: Clearance of a dialyzer under varying operating conditions. Artif Organs 1986;10:219–225.

11 Sigdell JE, Tersteegen B: Studies concerning the optimization of dialysate consumption. Nephron 1995;71:401–406.
12 Besarab A, Sherman R: The relationship of recirculation to access blood flow. Am J Kidney Dis 1997;29:223–229.
13 Leypoldt JK: Solute fluxes in different treatment modalities. Nephrol Dial Transplant 2000; 15(suppl 1):3–9.

John K. Leypoldt, PhD, Dialysis Program, University of Utah,
85 N. Medical Drive East Room 201, Salt Lake City, Utah 84112–5350 (USA)
Tel. +1 801 585 3812, Fax +1 801 581 4750, E-Mail Ken.Leypoldt@hsc.utah.edu

Ronco C, La Greca G (eds): Hemodialysis Technology.
Contrib Nephrol. Basel, Karger, 2002, vol 137, pp 138–145

Sterilization Procedures and Biocompatibility

Alberto Rodríguez-Benot, Rafael Santamaría, Alejandro Martín-Malo, Pedro Aljama

Servicio de Nefrología, Hospital Universitario Reina Sofía, Córdoba, Spain

Hemodialysis devices that enter in direct contact with blood require previous sterilization. However, certain agents used for this purpose may trigger unwanted reactions of clinical relevance (such as anaphylactic reactions) if they are not properly removed prior to the start of the hemodialysis session. Thus, the ideal sterilizing agent should have effective antimicrobial activity without inducing deleterious effects in the organism, fulfilling the broad concept of biocompatibility [1]. Biocompatibility of hemodialysis is mainly referred to the reactions induced by extracorporeal materials in contact with the blood, and the device most widely studied from this point of view is the hemodialysis membrane. Nevertheless, data regarding biocompatibility of other aspects as dialysate purity, tubing materials, leachables from the extracorporeal circuit, sterilizing agents or disinfection of reused dialyzers are scarce. In addition, the absence of a definite or unique marker of biocompatibility makes the understanding of those phenomena and their potential influence on clinical outcomes more complex.

Sterilization Systems and Biocompatibility

Several mechanisms have been involved in the biocompatibility of sterilization procedures. First, sterilants released from dialyzers and tubing may act as allergens and elicit an immune response with antibody formation and activation of complement cascade. This could be the case for ethylene oxide. Second, both physical and chemical properties of materials can be modified by radiation, promoting changes in the performance of the dialyzer and also inducing cellular activation upon contact of blood cells with the surface of modified structures. Third, chemical compounds, under particular conditions such as high temperature or ionizing radiation may became degraded and release sub-products capable of inducing biological responses (including carcinogenic effects).

The current sterilization procedures used for hemodialyzers are exposure to ethylene oxide gas (ETO), ionizing radiation with gamma rays and high temperature application with steam. Also, disinfectants such as formaldehyde, hydrogen peroxide, peracetic acid and glutharaldehyde are employed as germicides in dialyzer reuse. Despite its widespread use, the ability of ETO of inducing anaphylactic reactions makes this gas the most bioincompatible sterilizing agent. Nevertheless, gamma radiation and steam are not exempt of undesirable side effects. In addition, repeated sterilization of the reused dialyzer may also lead to bioincompatibility reactions.

Ethylene Oxide

Ethylene oxide (ETO) is a low-temperature colorless and flammable gas widely used for sterilizing medical equipment. ETO is effective against the majority of microorganisms, including viruses. The bactericidal, fungical and sporocide activity is due to its alkylating properties. ETO may react with H_2O and other compounds yielding adducts with esters, amides, amines and mercaptanes [2]. These major reactions are of importance for sterilization but also for hapten formation. ETO and its derivates are irritants for skin and mucosae, and may cause contact allergic reactions, hemolysis, coagulation abnormalities, dermatitis and respiratory tract dysfunction particularly in exposed workers [2, 3].

First reports of acute intradialytic anaphylactoid reactions in dialysis patients appeared in the 1970s [4], and after the introduction of hollow-fiber dialyzers the incidence of reactions was markedly enhanced [5]. Daugirdas et al. [6] reported 21 severe reactions (including four respiratory arrests and one death) during 260,000 dialysis sessions in a local population. A rate of five deaths per year has been reported in the collective US dialysis patient population [7]. These authors recognized a remarkable difference between flat-plate and hollow fiber dialyzers (0.2 and 4.3 induced reactions, respectively, per 100,000 dialyzers sold). This difference was attributed to the polyurethane (PU) used as potting agent in the manufacture of capillary dialyzers, that acts as a reservoir for ETO, allowing its slow release along the dialysis session [8]. Similar reactions have also been described in patients exposed to hemofiltration, plasma separation (with membranes other than cuprophan) [9] and in plasma donors repeatedly exposed to ETO-sterilized tubing [2].

The underlying pathogenesis of these hypersensitivity reactions has been explained by two hypotheses. Dolovich et al. [10], using a radioallergosorbent test (RAST), described specific IgE antibodies against ETO conjugated with albumin in dialysis patients showing hypersensitivity reactions. This finding, confirmed by other authors [11], explained the previous observation of Poothullil et al. [4], who described sensitization to ETO by skin-prick test using ETO conjugated with human serum albumin. The second hypothesis was suggested by Hakim et al. [12] based on the observation of anaphylactoid 'first-use reaction' in patients dialyzed with hollow-fiber membranes. Patients with hypersensitivity reactions showed enhanced activation of the alternate complement pathway as compared to nonreactive patients. This aspect is controversial and it has not been confirmed by other authors [13]. Although ETO is related to complement activation, more recent studies using ETO RAST or basophil degranulation tests implicate ETO hypersensitivity as the major pathogenic cause of its bioincompatibility [2, 14].

Presensitization of the patient by medical equipment as infusion lines, plastic bags or syringes sterilized with ETO may explain hypersensitivity reactions observed during the first dialysis with ETO treated membranes. Clinical presentation of ETO reaction is variable and includes pruritus, erythema, urticaria and angioedema, dyspnea due to bronchospasm, abdominal pain, vomiting, diarrhea, central nervous system symptoms, hypotension and shock [15]. Blood tests disclose eosinophilia and specific anti-ETO IgE (RAST).

Despite its relative bioincompatibility, ETO is by far the most used agent because is inexpensive, materials are unaffected by the sterilizing procedure, and it can be applied directly into devices ready for shipping due to its highly diffusive feature. Thorough rinsing of new dialyzers and lines with gentle saline solution (2 liters) generally avoids ETO exposure to the patient. However, in ETO-hypersensitive patients it is advised to avoid this sterilant and use only steam or gamma-irradiated dialyzers. It has been reported that clinical reactions disappeared when the method of dialyzer sterilization was changed from ETO to gamma radiation, even if ETO-sterilized tubing and needles are used [16], probably because of the very low level of residual ETO in these devices. Furthermore, in Japan, where steam and gamma radiation have progressively replaced ETO as sterilizing agents (fig. 1), hypersensitivity reactions have almost disappeared [2, 17]. Wide regional differences in the use of sterilants are found; in Europe and USA ETO is still the most used agent, although a slow-decline rate in ETO favoring steam utilization is turning up (fig. 1) [17]. By contrast, in Japan ETO-sterilized dialyzers have almost disappeared since 1993, gamma radiation being the predominant sterilizing procedure [17].

Finally, a meaningful argument to discontinue the use of ETO is the potential mutagenic and carcinogenic properties of this sterilizing agent. In the

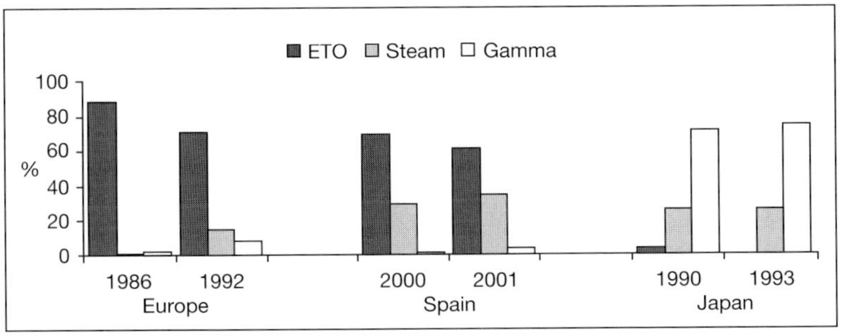

Fig. 1. Use of sterilizing agents in Europe and Japan; a progressive decrease of ETO is observed in Europe. Ethylene oxide (black bars); gamma-rays radiation (grey bars); steam (white bars). Data from reference [17] and from unpublished data (Spain).

nondialysis population exposed to ETO, increased rates of leukemia [18], chromosomal defects [19] and abortion [20] have been reported. Although long-term effects of ETO exposure in dialysis patients are not available from the literature, a cautious attitude should be adopted.

Gamma Rays and Steam

Ionizing radiation with gamma rays and steam are effective sterilizing methods used widely in medical devices. They largely overcome the negative effects of ethylene oxide and are in general more biocompatible. Gamma rays are generated by ^{60}cobalt and applied at a dose of 2–2.5 Mrad. However, gamma irradiation is not exempt of negative reactions. Polyurethane is used as potting material in hollow-fiber dialyzers; when PU is irradiated, a carcinogen, 4,4′-methylenedianiline (MDA) is produced and eluted from the dialyzer. MDA levels rise with increasing irradiation doses. Although it was found that MDA is formed only in a few ppm, a nonsignificant risk level for the patient, unknown compounds other than MDA are also formed, which can be potentially toxic and mutagenic [21]. Interestingly, MDA is not produced from PU when autoclave steam sterilization is performed.

Steam sterilizers usually employ prevacuum high-temperature steam, applied for 20 min at 121°C, followed by venting, cooling and drying [17]. The main concern of steam sterilization is membrane damage, since not all these materials are resistant to high temperatures and may became degraded [17, 22]. Steam sterilization does not produce chemical residues and to our knowledge no bioincompatible reactions have been described with its use.

Several studies comparing biocompatibility of such methods are available from the literature. Müller et al. [23] investigated biocompatibility profiles in patients dialyzed with polysulfone membranes sterilized with ETO and steam. As compared with ETO sterilization, steam was associated with a lower degree of leukopenia and thrombopenia, lower levels of C3a and C5a and a decrease in neutrophil elastase. On the other hand, a study [24] comparing granulocyte elastase and lysozyme in gamma-radiated versus ETO-sterilized membranes concluded that granulocyte activation during hemodialysis occurred independently of the sterilization procedure of dialyzers and blood lines. However, in this study steam was not tested and the membranes (cuprophan and polyacrylonitrile) were different from the previous study. Likewise, C5a anaphylatoxin generation and leukopenia are directly related to the composition of the membrane [25], which minimizes the possible role of the sterilant. It has also been reported that steam-sterilized polysulfone induces a lower cytokine (IL-1β) release than ETO-sterilized membrane [26]. Taking these considerations into account, it seems that the impact of the sterilization methods on biocompatibility is only found out in high biocompatible membranes [23]. In addition, ETO and steam-sterilized polysulfone membranes do not have different diffusive transport capabilities [27]. Recently, new markers of hemodialysis biocompatibility such as cell apoptosis [28, 29] have been reported; however, their relationship with sterilizing procedures have not yet been explored.

Thus, steam appears to be the more biocompatible sterilization method and the procedure of choice; however, is more expensive than ETO, and unfortunately the majority of membranes cannot be sterilized by steam, since these materials degrade when exposed to excessive temperature [22].

Sterilants and Dialyzer Reuse

Dialyzer reuse is performed because it reduces costs, decreases 'first-use' syndrome and improves biocompatibility of membranes. Major disadvantages are risk of infection, exposure to germicides and decreased dialyzer performance [30]. Sterilants (formaldehyde, peracetic acid and glutharaldehyde) may be released from reused dialyzers. Although predialysis thorough rinsing can reduce this release, leaching of formaldehyde and peracetic acid during dialysis has been described [31]. In fact, anti-N-like antibodies can be produced when residual formaldehyde levels are high, and these have been associated with hemolytic reactions [32]. Formaldehyde has also other potential risks due to its carcinogenic activity (not documented in intravenous administration in dialysis) and chromosomal abnormalities have been observed in patients when dialyzers are reused [33]. However, anaphylactoid reactions occur in a similar extent when polysulfone or cellulosic dialyzers were reused with peracetic acid [34]. Moreover, an association between the use of renalin (peracetic acid-peroxide hydrogen-acetic acid mixture) and increased mortality has been reported [35], in agreement with other authors [36] who also found higher mortality with renalin and glutaraldehyde when compared with formalin or with no reuse. But caution must be adopted since this different mortality has not always been found, and may be influenced by other variables such as type of membrane, dialysis adequacy, comorbid conditions and multicentric variability [37]. As an alternative to germicides, sterilization of dialyzers with heat and citric acid appears to be increasing in recent years [38, 39].

In summary, agents and procedures used for sterilizing hemodialyzers differ largely in their biocompatibility properties. Anaphylactoid reactions, complement activation, IgE-mediated hypersensitivity, membrane degradation and potential mutagenic effects are the main unwanted bioincompatible reactions. Ethylene oxide, the mainly used sterilizing agent, is also the most bioincompatible. Gamma radiation, and particularly steam, are more biocompatible and safe, although more expensive and not always feasible. Of special importance is the controversial negative effect on mortality when reprocessed dialyzers are employed. Further efforts should be made in clarifying and disclosing other possible long-term effects of sterilizing agents used in the hemodialysis process.

Acknowledgement

This work was supported in part by the Fundación Nefrológica of Córdoba.

References

1 Klinkmann H, Davison AM (eds): The Consensus Conference on Biocompatibility. Nephrol Dial Transplant 1994;9(suppl 2):1–186.

2 Bommer J, Ritz E: Ethylene oxide (ETO) as a major cause of anaphylactoid reactions in dialysis: A review. Artif Organs 1987;11:111–117.

3 Kessler M, Cao Huu T, Mariot A, Chanliau J: Hemodialysis-associated complications due to sterilizing agents ethylene oxide and formaldehyde. Contr Nephrol. Basel, Karger, 1988, vol 62, pp 13–23.

4 Poothullil J, Shimizu A, Day RP, Dolovich J: Anaphylaxis from the product(s) of ethylene oxide gas. Ann Intern Med 1975;82:58–60.

5 Ing TS, Daugirdas JT, Popli S, Ghandi VC: First-use syndrome with cuprammonium cellulose dialyzers. Int J Artif Organs 1984;6:235–239.

6 Daugirdas JT, Ing TS, Roxe DM, Ivanovich PT, Krumlovsky F, Popli S, McLaughlin MM: Severe anaphylactoid reactions to cuprammonium cellulose hemodialyzers. Arch Intern Med 1985; 145:489–494.

7 Villaroel F, Clarkowski AA: A survey on hypersensitivity reactions in hemodialysis. J Artif Organs 1985;9:231–238.

8 Ing TS, Daugirdas JT: Extractable ethylene oxide from cuprammonium cellulose plate dialyzers: Importance of potting compound. ASAIO Trans 1986;32:108–110.
9 Nicholls AJ, Platts MM: Anaphylactoid reactions due to hemodialysis, haemofiltration or membrane plasma separation. Br Med J 1982;285:1607–1609.
10 Dolovich J, Marshall CP, Smith EK, Shimizu A, Pearson FC, Sugona MA, Lee W: Allergy to ethylene oxide in chronic hemodialysis patients. Artif Organs 1984;8:334–337.
11 Rumpf KW, Seubert S, Seubert A, Lowitz HD, Valentin R, Rippe H, Igpren H, Sheler F: Association of ethylene-oxide-induced IgE antibodies with symptoms in dialysis patients. Lancet 1985;ii: 1385–1387.
12 Hakim RM, Breillatt HJ, Lazarus JM, Port FK: Complement activation and hypersensitivity reactions to dialysis membranes. N Engl J Med 1984;311:878–882.
13 Lemke HD, Heidland A, Schaefer RM: Hypersensitivity reactions during hemodialysis: Role of complement fragments and ethylene oxide antibodies. Nephrol Dial Transplant 1990;5:264–269.
14 Ing TS, Wong FK, Cheng YL, Potempa LD: The 'first-use syndrome' revisited: A dialysis centre's perspective. Nephrol Dial Transplant 1995;10(suppl 10):39–44.
15 Tielemans C, Gastaldello K, Goldman M, Vanherweghem JL: Acute haemodialysis membrane-associated reactions. Nephrol Dial Transplant 1996;11(suppl 2):112–115.
16 Rockel A, Wahn V, Hertel J, Fiegel P: Ethylene oxide hypersensitivity in dialysis patients. Lancet 1986;i:382–383.
17 Hoenich NA, Woffindin C, Ronco C: Haemodialysers and associated devices; in Jacobs C, Kjellstrand CM, Koch KM, Winchester JF (eds): Replacement of Renal Function by Dialysis, ed 4. Kluwer Academic Publishers, Dordrecht, 1996, pp 216–230.
18 Hogstedt C, Malquist N, Waldman B: Leukemia in workers exposed to ethylene oxide. JAMA 1979;242:1132–1133.
19 Garry VF, Hozier J, Jacobs D, Wade RL, Gray DG: Ethylene oxide: Evidence of human chromosomal effects. Environ Mutagen 1979;1:375–382.
20 Hemminki K, Mutanen P, Soloniemi I, Niemi ML, Vainio H: Spontaneous abortions in hospital staff engaged in sterilizing instruments with chemical agents. Br Med J 1981; 285:1461–1463.
21 Shintani H: Formation and elution of toxic compounds from sterilized medical products: Methylenedianiline formation in polyurethane. J Biomater Appl 1995;10:23–58.
22 Klinkmann H, Vienken J: Membranes for dialysis. Nephrol Dial Transplant 1995;10(suppl 3): 39–45.
23 Muller TF, Seitz M, Eckle I, Lange H, Kolb G: Biocompatibility differences with respect to the dialyzer sterilization method. Nephron 1998;78:139–142.
24 Horl WH, Riegel W, Schollmeyer P: Effect of gamma radiation versus ethylene oxide sterilization of dialyzers and blood lines on plasma levels of granulocyte elastase in hemodialyzed patients. Clin Nephrol 1985;24:232–236.
25 Martín-Malo A, Velasco F, Rojas R, Castillo D, Rodriguez M, Torres A, Aljama P: Fibrinolytic activity during hemodialysis: A biocompatibility-related phenomenon. Kidney Int 1993;41(suppl): 213–216.
26 Aucella F, Vigilante M, Grandone E, Colaizzo D, Margaglione M, Modoni S, Orlandini G, Stallone C: Reduction of mononuclear cytokine production in hemodialysis patients treated with steam-sterilized low-flux polysulphone membranes. Int J Artif Organs 1998;21:210–215.
27 Schaefer RM, Kulzer P, Gilge U, Shaefer L, Heidland A: Clinical evaluation of the new, steam-sterilized polysulfone high-flux dialyzer. Clin Nephrol 1994;42(suppl 1):21–25.
28 Carracedo J, Ramírez R, Martín-Malo A, Rodríguez M, Aljama P: Nonbiocompatible hemodialysis membranes induce apoptosis in mononuclear cells: the role of G proteins. J Am Soc Nephrol 1998;9:46–53.
29 Martin-Malo A, Carracedo J, Ramirez R, Rodriguez-Benot A, Soriano S, Rodriguez M, Aljama P: Effect of uremia and dialysis modality on mononuclear cell apoptosis. J Am Soc Nephrol 2000; 11:936–942.
30 Cheung AK, Agodoa LY, Daugirdas JT, Depner TA, Gotch FA, Greene T, Levin NW, Leypoldt JK: Effects of hemodialyzer reuse on clearances of urea and beta2-microglobulin. The Hemodialysis (HEMO) Study Group. J Am Soc Nephrol 1999;10:117–127.

31 Stragier A, Wenderickx D, Jadoul M: Rinsing time and disinfectant release of reused dialyzers: Comparison of formaldehyde, hypoclorite, warexin and renalin. Am J Kidney Dis 1995;26: 549–553.
32 Vanholder R, Noens L, De Smet R, Ringoir S: Development of anti-N-like antibodies using formaldehyde reuse in spite of adequate predialysis rinsing. Am J Kidney Dis 1988;11:477–480.
33 Kessler M, Cao HT, Mariot A, Chanliau J: Hemodialysis-associated complications due to sterilizing agents ethylene oxide and formaldehyde. Contrib Nephrol. Basel, Karger, 1988, vol 62, pp 13–23.
34 Pegues DA, Beck-Sague CM, Woolen SW, Greenspan B, Burns SM, Bland LA, Arduino MJ, Favero MS, Mackow RC, Jarvis WR: Anaphylactoid reactions associated with reuse of hollow-fiber hemodialyzers and ACE inhibitors. Kidney Int 1992;42:1232–1237.
35 Feldman HI, Kinosian M, Bilker WB, Simmons C, Holmes JH, Pauly MV, Escarce JJ: Effect of dialyzer reuse on survival of patients treated with hemodialysis. JAMA 1996;276:620–625.
36 Held PJ, Wolfe RA, Gaylin DS, Port FK, Levin NW, Turenne MN: Analysis of the association of dialyzer reuse and patient outcomes. Am J Kidney Dis 1994;23:692–708.
37 Port FK, Wolfe RA, Hulbert-Shearon TE, Daugirdas JT, Agodoa LY, Jones C, Orzol SM, Held PJ: Mortality risk by hemodialyzer reuse practice and dialyzer membrane characteristics: Results from the USRDS Dialysis Morbidity and Mortality Study. Am J Kidney Dis 2001;37:276–286.
38 Schoenfeld P, McLaughlin MD, Mendelson M: Heat disinfection of polysulfone dialyzers. Kidney Int 1995;47:638–642.
39 Levin NW, Parnell SL, Prince HN, Gotch F, Polashegg HD, Levin R, Alto A, Kaufman AM: The use of heated citric acid for dialyzer reprocessing. J Am Soc Nephrol 1995;6:1578–1585.

Pedro Aljama, Servicio de Nefrología, Hospital Universitario Reina Sofía,
Avda. Menéndez Pidal s/n, E–14004 Córdoba (Spain)
Tel. +34 957010440, Fax +34 957010307, E-Mail paljama@hrs.sas.junta-andalucia.es

Ronco C, La Greca G (eds): Hemodialysis Technology.
Contrib Nephrol. Basel, Karger, 2002, vol 137, pp 146–157

Computerized Selection of Membranes and Hemodialyzers

Claudio Ronco[a], *Paolo M. Ghezzi*[b], *Nicholas A. Hoenich*[c,d], *Piergiuseppe Delfino*[b]

[a] Department of Nephrology, St. Bortolo Hospital, Vicenza, Italy,
[b] Department of Nephrology, S. Croce Hospital, Cuneo, Italy;
[c] Department of Nephrology, School of Clinical Medical Sciences and Medical School, University of Newcastle, UK;
[d] Renal Research Institute, New York, N.Y., USA

Introduction

Renal replacement therapy is initiated when a substantial or total loss of ability of the human kidneys to remove water, excrete metabolic waste products or maintain body homeostasis occurs. The most commonly used replacement method is hemodialysis, which involves passing patient's blood through an artificial kidney or hemodialyzer containing a semipermeable membrane. Blood flows on one side of the membrane, the other side of which is bathed by a dilute electrolyte solution (dialysis fluid). The processes which occur within the hemodialyzer may be summarized as: (1) Equilibration of blood and dialysis fluid electrolyte composition; (2) elimination of metabolites elevated as a consequence of renal insufficiency by diffusion into the dialysis fluid. Convective mass transport due to ultrafiltration or fluid removal also takes place and contributes to the overall solute removal; (3) removal of water from the plasma, thence from the body by ultrafiltration. This occurs as a result of the hydrostatic pressure difference between the blood and the dialysis fluid. The hydrostatic pressure gradient may be supplemented by an osmotic pressure gradient induced by the inclusion of glucose in the dialysis fluid. Therefore, it appears evident that the choice of the hemodialyzer is of crucial importance to achieve the above-mentioned tasks.

Published in Contrib Nephrol. Basel, Karger, 2001, vol 133, pp 119–130.

In chemical engineering the hemodialyzer may be considered as a simple mass exchanger [1]. Its functionality will depend on the membrane that it contains, the geometric arrangement of the membranes and the fluid dynamic conditions on either side of the membrane during its use. In clinical terms the device is required to meet clinically important requirements. The ideal dialyzer must also contain the ideal membrane. The ideal membrane must have a high permeability for a range of molecular weights but, at the same time, the loss of vital solutes must be negligible. The membrane's ultrafiltration (or convective transport properties) must be controllable and reproducible. Membranes incorporated in hemodialyzers and associated devices represent the largest contact area with blood and they must be biocompatible. As the membranes are normally used wet, their physical and mechanical properties must be such as to ensure negligible leak rate during production and use, and they should be able to be sterilized by a variety of processes without alteration in their diffusive or convective transport properties or their biocompatibility [2–6].

Many of these requirements cannot be achieved, others are mutually exclusive and in consequence all currently used designs represent a compromise and are the manufacturers' interpretation of the ideal requirements. This differing interpretation coupled with market forces are responsible for the wide range of devices in commercial production [7–15].

Starting from this consideration, we have recently undertaken the effort of listing and categorizing the existing hemodialyzers in a database that should represent an important aid to help the clinician in the final selection of the most adequate device.

The Dialyzer Database

The database is contained in an interactive CD-ROM [16] and brings together a wealth of information unique in its form. It collects the most recent data on the membranes and filters currently on the market: to ensure a continuity of the database, a yearly update is scheduled.

In spite of a prolonged and extensive experience with hemodialyzer testing, the authors have decided not to provide personal results, but to include in the database only the data concerning a specific hemodialyzer that have been officially published in a brochure by the producer. For this reason, the authors are not responsible for possible inaccuracies of data and report in the last column of the spreadsheet the original publication from which the data were obtained. Furthermore, several values are accompanied by a note explaining the conditions in which the value was obtained. Under these circumstances, the values reported in the database and the derived calculations can only be intended as indicative and

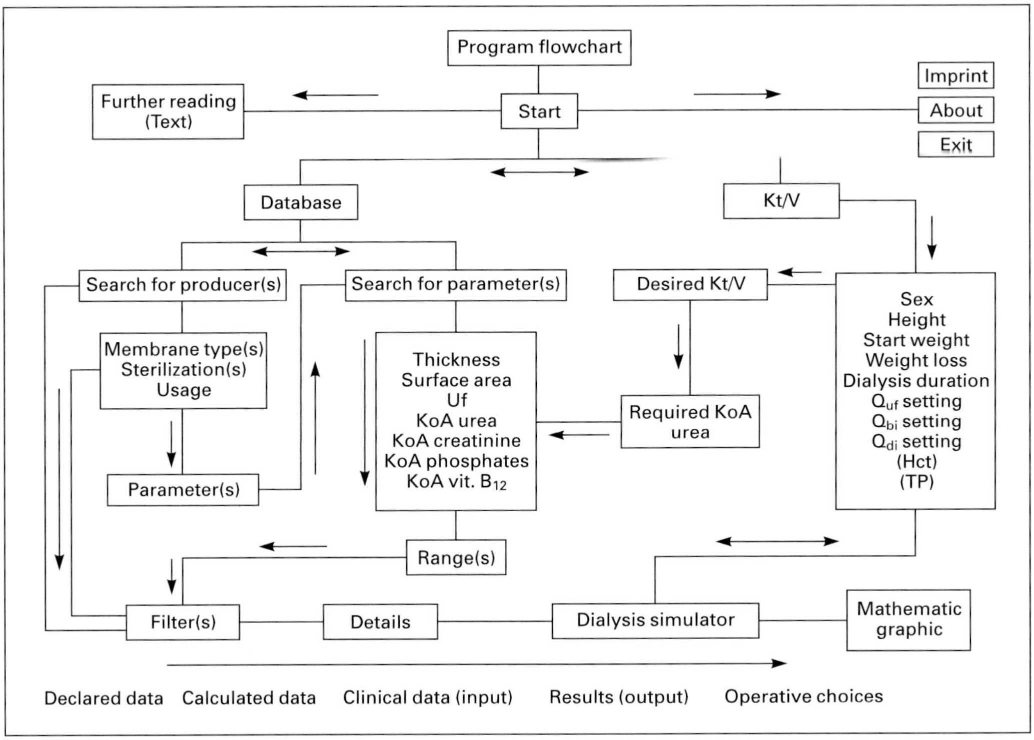

Fig. 1. Flowchart of the filters and membranes for hemodialysis program.

cannot be used as absolute values for prescription and patient care. Nevertheless, the number of parameters and the quality of the information provided by the program can definitely be of enormous help in the selection of the appropriate hemodialyzer, the identification of the most adequate operational parameters and the expansion of the knowledge relevant to the field of hemodialysis.

The program offers various possibilities including a guided search for the desired hemodialyzer by different searching keys, a selection of the hemodialyzers adequate to achieve a target Kt/V, a simulated dialysis treatment in virtual or real patients, complete background information on hemodialyzer structure and function (fig. 1).

Dialyzer Search

Users can perform hemodialyzer search entering information such as producer, membrane material, sterilization type, surface area or ultrafiltration coefficient.

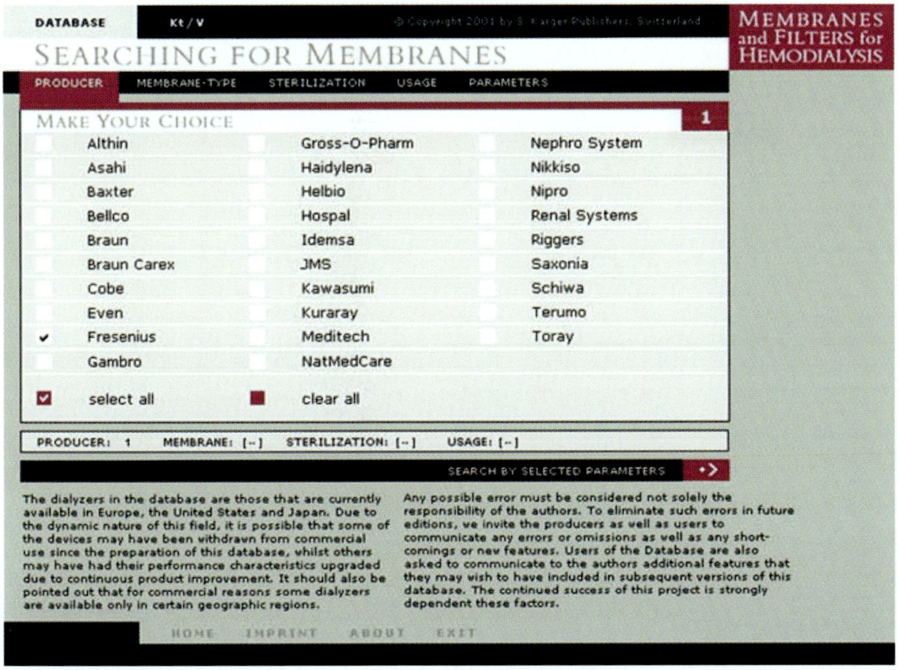

2

Fig. 2. Search by producer.

The search by producer (fig. 2) is guided by a window containing the actual producers list. Once one of these producers is selected, the database immediately sort out the hemodialyzers produced or commercialized by that company (fig. 3).

The search by membrane type is guided by a window containing the existing membranes (fig. 4). Today a wide range of membranes are available for the treatment of renal failure. Due to the dynamic nature of the industry and manufacturers' desire to meet changing clinical requirements, new membranes are continually being developed and introduced into clinical practice. Beyond the classical subdivision of membranes, i.e. cellulose-based and synthetic, further subdivisions are necessary to take account of the developments that have taken place. Once one membrane type is selected, all the hemodialyzers containing that membrane are listed by the program.

The search by sterilization type allows to identify all the hemodialyzers sterilized with a given process (fig. 5).

The search by usage mostly allows the separation of dialyzers into two main categories: the high-flux dialyzers usable in high-flux dialysis or hemodiafiltration, and the low-flux dialyzers mostly usable in standard hemodialysis (fig. 6). Clearly,

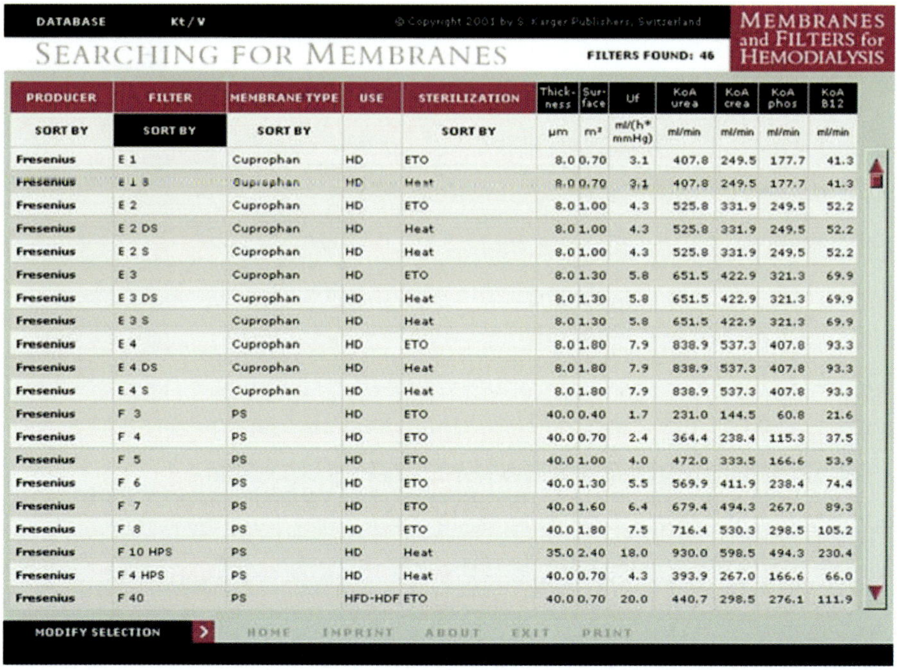

PRODUCER	FILTER	MEMBRANE TYPE	USE	STERILIZATION	Thick-ness	Sur-face	Uf	KoA urea	KoA crea	KoA phos	KoA B12
SORT BY	SORT BY	SORT BY		SORT BY	µm	m²	ml/(h* mmHg)	ml/min	ml/min	ml/min	ml/min
Fresenius	E 1	Cuprophan	HD	ETO	8.0	0.70	3.1	407.8	249.5	177.7	41.3
Fresenius	E 1 S	Cuprophan	HD	Heat	8.0	0.70	3.1	407.8	249.5	177.7	41.3
Fresenius	E 2	Cuprophan	HD	ETO	8.0	1.00	4.3	525.8	331.9	249.5	52.2
Fresenius	E 2 DS	Cuprophan	HD	Heat	8.0	1.00	4.3	525.8	331.9	249.5	52.2
Fresenius	E 2 S	Cuprophan	HD	Heat	8.0	1.00	4.3	525.8	331.9	249.5	52.2
Fresenius	E 3	Cuprophan	HD	ETO	8.0	1.30	5.8	651.5	422.9	321.3	69.9
Fresenius	E 3 DS	Cuprophan	HD	Heat	8.0	1.30	5.8	651.5	422.9	321.3	69.9
Fresenius	E 3 S	Cuprophan	HD	Heat	8.0	1.30	5.8	651.5	422.9	321.3	69.9
Fresenius	E 4	Cuprophan	HD	ETO	8.0	1.80	7.9	838.9	537.3	407.8	93.3
Fresenius	E 4 DS	Cuprophan	HD	Heat	8.0	1.80	7.9	838.9	537.3	407.8	93.3
Fresenius	E 4 S	Cuprophan	HD	Heat	8.0	1.80	7.9	838.9	537.3	407.8	93.3
Fresenius	F 3	PS	HD	ETO	40.0	0.40	1.7	231.0	144.5	60.8	21.6
Fresenius	F 4	PS	HD	ETO	40.0	0.70	2.4	364.4	238.4	115.3	37.5
Fresenius	F 5	PS	HD	ETO	40.0	1.00	4.0	472.0	333.5	166.6	53.9
Fresenius	F 6	PS	HD	ETO	40.0	1.30	5.5	569.9	411.9	238.4	74.4
Fresenius	F 7	PS	HD	ETO	40.0	1.60	6.4	679.4	494.3	267.0	89.3
Fresenius	F 8	PS	HD	ETO	40.0	1.80	7.5	716.4	530.3	298.5	105.2
Fresenius	F 10 HPS	PS	HD	Heat	35.0	2.40	18.0	930.0	598.5	494.3	230.4
Fresenius	F 4 HPS	PS	HD	Heat	40.0	0.70	4.3	393.9	267.0	166.6	66.0
Fresenius	F 40	PS	HFD-HDF	ETO	40.0	0.70	20.0	440.7	298.5	276.1	111.9

3

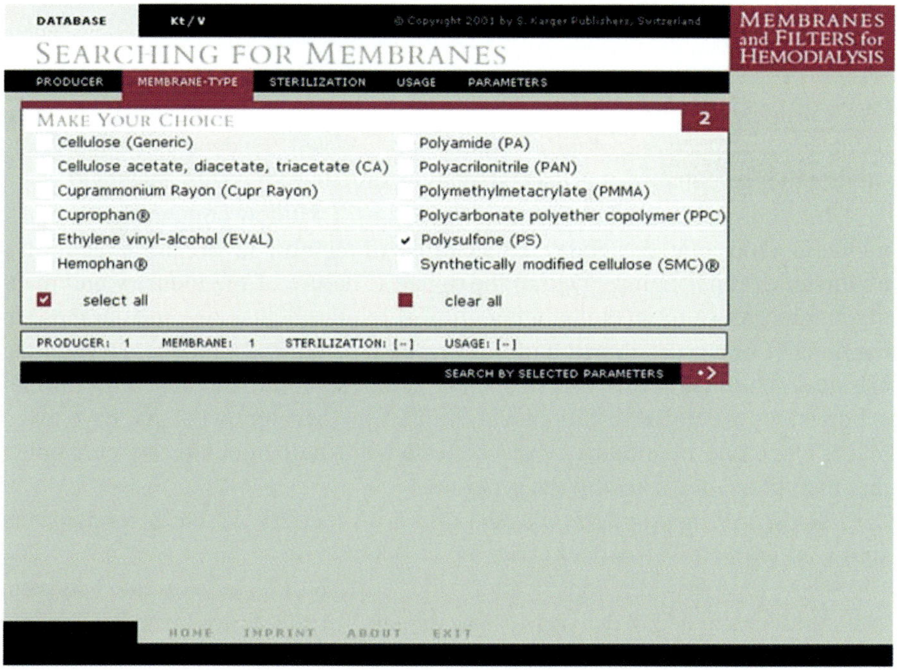

4

current membranes considerably overlap in their performance in respect of solute transport and biocompatibility and the historic divisions between the two categories have become less prominent. It would be tempting to devise a classification of membranes based upon performance. However, to date no precise definitions have been formed. Membranes may nevertheless be categorized into *low flux* with ultrafiltration coefficients of <10 ml/h/mm Hg, and negligible transmembrane removal of compounds such as β_2-microglobulin, *mid flux* with ultrafiltration coefficients between 10 and 20 ml/h/mm Hg and allowing some removal of β_2-microglobulin, and *high flux* with ultrafiltration coefficients in excess of 40 ml/h · mm Hg and permitting removal of β_2-microglobulin.

Finally, the search can be carried out *by different parameters* including membrane thickness, ultrafiltration capacity, and efficiency as expressed by KoA of different molecules (fig. 7). All these parameters can be indicated as a fixed value or as a range up to ±20% (default value) or ± variable value.

A cross-linked selection of parameters can therefore be carried out such that a restricted number of hemodialyzers are sorted by the program with the

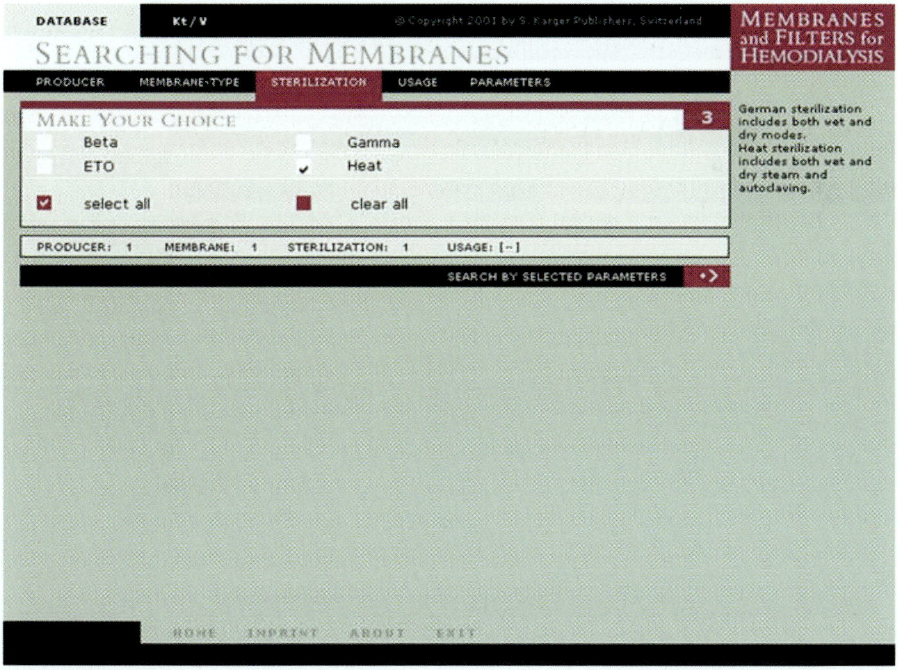

5

Fig. 3. Example of filters sorted by the program based on the producer search key.
Fig. 4. Search by membrane type.
Fig. 5. Search by type of sterilization.

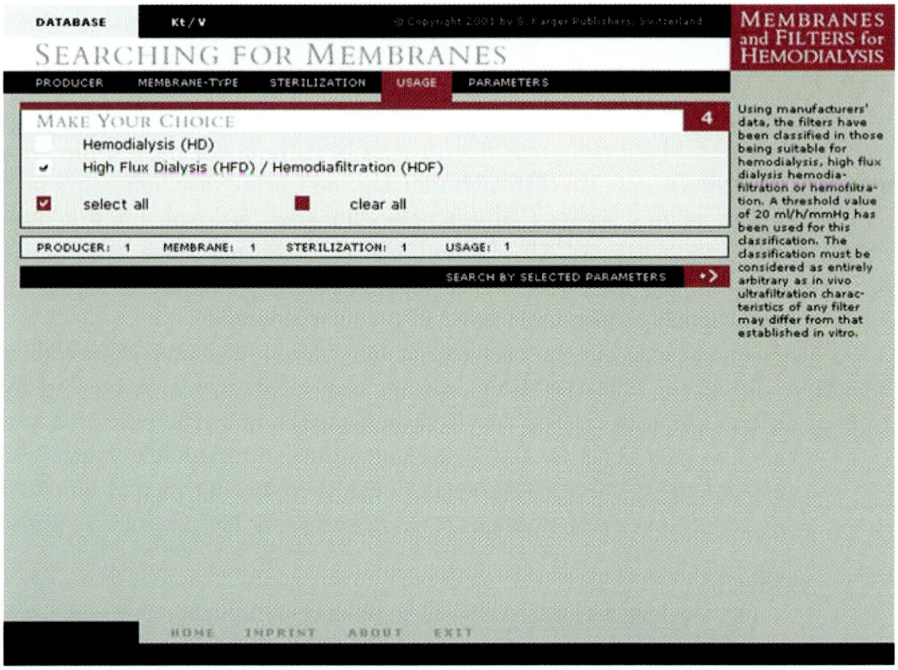
DATABASE
Kt/V
© Copyright 2001 by S. Karger Publishers, Switzerland
MEMBRANES and FILTERS for HEMODIALYSIS
SEARCHING FOR MEMBRANES
PRODUCER
MEMBRANE-TYPE
STERILIZATION
USAGE
PARAMETERS
MAKE YOUR CHOICE
4
Hemodialysis (HD)
High Flux Dialysis (HFD) / Hemodiafiltration (HDF)
select all
clear all
PRODUCER: 1
MEMBRANE: 1
STERILIZATION: 1
USAGE: 1
SEARCH BY SELECTED PARAMETERS
Using manufacturers' data, the filters have been classified in those being suitable for hemodialysis, high flux dialysis hemodia-filtration or hemofiltra-tion. A threshold value of 20 ml/h/mmHg has been used for this classification. The classification must be considered as entirely arbitrary as in vivo ultrafiltration charac-teristics of any filter may differ from that established in vitro.
HOME
IMPRINT
ABOUT
EXIT

6

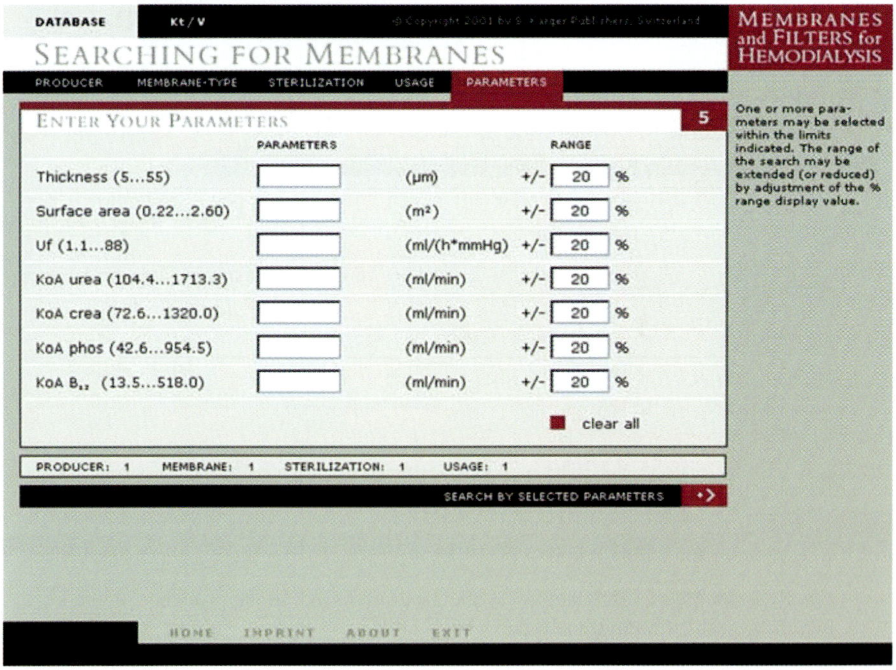
DATABASE
Kt/V
© Copyright 2001 by S. Karger Publishers, Switzerland
MEMBRANES and FILTERS for HEMODIALYSIS
SEARCHING FOR MEMBRANES
PRODUCER
MEMBRANE-TYPE
STERILIZATION
USAGE
PARAMETERS
ENTER YOUR PARAMETERS
5
PARAMETERS
RANGE
Thickness (5...55) (µm) +/- 20 %
Surface area (0.22...2.60) (m²) +/- 20 %
Uf (1.1...88) (ml/(h*mmHg) +/- 20 %
KoA urea (104.4...1713.3) (ml/min) +/- 20 %
KoA crea (72.6...1320.0) (ml/min) +/- 20 %
KoA phos (42.6...954.5) (ml/min) +/- 20 %
KoA B12 (13.5...518.0) (ml/min) +/- 20 %
clear all
PRODUCER: 1
MEMBRANE: 1
STERILIZATION: 1
USAGE: 1
SEARCH BY SELECTED PARAMETERS
One or more para-meters may be selected within the limits indicated. The range of the search may be extended (or reduced) by adjustment of the % range display value.
HOME
IMPRINT
ABOUT
EXIT

7

requested characteristics. For each dialyzer found, a window including all the details is provided by the program together with the calculated values of diffusive permeability for various solutes (fig. 8).

Dialysis Simulator

As videogames have become so popular and golf or flight simulators have occupied several megabytes in our computer, we decided that a dialysis simulator could be useful to complement the hemodialyzer database. The simulator allows the user to select a hemodialyzer by different searching keys and theoretically predict its performance in relation to different operational parameters (fig. 9).

Real or hypothetical parameters may be entered by the user and the program will sort out the performance characteristics of the dialyzer including solute clearances and Kt/V (fig. 10). The program includes a graphic function in which the dialyzer clearance for urea at different blood flows can be simply obtained

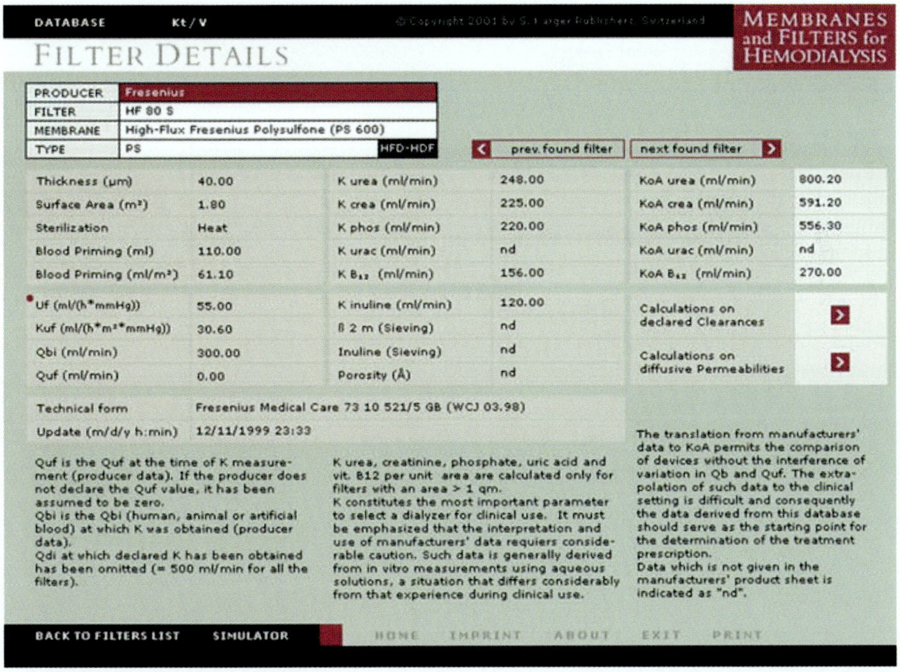

8

Fig. 6. Search by usage.

Fig. 7. Search by parameters.

Fig. 8. For each dialyzer, a window including all the details is provided by the program together with the calculated values of diffusive permeability for various solutes.

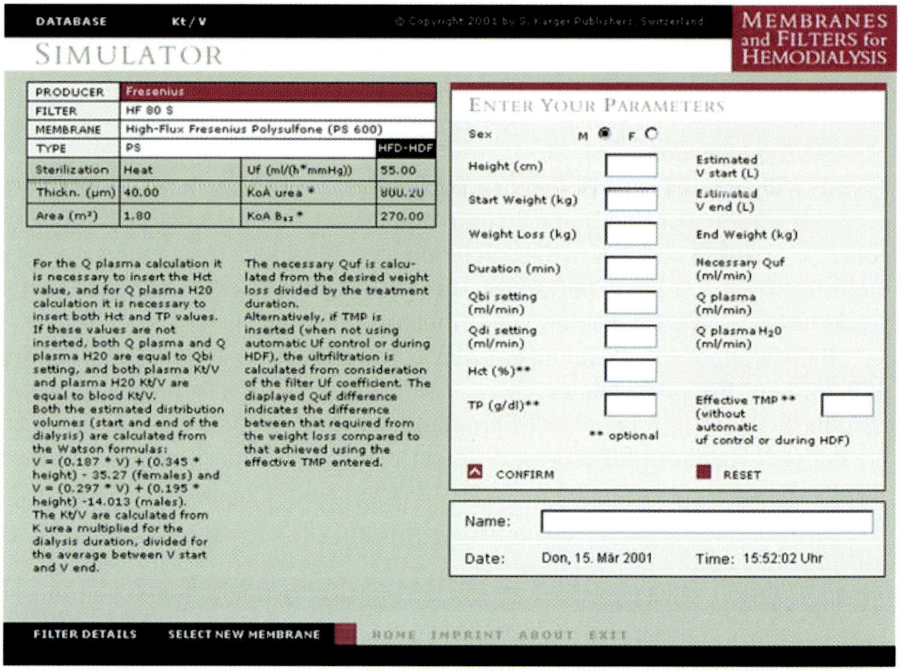
DATABASE
Kt/V
SIMULATOR
MEMBRANES and FILTERS for HEMODIALYSIS
PRODUCER Fresenius
FILTER HF 80 S
MEMBRANE High-Flux Fresenius Polysulfone (PS 600)
TYPE PS HFD-HDF
Sterilization Heat
Uf (ml/(h*mmHg)) 55.00
Thickn. (µm) 40.00
KoA urea *
Area (m²) 1.80
KoA B12 * 270.00
For the Q plasma calculation it is necessary to insert the Hct value, and for Q plasma H20 calculation it is necessary to insert both Hct and TP values. If these values are not inserted, both Q plasma and Q plasma H20 are equal to Qbi setting, and both plasma Kt/V and plasma H20 Kt/V are equal to blood Kt/V. Both the estimated distribution volumes (start and end of the dialysis) are calculated from the Watson formulas: V = (0.187 * V) + (0.345 * height) - 35.27 (females) and V = (0.297 * V) + (0.195 * height) -14.013 (males). The Kt/V are calculated from K urea multiplied for the dialysis duration, divided for the average between V start and V end.
The necessary Quf is calculated from the desired weight loss divided by the treatment duration. Alternatively, if TMP is inserted (when not using automatic Uf control or during HDF), the ultrfiltration is calculated from consideration of the filter Uf coefficient. The diaplayed Quf difference indicates the difference between that required from the weight loss compared to that achieved using the effective TMP entered.
ENTER YOUR PARAMETERS
Sex M F
Height (cm)
Estimated V start (L)
Start Weight (kg)
Estimated V end (L)
Weight Loss (kg)
End Weight (kg)
Duration (min)
Necessary Quf (ml/min)
Qbi setting (ml/min)
Q plasma (ml/min)
Qdi setting (ml/min)
Q plasma H2O (ml/min)
Hct (%)**
TP (g/dl)**
Effective TMP ** (without automatic uf control or during HDF)
** optional
CONFIRM
RESET
Name:
Date: Don, 15. Mär 2001
Time: 15:52:02 Uhr
FILTER DETAILS
SELECT NEW MEMBRANE
HOME IMPRINT ABOUT EXIT

9

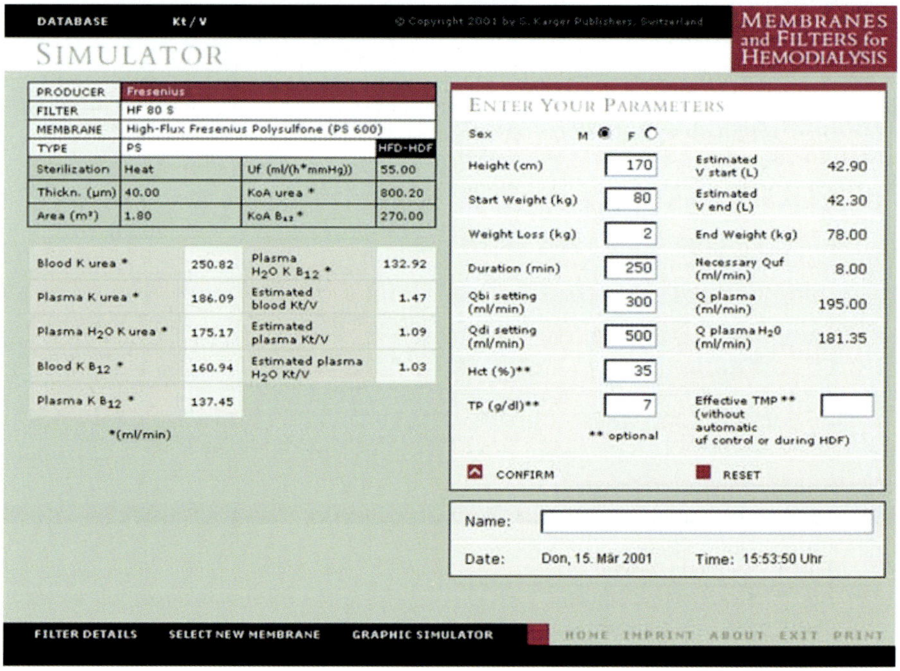
DATABASE
Kt/V
SIMULATOR
MEMBRANES and FILTERS for HEMODIALYSIS
PRODUCER Fresenius
FILTER HF 80 S
MEMBRANE High-Flux Fresenius Polysulfone (PS 600)
TYPE PS HFD-HDF
Sterilization Heat
Uf (ml/(h*mmHg)) 55.00
Thickn. (µm) 40.00
Area (m²) 1.80
KoA B12 * 270.00
Blood K urea * 250.82
Plasma H2O K B12 * 132.92
Plasma K urea * 186.09
Estimated blood Kt/V 1.47
Plasma H2O K urea * 175.17
Estimated plasma Kt/V 1.09
Blood K B12 * 160.94
Estimated plasma H2O Kt/V 1.03
Plasma K B12 * 137.45
*(ml/min)
ENTER YOUR PARAMETERS
Sex M F
Height (cm) 170
Estimated V start (L) 42.90
Start Weight (kg) 80
Estimated V end (L) 42.30
Weight Loss (kg) 2
End Weight (kg) 78.00
Duration (min) 250
Necessary Quf (ml/min) 8.00
Qbi setting (ml/min) 300
Q plasma (ml/min) 195.00
Qdi setting (ml/min) 500
Q plasma H2O (ml/min) 181.35
Hct (%)** 35
TP (g/dl)** 7
Effective TMP ** (without automatic uf control or during HDF)
** optional
CONFIRM
RESET
Name:
Date: Don, 15. Mär 2001
Time: 15:53:50 Uhr
FILTER DETAILS
SELECT NEW MEMBRANE
GRAPHIC SIMULATOR
HOME IMPRINT ABOUT EXIT PRINT

10

by moving the cursor in a bidimensional graph (fig. 11). Corrected values can then be achieved if the dialysate flow rate or other parameters are modified.

In summary, a complete set of simulated hemodialysis sessions can be carried out within minutes and the most suitable parameters and hemodialyzers can be selected according to the desired results.

Search by Target Kt/V

The user may wish to make a search of the ideal hemodialyzer utilizing a target Kt/V as a main parameter of interest. In this case, the characteristics of the patient (virtual or real) must be entered together with the potential operational parameters prescribed by the physician (fig. 12). Some parameters such as total protein and hematocrit are also useful to achieve an accurate result although they are not mandatory and they are considered optional by program.

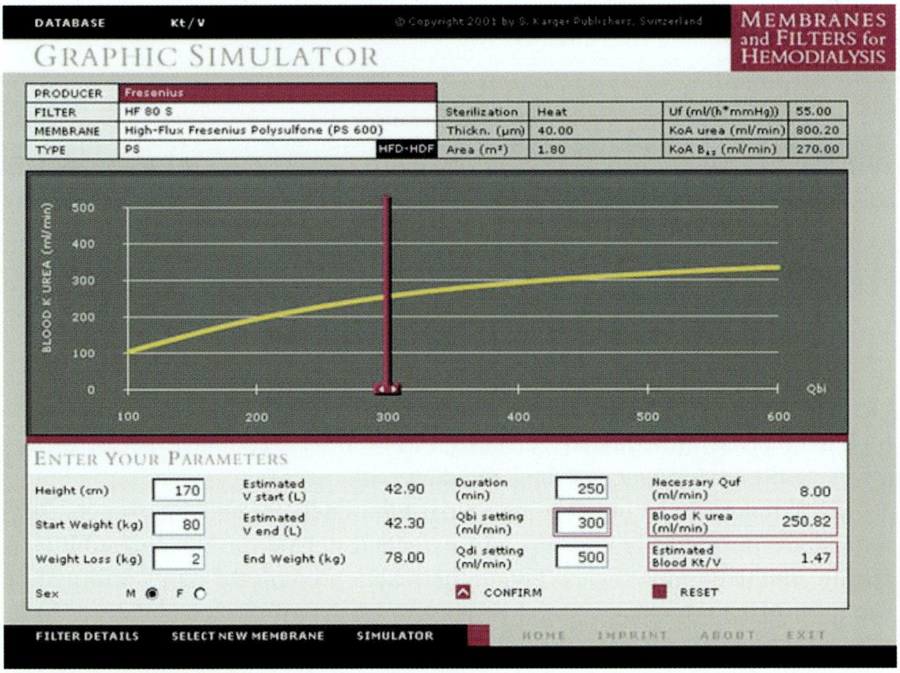

11

Fig. 9. Dialysis simulator: the simulator allows the user to select a hemodialyzer by different searching keys and theoretically predict its performance in relation to different operational parameters.

Fig. 10. Real or hypothetical parameters may be entered by the user and the program will sort out the performance characteristics of the dialyzer including solute clearances and Kt/V.

Fig. 11. Graphic function of the simulator in which the dialyzer clearance for urea can be obtained at different blood flows.

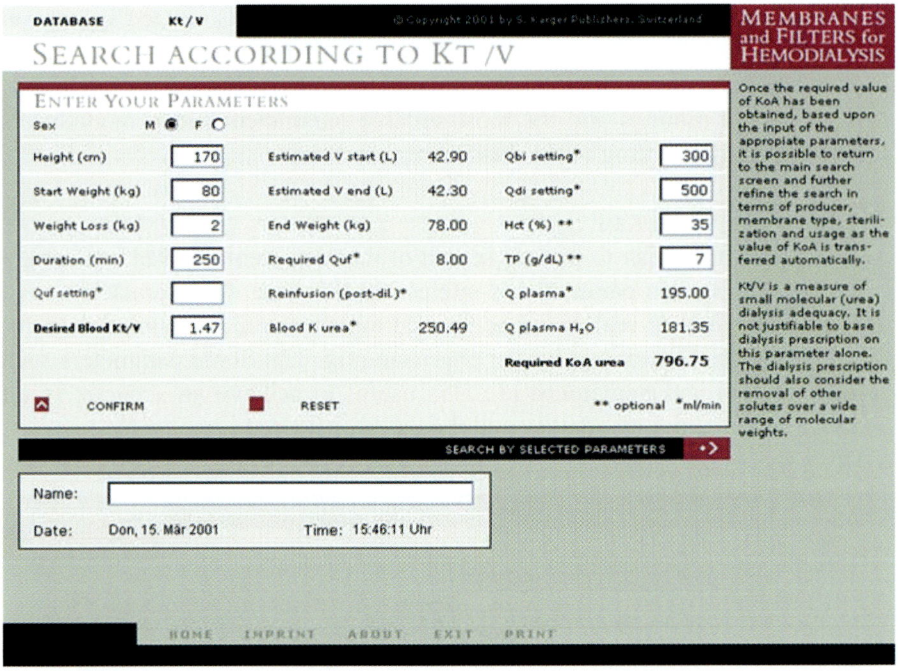

12

Fig. 12. Search by target Kt/V.

Hemodialyzers, Theory and Practice

The CD-ROM is finally completed by a more than 200-page review on hemodialyzers. The review includes a detailed analysis of the structural parameters involved in hemodialyzer design as well as a complete list of factors affecting the performance of the hemodialyzers.

Different types of membranes, sterilization methods and dialyzer configurations are discussed in the text. An extended debate on biocompatibility is finally completing the review giving the reader a complete set of information useful to make a meticulous and competent choice of the hemodialyzer to be used in a selected patient.

Conclusions

The collection of the enormous amount of data contained in this piece of work has been difficult and time-consuming. The elaboration of the program has required a lot of attention and dedication. The authors are indebted with all persons who made possible this enterprise. The final judgement will be given by the users and the success of this undertaking will only be determined by the level of their satisfaction.

We hope that the companies involved in the production and commercialization of the hemodialyzers in the world will become active partners in helping the authors in the difficult task of maintaining the database updated and complete.

References

1 Kiil F: Development of a parallel-flow artificial kidney in plastics. Acta Chir Scand 1960; 253(suppl):S142–S146.

2 Malchesky PS, Mrava GI, Nose Y: A totally disposable presterilized dialyzer. Arch Intern Med 1971;127:278–283.

3 Kolff VJ, Watshinger B: Further development of a coil kidney. J Lab Clin Med 1956;7:969–974.

4 Nakagawa S, Koshikawa S, Ishida Y, Uematsu M, Ishibashi K: Development of flat type hollow-fibre dialyzer (NF-01) achievement of better performance than cylinder type with same membrane area; in Frost TH (ed): Technical Aspects of Renal Dialysis. Tunbridge Wells, Pitman Medical, 1977, pp 29–37.

5 Sigdell JE: Hollow fiber dialyzers on the market. Artif Organs 1988;12:4–11.

6 Sigdell JE: Comparison of the hollow dialyzers. Artif Organs 1981;5:4–9.

7 Ghezzi PM, Ronco C: Membrane e filtri per emodialisi. Milano, Wichtig, 1995.

8 Van der Velde C, Leonard EF: Theoretical assessment of the effect of flow maldistributions on the mass transfer efficiency of artificial organs. Med Biol Eng Comput 1985;23:224–229.

9 Hoenich N, Ronco C: Dialyzers evaluation; in Winchester J, Koch K, Jacobs C, Kjellestrand C (eds): Replacement of Renal Function by Dialysis. Dordrecht, Kluwer Academic, 1996, pp 256–270.

10 Babb AL, Farrell PC, Uvelli DA, Scribner BH: Hemodialyzer evaluation by examination of solute molecular spectra. Trans Am Soc Artif Intern Organs 1972;18:98–105.

11 La Greca G, Ronco C: Cellulose triacetate: Evolution of a dialysis membrane. Milano, Wichtig, 1994.

12 Ronco C, Brendolan A, Crepaldi C, et al: Technical and clinical evaluation of a new asymmetric polysulfone membrane (Biosulfane). Int J Artif Organs 1993;8:573–584.

13 Ronco C, Brendolan A, Feriani M, et al: A new scintigraphic method to characterize ultrafiltration in hollow-fiber dialyzers. Kidney Int 1992;41:1383–1393.

14 Ronco C, Ballestri M: New developments in hemodialyzers. Blood Purif 2000;18:267–275.

15 Ronco C, Scabardi M, Goldoni M, Brendolan A, Crepaldi C, La Greca G: Impact of spacing filaments external to hollow fibers on dialysate flow distribution and dialyzer performance. Int J Artif Organs 1997;5:261–266.

16 Ronco C, Ghezzi PM, Hoenich NA, Delfino G: Membranes and Filters for Hemodialysis. CD-ROM. Basel, Karger, 2001.

Claudio Ronco, MD, Divisione di Nefrologia, Ospedale San Bortolo,
Viale Rodolfi, I–36100 Vicenza (Italy), E-Mail cronco@goldnet.it

Ronco C, La Greca G (eds): Hemodialysis Technology.
Contrib Nephrol. Basel, Karger, 2002, vol 137, pp 158–164

Adsorbents: From Basic Structure to Clinical Application

Claudio Ronco[a], *Valeria Bordoni*[a], *Nathan W. Levin*[b]

[a] Department of Nephrology, St. Bortolo Hospital, Vicenza, Italy
[b] Renal Research Institute, New York, N.Y., USA

The analysis of adsorbent material for the possible use in clinical extracorporeal therapies is a fascinating issue. It is also important to understand the basic concepts of the process of adsorption to move from the basic structure of the sorbents to their clinical application [1–5].

The mixing of chemicals to form a mixture is a spontaneous, natural process accompanied by an increase in entropy or randomness. The inverse process of separation of that mixture into its constituent species is not a spontaneous process and requires an expenditure of energy. If the mixture comes as two or more immiscible phases, we can use gravity, pressure or electrical fields, but if it exists in a single homogeneous phase different processes must applied such as:

- Separation by phase addition or creation (distillation, crystallization, desublimation).
- Separation by barrier (reverse osmosis, dialysis, microfiltration, ultrafiltration).
- Separation by solid agent (adsorption, chromatography, ion exchange).
- Separation by external field or gradient (electrodialysis, electrophoresis).

In clinical settings, blood purification techniques mostly rely on the second and the third group of processes. While, however, diffusion and convection are mostly used for membrane filtration processes, adsorption is generally employed in blood detoxification techniques such as hemoperfusion. Diffusion may be limited by the diffusion coefficients of the molecules or by other factors such as temperature, surface area and distance. Convection on the other hand is mostly limited by the sieving properties of the membrane and the flux of solvent obtained in response to a positive pressure gradient. When these processes are inadequate to remove the wanted molecules from patient's blood,

Table 1. Evolution of knowledge and clinical use of sorbents

1850 First inorganic allumosilicates (zeolites) used to exchange NH_4 and Ca
1910 Water softeners using zeolites display instability in presence of mineral acids
1935 Adams and Holmes synthetize the first organic polymer ion exchange resin
1950 Application of synthetic porous polymers (styrene or acrylic acid based) (spherical beeds: trade names of Amberlyte, Duolite, Dowex, Ionac and Purolite)
1960 manipulation of physical-chemical characteristics (commercial use)
1970 Application in blood purification techniques such as hemoperfusion
1980–2000 improved design and coating for better hemocompatibility of adsorbent materials

the use of adsorbents may become the alternative pathway for blood purification. Hemoperfusion is in fact a technique in which patient's blood is circulated through a unit containing a sorbent material. Blood purification is obtained by absorption of molecules on to the sorbent particles. Sorbents can be synthetic or natural. In the past, problems related to hemoperfusion were mostly due to the incompatibility of the biomaterial used as a sorbent. In fact, the first sessions of hemoperfusion were accompanied by chills, fever, cutaneous rash, thrombocytopenia, leukopenia and aluminum load.

There is, however, a rationale for the use of sorbents in ESRD: the limited efficiency of membrane separation processes (HD), the possible selectivity or size exclusion of adsorptive processes, and finally the possibility of placing the sorbent in direct contact with blood increasing enormously the efficiency of the system. The sorbent, however, must be hemocompatible or adequately coated; size-dependent, nonselective adsorption may cause unwanted losses and a completely different kinetics for middle-to-large molecules could be expected in comparison to that commonly observed in hemodialysis.

To make an adequate adsorbent therapy one needs an effective and safe sorbent material, an adequately designed sorbent cartridge and finally an optimal utilization of the available surface of the sorbent.

Sorbent Materials

The evolution in knowledge and clinical use of sorbents can be summarized in table 1. Sorbents can be divided practically into two categories: natural and synthetic.

The natural sorbents such as zeolites (alumino silicates) are inorganic porous polymers with porosity deriving from their crystal structure (today they can be synthetically modified to control the structure of the internal pore

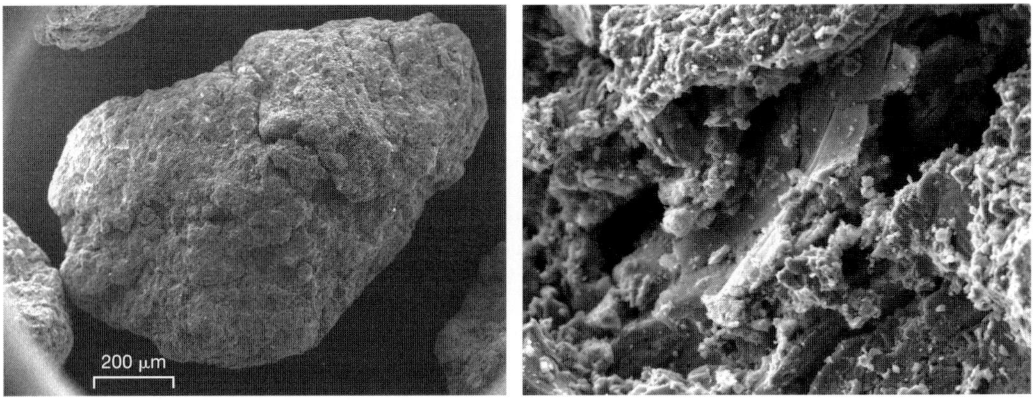

Fig. 1. Scanning electron microscopic view of a natural sorbent (uncoated charcoal) at different magnifications.

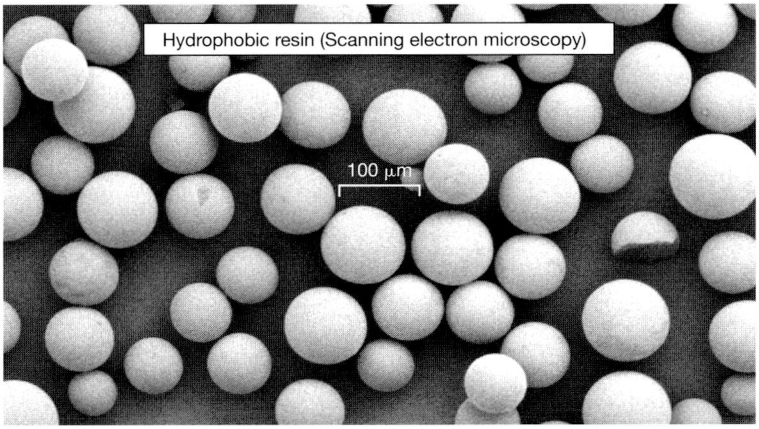

Fig. 2. Scanning electron microscopic view of a synthetic polymer in granules.

system). Other typical sorbents such as porous carbons, are cellulose-derived organic polymers prepared by controlled thermal oxidation (fig. 1).

Synthetic sorbents are constituted by different polymers of synthetic origin. Almost all polymerizable monomers can be built up into large molecules via a multitude of reactions. Difunctional monomers tend to aggregate in linear polymeric structures while high functional monomers tend to polymerize in cross linked structures. Divinylbenzene is generally used as a potent crosslinker (fig. 2).

Sorbents may be granules, spheres, cylindrical pellets, flakes and powder. They are solid particles with single particle diameter between 50 μm and 1.2 cm. Surface area to volume ratio is extremely high in sorbent particles with a surface area varying from 300 to 1,200 m^2/g. They can also be defined as (a) macroporous = pore size >500 Å (50 nm); (b) mesoporous = pore size 20–500 Å, and (c) microporous = pore size <20 Å.

Requirements

A suitable sorbent material must have high selectivity/affinity to enable sharp separation and high capacity to minimize the amount of sorbent employed to make a commercial product. The sorbent should have favorable kinetics and transport properties for rapid sorption of the target solutes, chemical and thermal stability, low solubility in the contacting fluid and mechanical strength to prevent crushing or erosion.

In a sorbent cartridge for clinical purposes, the material must have free flowing tendency for ease of filling and emptying of the packed bed, high resistance to fouling for long adsorption life, and maximal biocompatibility with no tendency to promote undesirable chemical reactions or side effects. Finally the sorbent must be cost effective and the possibility of regeneration should be explored for possible multiple use. Unwanted losses of hormones, proteins and drugs must be identified and addressed as potential side effects. Adequate anticoagulation should also be scheduled to prevent clotting or platelet losses.

Mechanism of Adsorption of Solutes in Porous Media

For the adsorption of a solute onto the porous surface of an adsorbent, the following steps are required: (a) external (interphase) mass transfer of the solute from the bulk fluid by convection through a thin film or boundary layer, to the outer surface of the sorbent; (b) internal (intraphase) mass transfer of the solute by pore diffusion from the outer surface of the adsorbent to the inner surface of the internal porous structure; (c) surface diffusion along the porous surface, and (d) adsorption of the solute onto the porous surface (fig. 3).

Efficiency of Adsorption

Porous polymers can be designed and constructed with varying internal surface selectivity and varying pore sizes so that molecules can be separated

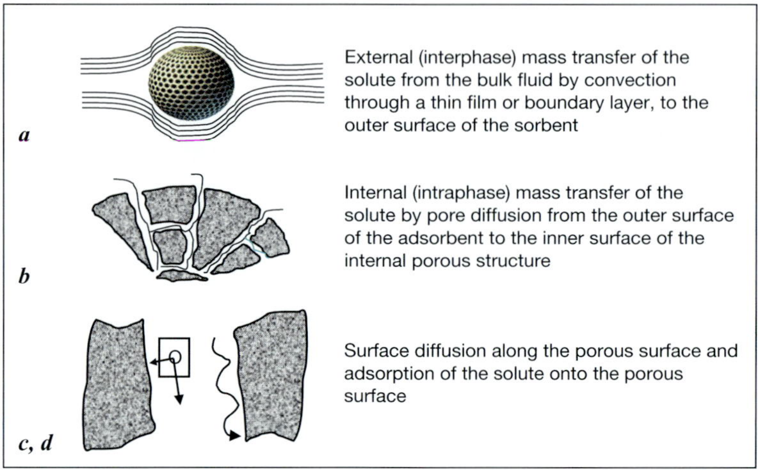

Fig. 3. Subsequent steps occurring in the process of adsorption: (***a***) interphase transport; (***b***) intraphase transport; (***c, d***) surface diffusion and adsorption on the porous surface.

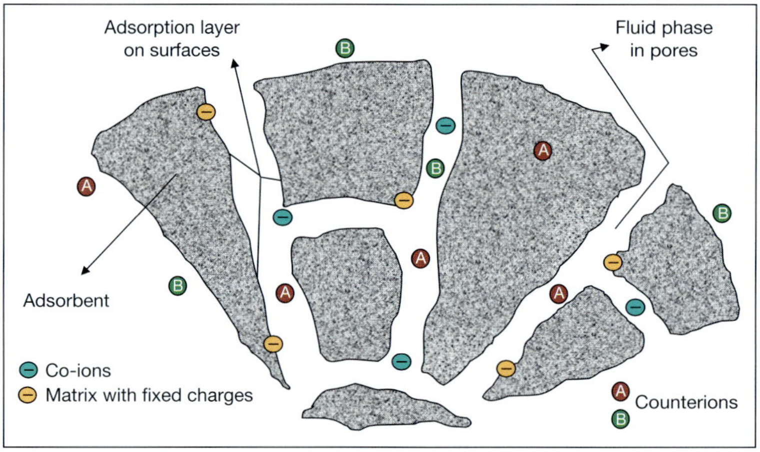

Fig. 4. Structure of sorbents and ion-exchange resins. Physical adsorption may occur thanks to van der Waals forces. Chemisorption mostly occurs due to chemical binding mechanisms.

from each other based upon size, geometry and individual binding properties (fig. 4).

To make a selective or partially selective process of adsorption, one needs to know the properties of the molecules to be separated or removed. If the information is lacking, the properties of the molecules under analysis can be

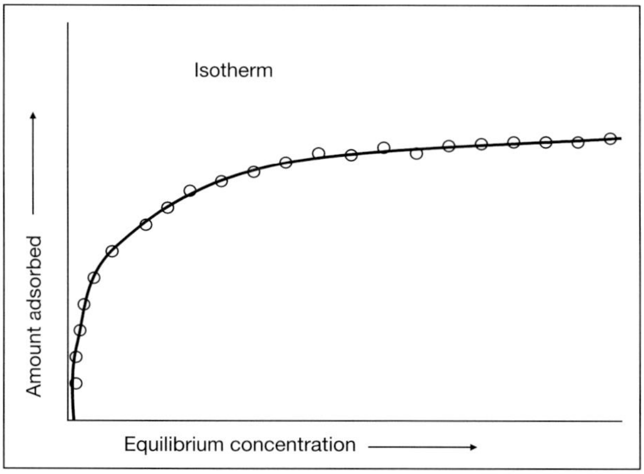

Fig. 5. Typical representation of an adsorption isotherm.

ascertained by combining a number of available analytical measurements to develop an understanding of the molecular distinctives or by trial and error through adsorption isotherms (fig. 5).

When a liquid mixture is brought into contact with a microporous solid, adsorption of certain components in the mixture takes place on the internal surface of the solid. The maximum extent of adsorption occurs when equilibrium is reached. No theory for predicting adsorption curves is universally embraced. Instead, laboratory experiments must be performed at fixed temperature (separation processes are energy intensive and affect entropy) for each liquid mixture and adsorbent to provide data for plotting curves called *adsorption isotherms*. Adsorption isotherms can be used to determine the amount of adsorbent required to remove a given amount of solute from the solvent.

To perform effective sorbent therapy it is important to ensure that blood flow is equally distributed within the packed sorbent particles so that all the sorbent material is adequately and effectively utilized. The flow distribution inside the cartridge of sorbent is one of the main issues concerning the performance and the reliability of the device. Any type of channeling phenomenon may affect the quantity of solute adsorbed per unit of sorbent and influences the saturation of the unit. Since blood is a non-Newtonian fluid, one must carry out an accurate analysis of the flow distribution taking into consideration different conditions of flows and blood viscosity. The flow distribution in packed beds can be theoretically modeled using equations of physical chemistry and transport. The structure of the packing is usually complex, and the resulting flow pattern is complicated. There are tortuous paths through the interstitial space of the bed, which consists of channels (pores) of various diameters. In well-packed beds, the diversity of channel diameters and velocities in the individual channels is small. Then the packed bed can be approximated as a bundle of tortuous capillary tubes. In practice, some wide-diameter channels and gaps in the packing structure may be present and the local flow velocity is relatively low. This may result in the undesirable phenomenon of channeling of the flow which may facilitate clotting.

Conclusions

The use of adsorbent materials in clinical dialysis has been proposed in the past. For various reasons including a poor compatibility with the patient's blood, sorbents were seldom utilized in the clinical routine. An improved knowledge of the manufacturing processes and the possibility of designing new sorbents with improved characteristics of biocompatibility, make today the use of sorbent possible and with an enormous potential. A new series of studies must therefore asses which additional advantages could be obtained by the use of sorbents either in the field of ESRD or in the field of acute renal failure [6–7].

References

1 Jost W: Diffusion in Solids, Liquids, Gases. Academic Press, New York, 1965.

2 Scheidegger AE: The Physics of Flow through Porous Media. McMillan, New York, 1960.

3 Samtleben W, Gurland HJ, Lysaght MJ, Winchester JF: Plasma exchange and hemoperfusion, in Jacobs C, Kjellstrand CM, Koch KM, Winchester JF (eds): Replacement of Renal Function by Dialysis. Kluwer Academic Publishers, Dordrecht, 1996, pp 472–500.

4 Ronco C, Brendolan A, Winchester JF, Golds E, Clemmer J, Polaschegg HD, Muller TE, La Greca G, Levin N: First clinical experience with an adjunctive hemoperfusion device designed specifically to remove β_2-microglobulin in hemodialysis. Blood Purif 2001;19:260–263.

5 Ronco C, Brendolan A, Winchester JF, Golds E, Clemmer J, Polaschegg HD, Muller TE, Davankov V, Tsyurupa M, Pavlova L, Pavlov M, La Greca G, Levin NW: First clinical experience with an adjunctive hemoperfusion device designed specifically to remove beta 2-microglobulin in hemodialysis. Contrib Nephrol. Karger, Basel, 2001, vol 133, pp 166–173.

6 La Greca G, Brendolan A, Ghezzi PM, De Smet R, Tetta C, Gervasio R, Ronco C: The concept of sorbents in hemodialysis. Int J Artif Organs 1998;21:303–308.

7 Tetta C, Bellomo R, Brendolan A, Piccinni P, Digito A, Dan M, Irone M, Lonnemann G, Moscato D, Buades J, La Greca G, Ronco C: Use of adsorptive mechanisms in continuous renal replacement therapies in the critically ill. Kidney Int 1999;56(suppl 72):S15–S19.

Dr. Claudio Ronco, Department of Nephrology,
St. Bortolo Hospital, I–36100 Vicenza (Italy)
Tel. +39 0444993869, Fax +39 0444920693, E-Mail cronco@goldnet.it

Ronco C, La Greca G (eds): Hemodialysis Technology.
Contrib Nephrol. Basel, Karger, 2002, vol 137, pp 165–169

Biocompatibility of Sorbent Systems

N.A. Hoenich

Department of Nephrology, School of Clinical Medical Sciences, Medical School, University of Newcastle, UK

Introduction

A sorbent may be defined as a material which retains molecular species contained in solution when such solution comes into contact with it. Retention occurs via two distinct physical processes: adsorption and absorption. The former being retention at the material surface, the latter within the sorbent bulk. Thus, for the highest adsorption capacity per unit volume or mass, an adsorbent should have a large surface area. Historically, uncoated activated carbons were used adsorbing molecules from blood. These materials were produced by the carbonisation of the raw material in an inert atmosphere and the activation of the carbonised product either by chemical in which the raw material is impregnated with an activating agent and carbonisation and activation take place in a single stage or using a physical process in which the carbonised material is treated with steam or carbon dioxide. Both these processes small pores initially develop followed by larger pores as activation continues. Such activation not only determines the porous structure but also the material hardness, i.e. the more activated the material, the more fine particles are produced during the manufacturing process. This process permits the attainment of materials with large surface areas within which a wide range of pores exist. Due to the techniques used in the production of these early materials, the final product was often irregular in shape and contained a wide distribution of particle sizes. Concern about the release of such fine particles into the circulation as well as the potential effects of blood coming into contact with rough surfaces led to the development coated materials in which the particles were coated with haemocompatible materials. Other materials used as sorbents include synthetic organic polymers in the form of resins which are also coated whilst more recently biospecific immunoadsorbents in which ligands have been immobilized onto the surface of the material have been developed. When used in the clinical setting, the sorbent is generally in the form of a packed bed encased into a cylinder with fittings to permit connection to blood tubing sets. The purpose of this paper is to discuss the biocompatibility of materials used in contact with blood for adsorption.

Clinical Application of Sorbents

Due to their ability to remove solutes over a wide range of molecular weight sorbents have been used in the treatment of both acute and chronic renal failure, liver failure, poisoning, as well as in the treatment of autoimmune diseases and hyperlipaemia. In the treatment of renal failure sorbents have been used orally, alone in the form of a haemoperfusion system or in conjunction with diffusive and convective therapies such as haemodialysis [1]. In addition to removal of metabolites, they have also been used to remove molecular species from the used dialysis fluid and from ultrafiltrate [2]. In the treatment of acute renal failure their use has been in patients with sepsis to eliminate circulating cytokines and other inflammatory mediators [3]. The first use of activated carbon or charcoal for the treatment of patients with chronic renal failure was reported in 1963 by Yatzidis [4] who used a carbon material designed for gas chromatography which was washed with deionised water and a heparin saline mixture before use. Treatments were carried out using 200 g of charcoal and lasted between 30 and 90 min. Orally administered sorbents such as charcoal and oxystarch have also been used in the treatment of uremia [5].

Definition of Biocompatibility in the Context of Materials

Sorbents in the context of haemoperfusion may be considered as biomaterials that are used to supplement or replace the functions of living tissue. Ideally, such a material should be able to exist within the physiological environment without any significant adverse effect to the body whilst the biological environment should not have a significant adverse effect on the material. If these requirements are met, then the material is said to be biocompatible. No material can be considered universally biocompatible for what is potentially an acceptable performance in one situation may be unacceptable in another. In a simplistic way, it is logical to assume that for the material to be considered biocompatible, it must elicit a minimal and appropriate response from the biological material in contact with it. Any material that comes into contact with blood, is subject to the activation of cellular components and humoral the nature and magnitude of which are governed primarily by protein deposition onto the material surface. In addition the prolonged contact of the material with a biological solution may result in the release of particulate matter, leaching, which can result in the development of defects in the material and damage to blood components.

Biocompatibility of Sorbents

Particle Embolization Leaching and Haemolysis

Early haemoperfusion devices were manufactured using uncoated materials. Despite thorough washing of the material, microparticles of 5–35 μm were persistently detected in blood samples and washing solutions taken from the outlet of the column. The clinical sequelae associated with this release was the formation of microembolii. This problem was eventually solved by the coating of the activated carbon granules with a semipermeable and potentially haemocompatible materials. In addition to the release of small particles or fines, the carbon particles were irregular in shape and had varying surface roughness. This resulted in poor fluid dynamic conditions within the column leading to cellular damage resulting in platelet activation, release of platelet factors and red cell damage causing haemolysis. Improvement in the production techniques, or the use of polymer microbeads that are carbonised and activated has resulted in the ability to produce spherical granules which has largely eliminated this problem and has improved the fluid dynamic flow characteristics of haemoperfusion columns [6]. Use of early haemoperfusion devices was also associated with pyrogenic reactions. One possible cause of these reactions may be a consequence of the release of contaminants from the sorbent, or activation of monocytes leading to the release of cytokines following contact with the material.

Cellular and Humoral Pathway Activation

The body's defense mechanisms in plasma consist of a series of interrelated biochemical pathways: the complement, coagulation, fibrinolytic and kinin systems. When blood comes into contact with foreign surfaces these pathways are activated (fig. 1). Use of early haemoperfusion devices utilizing uncoated charcoal resulted in a marked platelet loss [7]. The introduction of microencapsulated materials has largely minimized this problem. Transient leucopaenia similar to that seen during haemodialysis also occurs during haemoperfusion. The leucopaenia is related to the activation of the complement system, and is a consequence of the up regulation of surface receptors responsible for adhesion. Material contact with blood also leads to the release of

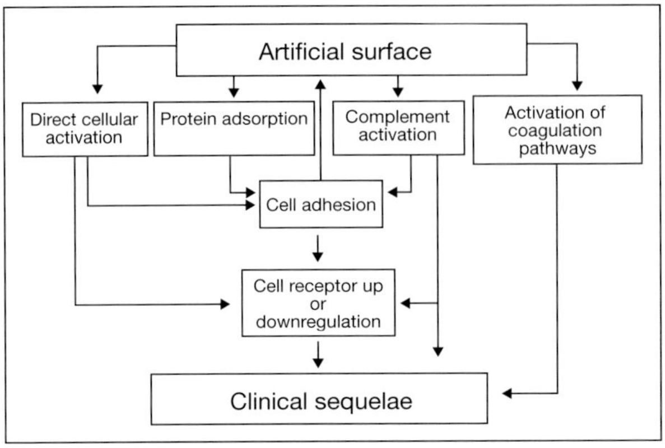

Fig. 1. Biological processes related to blood material contact.

cytokines such as Interleukin 1 and in the context of haemodialysis a hypothesis has been suggested that such release from monocytes is responsible for a series of adverse effects [8].

The recognition of foreign surfaces by the body's immune system results in the deposition of complement fragments such as C3b onto the material surface, this in turn leads to the production of split products or anaphylatoxins that are released into the circulation (C3a, and C5a). The cleavage of C5 to form C5a also produces C5b which complexes with other components of the complement system to form C5b-9 or the membrane attack complex (MAC) involved in cellular activation.

Blood contact with a foreign surface also initiates the coagulation pathway resulting in platelet activation; such activation being implicated in the formation of platelet microaggregates. Adsorption or activation of the coagulation factors has also been noted during haemoperfusion and a reduction in fibrinogen concentration and fibronectin are present even with new polymer coated materials [9]. Columns containing negatively charged dextran sulfate beads have been implicated in the activation of the kinin system resulting in anaphylactoid-like reactions [10].

Concluding Comments

The biocompatibility of materials such as uncoated charcoal and resins used historically in haemoperfusion were poor resulting in activation of cellular and humoral pathways. The coating of sorbent materials and the use of techniques to eliminate surface roughness of the particles enhances biocompatibility and this coupled with the availability of bioselective adsorbents, e.g. for the removal of β_2-microglobulin is likely to see increased utilization of this modality of treatment.

References

1 Botella J, Ghezzi PM, Sanz-Moreno C: Adsorption in hemodialysis. Kidney Int 2000;76(suppl): S60–S65.

2 Bigsby RJ, Rider RJ, Blount GN: The design of an optimized portable artificial kidney system using recirculation and regeneration of dialysate. Proc Inst Mech Eng [H] 1998;212:373–381.

3 Tetta C, Cavaillon JM, Schulze M, Ronco C, Ghezzi PM, Camussi G, Serra AM, Curti F, Lonnemann G: Removal of cytokines and activated complement components in an experimental model of continuous plasma filtration coupled with sorbent adsorption. Nephrol Dial Transplant 1998;13:1458–1464.

4 Yatzidis H, Oreopoulos D: Early clinical trials with sorbents. Kidney Int 1976;7(suppl): S215–S217.

5 Manis T, Zeig S, Feinstein EI, Lum G, Friedman EA: Oral sorbents in uremia and diabetes: Charcoal-induced hypolipidemia. Trans Am Soc Artif Intern Organs 1979;25:19–23.

6 Ronco C, Ghezzi PM, Morris A, Rosales L, Wang E, Zhu F, Metry G, De Simone L, Rhamati S, Adhikarla R, Bashir A, Manzoni C, Spittle M, Levin NW: Blood flow distribution in sorbent beds: Analysis of a new sorbent device for hemoperfusion. Int J Artif Organs 2000;23:125–130.

7 Tangerman A, Snel P, van Schaik A, van Tongeren JH: Acid citrate dextrose reduces platelet retention during in vitro and in vivo dog hemoperfusion: A comparative study of different charcoal adsorbers. Artif Organs 1981;5:357–362.

8 Dinarello CA, Koch KM, Shaldon S: Interleukin-1 and its relevance in patients treated with hemodialysis. Kidney Int 1988;24(suppl):S21–S26.

9 Lohmann J, Pott G, Voss B, Gerlach U: Drug intoxication: Influence of hemoperfusion on human plasma fibronectin. Klin Wochenschr 1983;61:369–372.

10 Kojima S: Low-density lipoprotein apheresis and changes in plasma components. Ther Apher 2001;5:232–238.

N.A. Hoenich, Department of Nephrology, School of Clinical Medical Sciences,
Medical School, University of Newcastle, Framlington Place,
Newcastle upon Tyne, NE 2 4 HH (UK)
Tel. +44 191 222 6998, Fax +44 191 222 0723, E-Mail nicholas.hoenich@ncl.ac.uk

Ronco C, La Greca G (eds): Hemodialysis Technology.
Contrib Nephrol. Basel, Karger, 2002, vol 137, pp 170–180

Sorbent Augmented Dialysis Systems

F.J. Winchester[a], C. Ronco[b], J. Salsberg[a], E. Yousha[a], J.A. Brady[a], L.D. Cowgill[c], M. Choquette[a], R. Albright[a], J. Clemmer[a], V. Davankov[e], M. Tsyurupa[e], L. Pavlova[e], M. Pavlov[e], G. Cohen[f], W. Hörl[f], F. Gotch[d], N.W. Levin[g]

[a]RenalTech International, New York, N.Y., USA; [b]Ospedale San Bortolo, Vicenza, Italy; University of California, [c]Davis, [d]San Francisco, Calif., USA; [e]Russian Academy of Sciences, Moscow, Russia; [f]University of Vienna, Austria; [g]Renal Research Institute, New York, N.Y., USA

Since the 1970s sorbent technology has been used to increase the efficiency of dialysis, for end-stage renal disease (ESRD). Regeneration of dialysate with sorbents has a well-defined role in providing portability and low volume dialysate [1], while charcoal (carbon) hemoperfusion has been studied in ESRD therapy, with modest increments in dialysis efficiency. Conventional carbon is limited by its pore structure and incompatibility with blood [2], and hence new sorbent development with improved pore dimensions, is gaining ground as a valuable adjunct to dialysis [3, 4]. Novel adsorptive carbons with larger pore diameters are also being synthesized for potential clinical use [5]. Newly recognized uremic toxins [6, 7], have resulted in several investigations on alternatives to standard or high-flux hemodialysis, to remove these molecules. These methods include hemodiafiltration with [8] or without [9, 10] dialysate regeneration using sorbents, as well as hemoperfusion using adsorbents such as charcoal [11] and resins [12]. In addition, as ESRD is increasingly being recognized as an inflammatory state, many investigators have concentrated on middle molecular weight substances, inflammatory mediators (CRP, cytokines) [13, 14] advanced glycosylation end products (AGEs), advanced lipoxygenation compounds (ALEs), carbonyl and oxidative stress [15] which may produce malnutrition [16], wasting and increased levels of β_2-microglobulin [17]. High efficiency hemodiafiltration may reduce some of these proteins, with the high cost of ultrapure replacement fluid; on-line generation or regeneration of replacement fluid may become practical in the future. Sorbent hemoperfusion for removal of these toxins is attractive in offering low cost and high efficiency removal for certain substances.

β_2-Microglobulin (11.8 kD) is the most studied small molecular weight protein toxin; it produces dialysis-related amyloidosis (DRA) [18]; it becomes glycosylated [19] and deposited in amyloid fibrils, and retained in a deep body pool [20], eventually causing bone cysts, severe carpal tunnel syndrome and crippling arthritis [21]. Cellulosic membranes and CAPD [22] do not remove β_2-microglobulin, while reuse of PMMA and other membranes impairs its mass transfer [23, 24]. Reduction of β_2-microglobulin concentrations in dialysis patients, is associated with improved survival [25]. Transplantation with normal renal function causes reduction in β_2-microglobulin concentrations.

Sorbents: Theory and Practice

Adsorption efficiency is dependent on the nature of the solute and the sorbent. Specific or nonspecific attractive forces between solute and sorbent are paramount to the adsorptive process. Specific adsorption relies on the presence of tailored ligands or antibodies that have high selectivity for their targets. Specific adsorbents have been used in the treatment of idiopathic thrombocytopenic purpura [26] and for removal of lipids in familial hypercholesterolemia [27]. Specific adsorbents, though highly selective, are often expensive and have a low capacity for toxin removal.

Nonspecific adsorbents, typically charcoal and resins, attract solutes through a variety of forces including hydrophobic interactions, ionic (or electrostatic) attraction, hydrogen bonding, and van der Waals interactions. Manipulating the pore structure increases the selectivity of nonspecific adsorbents for particular solutes, by a process similar to size-selective chromatography. In this case, solute molecules are separated according to their size by their ability to penetrate the pores of the sorbent bead. For targeting middle molecular weight uremic toxins (MW 4–30 kD), pores between 4 and 10 nm allow entry to the bead, while excluding larger proteins, such as albumin (MW = 69 kD) [28]. Ion-exchange groups can also significantly increase the affinity of resin sorbents for bilirubin [29] and endotoxin [30].

Adsorption surface area for resins and charcoals is often quite high, in excess of 500 m^2/g adsorbent. These materials are also relatively cheap to produce and are used in several commercial applications. Until recently, poor hemocompatibility, as evidenced by thrombocytopenia and neutropenia [31], has been the major clinical limitation of these materials. Newer resin adsorbents appear to have solved this issue with the addition of a hemocompatible coating [32].

Sorbent Systems

Various sorbent systems are given in table 1. These consist of carbon or resin hemoperfusion systems, dialysate regeneration systems, sorbent column and suspension systems, plasma filtration adsorption systems and ultrafiltrate regeneration processes. Some of these systems will be described below.

HemoTherapies Unit

The HemoTherapies Unit for Liver Dialysis is a liver-assist device that employs hemodiadsorption (dialysis of blood against powdered sorbents) to selectively remove small molecular weight toxins in hepatic failure. The device is indicated for treatment of acute hepatic encephalopathy due to decompensation of chronic liver disease or fulminant hepatic failure. Controlled, prospective and randomized studies have been conducted at several centers, with treatment for 6 h daily over 1–5 days. A physiologic and neurologic improvement of patients with acute hepatic encephalopathy; of 31 treated patients, 51.6% survived. The Plasma Filtration Unit (PFU) combines hemodiadsorption with push-pull sorbent-based pheresis (the PFU add-on module, has powdered sorbent surrounding plasma filter hollow fibers). At blood flow rates of 200 ml/min, the system clears creatinine and aromatic amino acids at 120–160 ml/min, unconjugated bilirubin at 20–40 ml/min, and cytokines at 15–25 ml/min. The PFU has been tested in a few patients with hepatic failure with grade 3–4 encephalopathy, as well as respiratory and renal insufficiency [33]. Treatment appeared to be safe, and include improved blood pressure, encephalopathy, and stable urine output. A decrease in plasma levels of bilirubin, aromatic amino acids, ammonium, creatinine, and IL-1 was seen. The PFU offers increased protein-bound toxin removal over hemodialysis membranes.

Dialysis Combined with Sorbent Systems

Peritoneal Dialysis

Sorbents have been investigated for their role in enhancing solute removal, but have since been abandoned, due to lack of clear-cut efficacy [34, 35]. Combination of zirconium, charcoal and urease have also been used to regenerate dialysate in the REDY® system [36]. Regeneration of peritoneal dialysis effluent with high flow has increased urea and creatinine clearances to as high as 58 and 48 ml/min, respectively [37].

Table 1. Sorbent systems available to augment the efficiency of dialysis

System	Sorbent	Advantages	Disadvantages	Manufacturer	Potential or defined indication
Hemoperfusion	carbon	augments removal of creatinine, uric acid, low end middle molecular weight toxins; poisons with (e.g. aluminum, iron) or without (e.g. phenobarbital) chelating agents	platelet and WBC losses; no removal of water, small molecular weight uremic toxins; no removal of small molecular weight proteins	various	uremia, poisoning
Dialysate regeneration system - REDY	urease, carbon, zirconium	portable low volume dialysate	saturation, requires reinfusion of calcium, etc.	Organon	uremia
BetaSorb device	nonionic resin	improved small molecular weight protein removal (e.g. β_2-microglobulin, leptin, TNF, IL-1, IL-6, IL-10, retinol binding protein, angiogenin, cytokines)	no removal of water, small molecular weight uremic toxins	RenalTech	uremia, sepsis, liver failure
Lixelle device	cellulosic bead with ligands	improved small molecular weight protein removal (e.g. β_2-microglobulin). Symptomatic improvement in dialysis related amyloidosis	platelet and WBC losses; no removal of water, small molecular weight uremic toxins	Kaneka	dialysis-related amyloidosis
Dialysate suspension sorbent systems with parallel plate cellulosic membrane dialyzer – liver dialysis unit	carbon/cationic resin	removal of bilirubin, ammonia, aromatic amino acids, poisons (e.g. acetaminophen)	5-kD cut-off of membrane limits small molecular weight protein removal	Hemotherapies	liver failure, poisoning

Table 1. (Continued)

System	Sorbent	Advantages	Disadvantages	Manufacturer	Potential or defined indication
Dialysate suspension sorbent systems with added plasma filter sorbent system – liver dialysis unit with plasma filtration module	carbon/cationic resin with additional plasma adsorptive carbon module	improved small molecular weight protein removal with plasma filtration removal; TNF, cytokines	needs novel detectors for hemolysis and particulate release into blood	Hemotherapies	liver failure, poisoning
Albumin dialysate, highly permeable membrane dialyzer with column sorbent systems, and dialysis – MARS unit	carbon/cationic resin	removal of protein bound and lipophilic toxins (bilirubin, bile acids, ammonia)	requires albumin dialysate, and complex apparatus	Teraklin	liver failure
Continuous plasma filtration adsorption system	plasma filter and Amberchrome CG300 nonionic resin, with reinfusion of treated filtrate	TNF, IL-8, C3a, platelet activating factor	requires apparatus for reinfusion of plasma	Bellco	uremia, sepsis
Polymyxin B immobilized on polystyrene based fibers	polymyxin B antibiotic immobilized by amidemethylation	removes endotoxin, anandamide	specific for endotoxin	Toray	sepsis, ARDS
Hemodiafiltration with regeneration of ultrafiltrate – HFR	carbon and styrenic hydrophobic resin (Selecta)	removes TNF, IL-1	apparatus to control ultrafiltrate reinfusion required	Bellco	regeneration of ultrafiltrate
Hemodiafiltration with regeneration of ultrafiltrate	hydrophobic resin	removes TNF, IL-1	apparatus to control ultrafiltrate reinfusion required	B Braun	regeneration of ultrafiltrate

Hemodialysis

Short-term studies of charcoal hemoperfusion in uremia [2] suggested that improvement in the following occurred: pericarditis, gastrointestinal symptoms and lethargy [38, 39], and cardiac function [40]. Longer-term studies have shown improvements in; mean nerve conduction velocity [41, 42], electromyogram patterns, pruritus, and pericarditis [41], and a substantial reduction in dialysis time without uremic symptoms [43]. One study did not confirm improvement in nerve conduction velocity [44]. Hypotension, flushing, fever, chills, nausea and headaches [45, 46] have been observed infrequently with intermittent prolonged charcoal hemoperfusion. Bioincompatibility was not of any clinical significance; falls in platelet and leukocyte count occurred indicating foreign surface interaction between blood cells and the charcoal particles is present.

Hemodialysis – Aluminum and Iron Removal

Introduced by Chang, the combination of chelating agent and combined hemodialysis and hemoperfusion was used for the treatment of aluminum poisoning in ESRD patients [47]. This was extended into the treatment of iron intoxication [48]. In the following study [49], removal of aluminoxamine and ferrioxamine by combined carbon hemoperfusion (AluKart, Erika, Freehold, N.J., USA) and cuprophane (Cuprophan F-120 or a Hemophan FH-160) or hemodialysis with a high-flux F-60 polysulfone membrane was studied. Six ESRD patients underwent treatment after infusion of 30 mg/kg of desferrioxamine during the preceding dialysis session. The plasma clearance of aluminoxamine and ferrioxamine fell from 194.3 and 164.2 ml/min at the start of dialysis to 76.6 and 68.5 ml/min, respectively, at the end of dialysis. With the high-flux dialysis membrane the plasma clearance of aluminoxamine and ferrioxamine remained constant at 81.5 and 60.0 ml/min, respectively. Aluminoxamine and ferrioxamine uptake, respectively, was 84 and 84% of that available for adsorption, during a 4-hour hemoperfusion cuprophane hemodialysis.

High-Flux Dialysis Combined with Plasma Filtration System

These systems combine plasma filtration membranes and a sorbent system containing carbon and Amberchrome CG300 along with dialysis. The filtered plasma is passed through the sorbents prior to reinfusion. α_2-Macroglobulin, TNF, IL-8, C3a and platelet-activating factor are removed [50]. Clinical studies have been encouraging [51].

Hemodiafiltration with Online Regeneration of Ultrafiltrate [52, 53]

Regeneration of ultrafiltrate in particular has some advantages since it allows the concomitant infusion of sodium, calcium, and bicarbonate and the sorption of toxic species without blood contact. An integrated two-step sorbent system has been developed combining carbon and hydrophobic resins to detoxify ultrafiltrate: sodium, calcium, phosphate, bicarbonate, uric acid, creatinine, and β_2-microglobulin were studied, in vitro and ex vivo. The studies showed the presence of immunomodulatory substances in the ultrafiltrate and a significant increase in the lipopolysaccharide-induced release of both IL-1 and TNF. Further studies are awaited [54].

REDY System

The REDY system combines activated carbon layered above zirconium and urease; the latter converts urea to ammonia which is adsorbed onto carbon. The system prepares individualized dialysate for chronic and acute renal failure patients. The system is readily adaptable to home hemodialysis, and negates the need for expensive plumbing in view of the low level of dialysate used (6–12 liters). The system can be reduced in size resulting in a continuously wearable hemodialysis system [55].

MARS System

The molecular adsorbents recirculating system (MARS™, Teraklin, Rostock, Germany) employs a polysulfone high permeability dialyzer with albumin on the dialysate side to aid transfer of protein-bound toxins such as bilirubin and bile acids across the membranes. Sorbent columns of charcoal and an anion exchanger remove hepatic toxins from the albumin dialysate, and a second dialyzer removes water-soluble toxins such as ammonium. Clinical results of daily MARS treatments of patients with hepatic failure are associated with neurologic and physical improvement in most patients with acute hepatic encephalopathy, improved outcome for patients with acute on chronic exacerbation of liver disease and hepatorenal syndrome.

Resin Hemoperfusion

Using nonspecific agents such as activated charcoal [56], hemoperfusion has been shown to enhance 'middle molecule', amino acid, and creatinine removal in dialysis patients. All sorbent systems are limited in sorption of water, urea and acidic species, and must be combined with dialysis.

A newly developed resin system (BetaSorb™, RenalTech, New York, N.Y., USA), containing 300 g of a hydrated cross-linked polystyrene divinylbenzene resin, of pore structure designed to remove molecules between 4 and 30 kD, has been studied in pilot clinical studies. The resin beads have a blood-compatible coating, confirmed in vivo in animals [27], and ex vivo in human volunteers [57]. In 2 dialysis patients, BetaSorb™ with high-flux hemodialysis reduced β_2-microglobulin by 70% in each separate session. Predialysis β_2-microglobulin was reduced by 29.6% in 1 patient over a period of 3 weeks. The device was well tolerated clinically, producing no changes in platelet or leukocyte counts during the procedure. No changes in total protein and albumin concentrations were observed.

In addition to removal of β_2-microglobulin, we also observed reductions in leptin (16 kD), angiogenin (homologous to degranulation inhibitory protein I (DIP I), 14.2 kD) [4] and retinol-binding protein (21 kD) [58]. In other studies, IL-1 (17 kD), IL-6 (26 kD), IL-10 (18 kD) and TNF (21.5–28 kD) were reduced by this resin [59–61].

A cellulosic resin to which ligands trapping β_2-microglobulin are attached (Kaneka Corporation, Osaka, Japan) has also been shown to reduce β_2-microglobulin concentrations during extracorporeal treatment. Removal of β_2-microglobulin was associated with partial regression of dialysis related amyloidosis over 6–13 months [62, 63]; small decreases in platelets and leukocytes occur. The device is approved for established DRA in Japan for one year of treatment. Its high cost has precluded more widespread use after the first year of treatment.

Discussion

Much more clinical experience is needed with the newly designed and introduced sorbent devices in uremia. The clinical outcomes resulting from the molecular species that can be adsorbed, unlike any sorbents previously introduced, must be studied carefully. Many clinical trials are planned or underway, and trials are being devised to answer important clinical outcome questions, such as improvement in infection, atherosclerosis, DRA and other dialysis-related complications. It is likely that adsorbents will solve many of the problems of conventional or high flux dialysis, and could represent a detoxification platform for treatment of other disease states, such as sepsis, hepatic failure, etc.

References

1 Roberts M: The status of sorbent technology in hemodialysis treatment. Clin Nephrol 1986;26(suppl 1):S44–S46.

2 Winchester JF, Ronco C: Hemoperfusion in uremia: An in-depth review. Adv Renal Replace Ther, in press.

3 Winchester JF, Ronco C, Brady JA, Brendolan A, Davankov V, Tsyurupa M, Pavlova L, Pavlov M, Clemmer J, Polaschegg HD, Muller TE, La Greca G, Levin NW: Rationale for combined hemoperfusion/hemodialysis in uremia. Contrib Nephrol. Karger, Basel, 2001, vol 133, pp 174–179.

4 Winchester JF, Ronco C, Brady JA, Cowgill LD, Salsberg J, Yousha E, Choquette M, Albright R, Clemmer J, Davankov V, Tsyurupa M, Pavlova L, Pavlov M, Cohen G, Horl W, Gotch F, Levin NW: The next step from high-flux dialysis: Application of sorbent technology. Blood Purif 2002;20:81–86.

5 Mikhalovsky S: The detoxication with bioselective carbon sorbents. Biomater Artif Cells Artif Organs 1989;17:157–160.
6 Dhondt A, Vanholder R, Van Biesen W, Lameire N: The removal of uremic toxins. Kidney Int 2000;58(suppl 76):S47–S59.
7 Haag-Weber M, Cohen G, Horl WH: Clinical significance of granulocyte-inhibiting proteins. Nephrol Dial Transplant 2000;15(suppl 1):15–16.
8 Marinez de Francisco AL, Ghezzi PM, Brendolan A, Fiorini F, La Greca G, Ronco C, Arias M, Gervasio R, Tetta C: Hemodiafiltration with online regeneration of the ultrafiltrate. Kidney Int 2000;58(suppl 76):S66–S71.
9 Ward RA, Schmidt B, Hullin J, Hillebrand GF, Samtleben W: A comparison of On-line hemodiafiltration and high-flux hemodialysis: A prospective clinical study. J Am Soc Nephrol 2000; 11:2344–2350.
10 Takenaka T, Itaya Y, Tsuchiya Y, Kobayashi K, Suzuki H: Fitness of Biocompatible high-flux hemodiafiltration for dialysis-related amyloidosis. Blood Purif 2001;19:10–14.
11 Samtleben W, Gurland HJ, Lysaght MJ, Winchester JF: Plasma exchange and hemoperfusion; in Jacobs C, Kjellstrand CM, Koch KM, Winchester JF (eds): Replacement of Renal Function by Dialysis. Dordrecht, Kluwer Academic Publishers, 1996, pp 472–500.
12 Ronco C, Brendolan A, Winchester JF, Golds E, Clemmer J, Polaschegg HD, Muller TE, La Greca G, Levin N: First clinical experience with an adjunctive hemoperfusion device designed specifically to remove β_2-microglobulin in hemodialysis. Blood Purif 2001;19:260–263.
13 Memoli B, Postiglione L, Cianciaruso B, Bisesti V, Cimmaruta C, Marzano L, Minutolo R, Cuomo V, Guida B, Andreucci M, Rossi G: Role of different dialysis membranes in the release of interleukin-6-soluble receptor in uremic patients. Kidney Int 2000;58:417–424.
14 Guth HJ, Gruska S, Kraatz G: The measurement of cytokine production capacity during dialysis: A new dynamic method for the evaluation of biocompatibility? Int J Artif Organs 2000;23: 675–679.
15 Inagi R, Miyata T: Oxidative protein damage with carbohydrates and lipids in uremia: 'Carbonyl stress'. Blood Purif 1999;17:95–98.
16 Don BR, Kaysen GA: Assessment of inflammation and nutrition in patients with end-stage renal disease. J Nephrol 2000;13:249–259.
17 Ferreira A, Drueke TB: Biological markers in the diagnosis of the different forms of renal osteodystrophy. Am J Med Sci 2000;320:85–89.
18 Gejyo F, Yamada T, Odani S, Nakagawa Y, Arakawa M, Kunitomo T, Kataoka H, Suzuki M, Hirasawa Y, Shirahama T, Cohen AS, Schmid K: A new form of amyloid protein associated with hemodialysis was identified as β_2-microglobulin. Biochem Biophys Res Commun 1985;129: 701–706.
19 Miyata T, Wada Y, Maeda K: β_2-Microglobulin modified with AGE products of the Maillard reaction in dialysis related amyloidosis; in Maeda K, Shinzato T (eds): Dialysis-Related Amyloidosis. Contrib Nephrol. Basel, Karger, 1995, vol 112:, pp 52–64.
20 Vincent C, Chanard J, Caudwell V, Lavaud S, Wong T, Revillard J-P: Kinetics of ^{125}I-β_2-microglobulin turnover in dialyzed patients. Kidney Int 1992;42:1434–1443.
21 Drueke TB: Beta-2-microglobulin and amyloidosis. Nephrol Dial Transplant 2000;15(suppl 1): 17–24.
22 Tan SY, Baillod R, Brown E, Farrington K, Soper C, Percy M, Clutterbuck E, Madhoo S, Pepys MB, Hawkins PN: Clinical, radiological and serum amyloid P component scintigraphic features of beta-2-microglobulin amyloidosis associated with continuous ambulatory peritoneal dialysis. Nephrol Dial Transplant 1999;14:1467–1471.
23 Westhuyzen J, Foreman K, Battistutta D, Saltissi D, Fleming SJ: Effect of dialyzer reprocessing with renalin on serum beta-2-microglobulin and complement activation in hemodialysis patients. Am J Nephrol 1992;12:29–36.
24 Leypoldt JK, Cheung AK, Deeter RB: Effect of dialyzer reuse: Dissociation between clearances of small and large solutes. Am J Kidney Dis 1998;32:295–301.
25 Koda Y, Nishi S, Miyazaki S, Haginoshita S, Sakurabayashi T, Suzuki M, Sakai S, Yuasa Y, Hirasawa Y, Nishi T: Switch from conventional to high-flux membrane reduces the risk of carpal tunnel syndrome and mortality of hemodialysis patients. Kidney Int 1997;52:1096–1101.

26 Snyder HW Jr, Cochran SK, Balint JP Jr, Bertram JH, Mittelman A, Guthrie TH Jr, Jones FR: Experience with protein A-immunoadsorption in treatment-resistant adult immune thrombocytopenic purpura. Blood 1992;79:2237–2245.
27 Bosch T, Lennertz A, Kordes B, Samtleben W: Low density lipoprotein hemoperfusion by direct adsorption of lipoproteins from whole blood (DALI apheresis): Clinical experience from a single center. Ther Apher 1999;3:209–213.
28 Davankov V, Pavlova L, Tsyurupa M, Brady J, Balsamo M, Yousha E: Polymeric adsorbent for removing toxic proteins from blood of patients with kidney failure. J Chromatogr [B] 2000; 739:73–80.
29 Mertens PR, Schonfelder T, Handt S, Kierdorf H, Marschall H, Busch N, Heintz B, Sieberth H: Long-term extracorporeal bilirubin elimination: A case report on cascade resin plasma perfusion. Blood Purif 1998;16:341–348.
30 Sato T, Orlowski JP, Zborowski M: Experimental study of extracorporeal perfusion for septic shock. ASAIO J 1993;39:M790–M793.
31 Pond SM: Extracorporeal techniques in the treatment of poisoned patients. Med J Aust 1991; 154:617–622.
32 Ronco C, Brendolan A, Winchester JF, Golds E, Clemmer J, Polaschegg HD, Muller TE, Davankov V, Tsyurupa M, Pavlova L, Pavlov M, La Greca G, Levin NW: First clinical experience with an adjunctive hemoperfusion device designed specifically to remove beta 2-microglobulin in hemodialysis. Contrib Nephrol. Basel, Karger, 2001, vol 133, pp 166–173.
33 Steczko J, Ash SR, Blake DE, Carr DJ, Bosley RH: Cytokines and endotoxin removal by sorbents and its application in push-pull sorbent-based pheresis: The BioLogic-DTPF System. Artif Organs 1999;23:310–318.
34 Lang HL, Nolph KD, McGary TJ: Enhancement of clearances by activated charcoal in an in vitro model of peritoneal dialysis. Clin Exp Dial Apheresis 1982;6:85–95.
35 Blumenkrantz MJ, Lewin AJ, Gordon A, Roberts M, Pecker EA, Coburn JW, Maxwell MH: Development of a sorbent peritoneal dialysate regeneration system: A progress report. Proc Eur Dial Transplant Assoc 1978;15:213–219.
36 Gordon A, Maxwell MH, Lewin AJ: Sorbent regeneration of peritoneal dialysate: An approach to ambulatory dialysis. J Dial 1976–77;1:145–164.
37 Roberts M, Ash SR, Lee DB: Innovative peritoneal dialysis: Flow-thru and dialysate regeneration. ASAIO J 1999;45:372–378.
38 Martin AM, Gibbins JK, Kimmitt J, Rennie F: Hemodialysis and hemoperfusion in the treatment of uremic pericarditis: A study of 13 cases. Dial Transplant 1979;8:135.
39 Odaka M, Kirasawa H, Kobayashi H, Ohkawa M, Soeda K, Tabata Y, Soma M, Sato H: Clinical and fundamental studies of cellulose coated bead-shaped charcoal haemoperfusion in chronic renal failure; in Sideman S, Chang TMS (eds): Hemoperfusion, Kidney and Liver Support and Detoxification. Washington, Hemisphere Publishing, 1980, p 45.
40 Trznadel K, Luciak M, Wyszogrodzka M: Effect of haemoperfusion on the left ventricular systolic function in patients with chronic uraemia. Acta Med Pol 1981;22:75.
41 Otsubo O, Kuzuhara K, Simada Y, Yamauchi Y, Ta~ahashi 1, Yamada Y, Otsubo K, Inou T: Treatment of uraemic peripheral neuritis by direct haemoperfusion with activated charcoal. Proc Eur Dial Transplant Assoc 1979;16:731.
42 Agishi T, Yamashita N, Ota K: Clinical results of direct charcoal hemoperfusion for endogenous and exogenous intoxication; in Sideman S, Chang TMS (eds): Hemoperfusion, Kidney and Liver Support and Detoxification, Washington, Hemisphere Publishing, 1980, p 255.
43 Chang TMS, Barre P, Kuruvilla S: Long-term reduced time hemoperfusion-hemodialysis compared to standard dialysis: A preliminary crossover analysis. Trans Am Soc Artif Intern Organs 1985;31:572.
44 Henderson IS, Kennedy AC: Long-term evaluation of charcoal haemoperfusion combined with dialysis for uraemic patients; in Paul JP, Gaylor JDS, Courtney JM, Gilchrist T (eds): Biomaterials in Artificial Organs. London, Macmillan Press, 1984, p 72.
45 Odaka M, Tabata Y, Kabayashi H, Nomura Y, Soma A, Hirasawa A, Sato H: Clinical experience of bead-shaped charcoal hemoperfusion in chronic renal failure and fulminant hepatic failure; in Chang TMS (ed): Artificial Kidney, Artificial Liver and Artificial Cells. New York, Plenum Press, 1978, p 79.

46 Bonomini V, Stefoni S, Feliciangeli G, Coli L, Scolari MP, Orsi C, Nanni Costa A, Prandini R, Galanti S: Shortened treatment time by combined hemodialysis and hemoperfusion. Contr Nephrol. Basel, Karger, 1985, vol 44, p 57.
47 Chang TMS, Barre P: Effect of desferrioxamine on removal of aluminum and iron by coated charcoal haemoperfusion and haemodialysis. Lancet 1983;ii:1051–1053.
48 Winchester JF: Management of iron overload in dialysis patients. Semin Nephrol 1986;4(suppl 1): 22–26.
49 Vasilakakis DM, D'Haese PC, Lamberts LV, Lemoniatou E, Digenis PN, De Broe ME: Removal of aluminoxamine and ferrioxamine by charcoal hemoperfusion and hemodialysis. Kidney Int 1992;41:1400–1407.
50 Ronco C, Brendolan A, Dan M, Piccinni P, Bellomo R, Wratten ML, Inguaggiato P, Tetta C: Use of sorbents in acute renal failure and sepsis. Contrib Nephrol. Basel, Karger, 2001, vol 133, pp 180–193.
51 Brendolan A, Irone M, Digno A, Cioffi M, Piccinni P, Dan M, Tetta C, Ronco C: Coupled plasma filtration-adsorption technique (CPAT) in sepsis-associated acute renal failure. J Am Soc Nephrol 1998;9:127A.
52 de Francisco AL, Pinera C, Heras M, Rodrigo E, Fernandez Fresnedo G, Ruiz JC, Tetta C, Arias M: Hemodiafiltration with on-line endogenous reinfusion. Blood Purif 2000;18:231–236.
53 Marinez de Francisco AL, Ghezzi PM, Brendolan A, Fiorini F, La Greca G, Ronco C, Arias M, Gervasio R, Tetta C: Hemodiafiltration with online regeneration of the ultrafiltrate. Kidney Int 2000;76(suppl):S66–S71.
54 Opal SM: Hemofiltration-absorption systems for the treatment of experimental sepsis: Is it possible to remove the 'evil humors' responsible for septic shock? Crit Care Med 2000;28:1681–1682.
55 Roberts M: The status of sorbent technology in hemodialysis treatment. Clin Nephrol 1986; 26(suppl 1):S44–S46.
56 Winchester JF, Ratcliffe JG, Carlyle E, Kennedy AC: Solute, amino acid, and hormone changes with coated charcoal hemoperfusion in uremia. Kidney Int 1978;14:74–81.
57 Bosch T, Wendler T, Duhr C, Brady J, Samtleben W: Ex vivo biocompatibility of a new β_2-microglobulin adsorbent during hemoperfusion with human whole blood. J Am Soc Nephrol 2000;11:257A.
58 Cohen G: Personal communication, 2002.
59 Brady JA, Potempska A, Ronco C, Yousha E, Muller T, Levin N: Ex vivo cytokine clearance with a new adsorbent material from endotoxin-stimulated whole blood. J Am Soc Nephrol 2000; 11:586A.
60 Kellum J: Pers commun, 2002.
61 Jaber B: Pers commun, 2002.
62 Homma N, Gejyo F, Hasegawa S, Teramura T, Ei I, Maruyama H, Arakawa M: Effects of a new adsorbent column for removing beta-2-microglobulin from circulating blood of dialysis patients; in Maeda K, Shinzato T (eds): Dialysis-Related Amyloidosis. Contrib Nephrol. 1995, vol 112, pp 164–171.
63 Hyodo T, Tiara T, Hiyama E, et al: The clinical study on the newer type (Lixelle Type S-15) of the direct hemoperfusion B2-MG adsorption column. J Am Soc Nephrol 2001;12:267A.

James F. Winchester, MD, Chief Medical Officer, RenalTech International, LLC,
320 East 65th St, #116, New York, NY 10021 (USA)
Tel. +1 (212) 717 8644, Fax +1 (212) 717 8643, E-Mail jamesw@renaltech.com

Ronco C, La Greca G (eds): Hemodialysis Technology.
Contrib Nephrol. Basel, Karger, 2002, vol 137, pp 181–188

Use of Adsorbents in ARF Therapy

C. Tetta[a], *R. Bellomo*[b], *M. Formica*[c], *S. Livigni*[d], *F. Mariano*[e], *M.L. Wratten*[a], *G. Carraro*[f], *C. Ronco*[g]

[a]Clinical and Laboratory Research Department, Bellco Spa, Mirandola, Italy; [b]Intensive Care Unit, Austin & Repatriation Medical Center, Melbourne, Australia; [c]UU.OO. Nephrology-Dialysis and [d]Intensive Care Unit, Turin North Emergency St. John Bosco, Turin; [e]Department of Area of Medicine, Nephrology and Dialysis Unit, CTO Hospital, Turin; [f]Nephrology and Dialysis II, AO Padua; [g]Nephrology and Dialysis, St. Bortolo Hospital, Vicenza, Italy

Sepsis is the leading cause of acute renal failure and mortality in intensive care units [1–3]. The pathogenesis of sepsis represents a complex mosaic of interconnected events. Components of the gram-negative bacterial cell wall, such as the lipid-A containing lipopolysaccharide (LPS), or other inflammatory nonbacterial stimuli trigger a global response that involves both cellular and humoral pathways. In sepsis and non-infectious systemic inflammatory response syndrome (SIRS), stimulus-receptor interaction activates different signal transduction pathways leading to exacerbated generation of cytokines, and phospholipase A2-dependent, arachidonic acid-derived platelet-activating factor, leukotrienes and thromboxanes. At the plasma level, activation of the complement (C3a, C5a, and their desarginated products) and coagulation pathways interacts with the process as products generated in the fluid phase may in turn trigger and sustain cell activation. Other agents play a role in the pathophysiology of sepsis such as surface-expressed and soluble adhesion molecules, kinins, thrombin, myocardial depressant substance(s), endorphin and heat shock proteins.

In physiological conditions, the biological activity of sepsis-associated mediators is under the control of specific inhibitors that may act at different levels. In sepsis, the homeostatic balance is altered. On the one hand, inflammatory mediators with autocrine or paracrine effects are spilled over into the circulation and generate systemic effects including endothelial damage, loss of permselectivity, and vasoparalysis. On the other hand, cell-associated cytokines in peripheral blood mononuclear cells are decreased and the capacity of these cells to produce in vitro tumor necrosis factor (TNFα) and interleukin-1β (IL-1β) in response to LPS is significantly reduced. The pathogenesis of sepsis might therefore be described as a severe, protracted imbalance between pro- and anti-inflammatory factors in the host. Hyporesponsiveness is not only present in monocytes, but it occurs in whole blood (lymphocytes, polymorphonuclear neutrophils). It is associated with increased plasma levels of IL-10 and prostaglandin E2 both potent inhibitors of cytokine generation. The mechanisms responsible for cell hyporesponsiveness in sepsis and SIRS are not clear. Protracted synthesis and release of IL-10, and IL-1 receptor antagonist (IL1ra), reduced expression of the p65/p50 complex (NFκB regulators) all appear to contribute. Cavaillon et al. [3] recently summarized the features of cell hyporesponsiveness. First, hyporesponsiveness is a cell- and stimulus-specific as well as dose-dependent phenomenon. It occurs only with circulating monocytes but not with polymorphonuclear neutrophils. As a matter of fact, the latter cells are primed by circulating pro-inflammatory cytokines. Reduced synthesis occurs for IL-1, TNFα, IL-8 but not for IL-1ra, suggesting that IL-1ra may proceed through pathways independent from the deactivation of the NFκB.

Continuous renal replacement therapies (CRRT) have made extracorporeal treatment possible also in septic patients even when they are hemodynamically unstable, in order to balance hypercatabolism and fluid overload. In addition to removing excess fluid and waste products in septic patients, the possibility that CRRT may remove bacterial LPS and other mediators introduced a new concept of blood purification. Synthetic high permeability membranes may extract substances soluble in plasma water by three mechanisms – convection, diffusion and adsorption – related to the type of experimental set-up, polymer and target compounds. The work by Hoffmann et al. [4] provided evidence for the convective effect of polysulfone-based membranes. These authors convincingly demonstrated that only activated complement components (C3a,C5a and their desarginated derivatives) were significantly eliminated, while very little removal could be observed for molecules such as cytokines (TNFα, IL-1). This was confirmed in studies by Tetta et al. [5] showing the very small extraction for different cytokines when using high permeability polysulfone membranes. However, with the present availability of polysulfone-based membranes by different manufacturers, one should carefully analyze the results in relationship to the type of polysulfone used (polymer, hydraulic permeability, diffusive properties, geometry of the dialyzers). Finally, although adsorption by the polymer has been implicated as an important adjunctive mechanism for solute extraction, it must be emphasized that this is true only for certain polymers, and when it occurs, it is instrumental in the first hour or so. In an in vivo study, De Vriese et al. [6] analytically showed the kinetics of plasma concentrations of

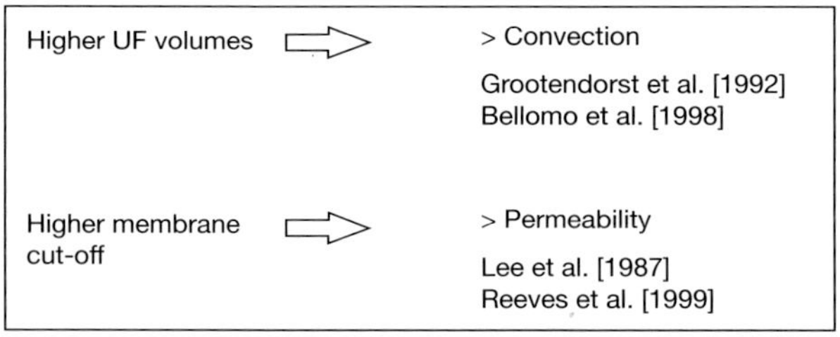

Fig. 1. Possible alternatives to conventional CRRT.

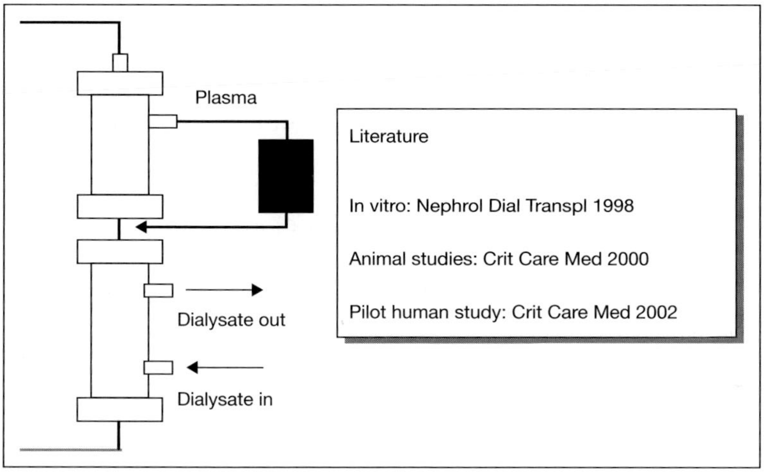

Fig. 2. Scheme of coupled plasma filtration adsorption (CPFA) and conventional CRRT.

different cytokines suggesting that adsorption occurs and may significantly reduce the plasma concentrations of cytokines only transiently.

The presently available technology opens two possibilities (fig. 1). On one side the increased (>35 ml/kg/h) ultrafiltration rate to reach what the 2000 Workgroup of the Acute Dialysis Quality Initiative defined as high volume CRRT. The second is to increase the removal of high-molecular-weight mediators by coupling plasma filtration with regeneration on high-gain adsorbing columns. We will briefly review the rationale based on the animal and clinical data for coupled plasma filtration adsorption (CPFA) in sepsis (fig. 2). Rather than only present work in which the authors have been directly implicated, we would like to provide the interpretation framework for considering a new technique as innovative.

Rationale for Plasma Filtration in Addition to Ultrafiltration

For several years, the concept of hemofiltration as a 'blood purification' technique has been controversial. It has been argued that the amounts of mediators detected in the ultrafiltrate is not sufficiently relevant to determine an effective body clearance. However, significant removal during the first hours of hemofiltration has been demonstrated for TNF, IL-6, C3a des Arg and IL-8, a cytokine possibly involved in the priming of polymorphonuclear neutrophils [7]. Depending on the membrane used particularly in relation to the type of polymer, and its porosity, either convection, adsorption or diffusion alone or in combination were found to be relevant for the removal. In the context of ARF during sepsis, it must be also remembered that metabolic compounds are accumulated as a consequence of the loss of renal function. Uremic toxins rapidly accumulate in the tissues and plasma and they may be responsible for the immune dysregulation associated with sepsis. Lonnemann et al. [8], using the Genius® machine, showed that cell hyporesponsiveness could be significantly reduced after a diffusive treatment and conventional high permeability polysulfone (Fresenius) membranes. From what is apparent from the literature and common practice, hemofiltration or even better hemodiafiltration do remove to a certain extent mediators provided a sufficient 'sepsis dose' is administered. On these premises, enough evidence supports the concept that conventional CRRT combining both diffusive and convective driving forces for solute extraction are associated with relevant biological and clinical effects. The question that arose some years ago was whether these effects were sufficient in magnitude and how long would it take for a clinically relevant benefit to manifest. As we stated above, the benefits of a major increase in the ultrafiltration rates (100 liters/12 h) were initially observed by Grootendorst et al. [9] and later confirmed in human studies [10]. However, such high-volume CRRT requires a dedicated machine and may only be attempted by experienced personnel. On the contrary, extensive experience and technology are available for plasma treatment due to the long-standing tradition of applications in apheresis also in intensive care medicine. Using an experimental model of acute endotoxemia in the rabbit, we showed that non-selective adsorption from plasma of cytokines and other proinflammatory mediators known to be produced in excess during sepsis could improve survival [11]. The simultaneous removal of peak concentrations of TNF and platelet-activating factor could also possibly prevent the formation of other biologically active substances, such as prostaglandins/leukotrienes, other cytokines, molecules up- or downregulating membrane receptors, selectins, and adhesion molecules, thus amplifying and perpetuating the immunologic disorders. The results that stemmed from these studies strongly supported the concept that a relationship would link the simultaneous removal of different mediators to improved survival. As stated above, the nonselective, simultaneous removal of

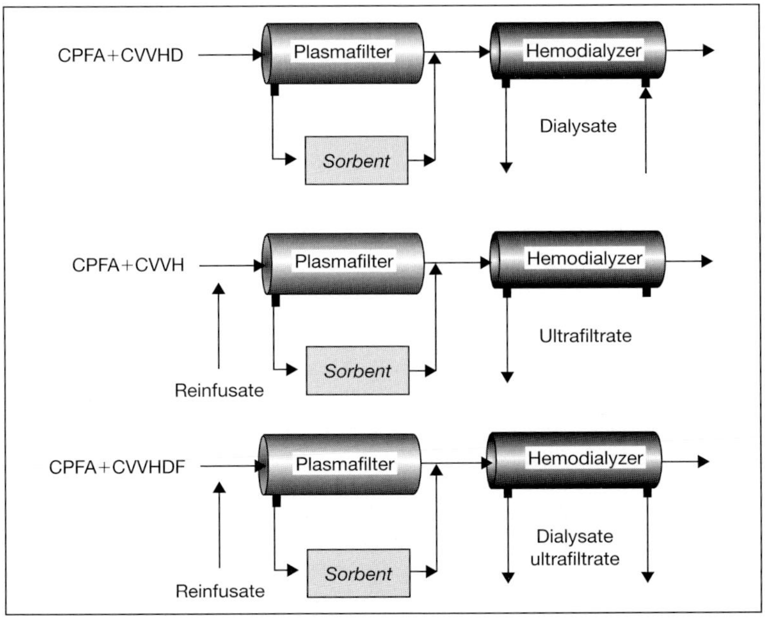

Fig. 3. CPFA may be used with pure diffusive (CVVHD), pure convective (CVVH) or mixed convective-diffusive (CVVHDF) treatments according to the clinical indication.

different mediators may not necessarily implicate that the goal of blood purification be achieved only on the basis of a significant reduction of the circulating cytokines. A much more effective strategy would be the impact on the functional responses of cells implicated in the pathogenesis of sepsis.

In a very recent study, we tested the hypothesis that nonselective removal of mediators could improve not only hemodynamics but could also restore leukocyte responsiveness in patients with septic shock [12]. CPFA was associated with the restoration of stable hemodynamics, particularly due to an increase in mean arterial pressure and to a significant reduction in norepinephrine requirement. CPFA also restored in vitro leukocyte responsiveness to LPS from *Escherichia coli*. The magnitude of these effects was significantly greater with CPFA than with CVVHDF. Plasma levels of TNFα and IL-10, however, were not significantly changed during CPFA or CVVHDF but they did not display concentration peaks [12]. Finally, CPFA may be associated with the different modes of CRRT such as CVVH, CVVHD, CVVHDF, depending on the clinical indications (fig. 3).

The ability of CPFA to restore immune cell responsiveness may be clinically beneficial. Several studies reported the suppression of cytokine

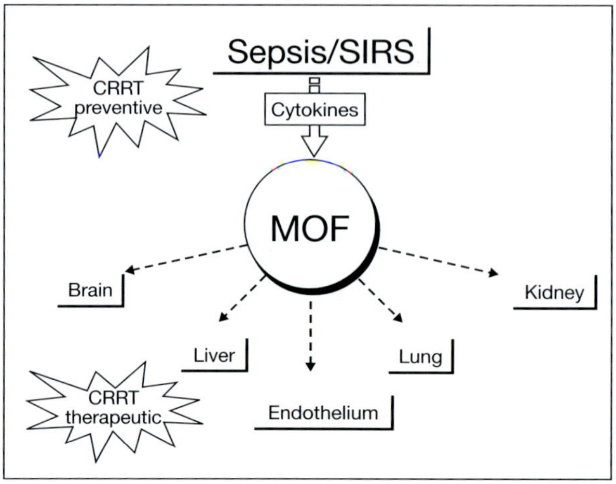

Fig. 4. In patients with sepsis/SIRS, the imbalance in pro-inflammatory and anti-inflammatory cytokine production may trigger a cascade of events leading to multiple organ failure (MOF). CRRT and possible new innovative approaches to blood purification may not only be considered as treatments for already established failing function of the kidneys and other organs, but could insure hemodynamic stability and leukocyte responsiveness in the very early stages of MOF development thus protecting the target organs.

production in leukocytes from septic patients. Postoperative sepsis has been shown to be associated with immediate monocyte defects that may affect both pro- and anti-inflammatory cytokine secretion, which suggests that immunosuppression is a primary, rather than a compensatory response to sepsis [3].

Recent preliminary clinical data suggest the benefit of early intervention with CPFA in patients with severe sepsis before ARF develops. The concept of 'blood purification' in critically ill patients may be more adequate if the supportive therapy allows the prevention of ARF. Maintaining renal function could be in fact an important hallmark for insuring the homeostatic balance in the different body fluids (fig. 4). Supportive therapies such as CPFA may be a better therapeutic option as it has a faster and more profound effect on both the hemodynamics and the leukocyte responsiveness than conventional CRRT as it has been shown in our pilot study [12]. CPFA was associated with the prompt restoration of hemodynamic stability, reduction of vasopressor requirement and perfusion of tissue microcirculation. However, several sessions of CPFA were needed to attain hemodynamic stability due to the rapid deterioration when CPFA was temporally interrupted even if followed by conventional CRRT (fig. 5).

In summary, the application of new therapies for the treatment of ARF in the clinical setting of multiple organ failure should be carefully examined. While

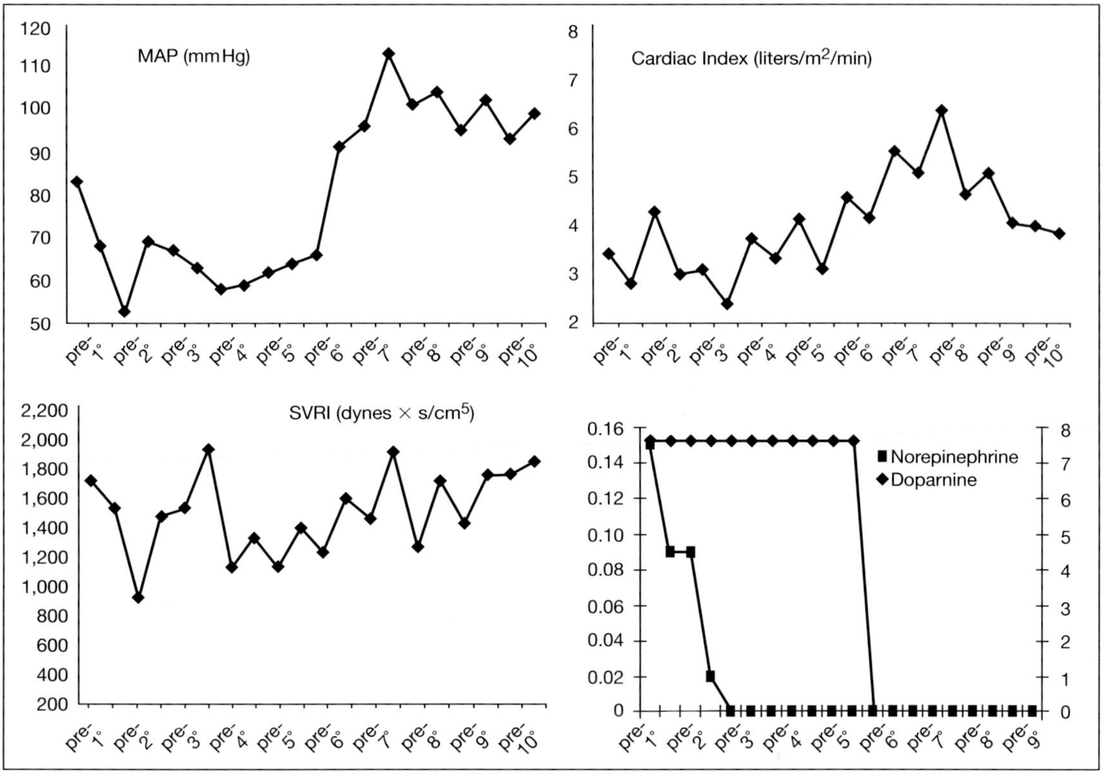

Fig. 5. Summary of different hemodynamic parameters and vasopressor requirement in a patient treated with several sessions of CPFA (abscissa).

the plasma levels of different cytokines are only 'the tip of the iceberg' [13], deeper insight into the complex scenario of sepsis needs to be addressed before the new technological approaches may be conclusively considered innovative. Mortality may not be an adequately powerful outcome since it depends upon various factors that are independent from CRRT. Nevertheless, a mechanistic interpretation of the effects of new extracorporeal technology is imperative and will need future, rigorous, randomized, controlled clinical studies.

References

1 Pinsky MR: Sepsis: A pro- and anti-inflammatory disequilibrium syndrome. Contrib Nephrol. Basel, Karger, 2001, vol 132, pp 354–366.

2 Adrie C, Pinsky MR: The inflammatory balance in human sepsis. Intens Care Med 2000;26: 364–375.

3 Cavaillon JM, Adib-Conquy M, Cloez-Tayarani I, Fitting C: Immunodepression in sepsis and SIRS assessed by ex vivo cytokine production is not a generalized phenomenon: a review. Endotoxin Res 2001;7:85–93.
4 Hoffmann JN, Hartl WH, Deppisch R, Faist E, Jochum M, Inthorn D: Hemofiltration in human sepsis: Evidence for elimination of immunomodulatory substances. Kidney Int 1995;48: 1563–1570.
5 Tetta C, Cavaillon JM, Schulze M, Ronco C, Ghezzi PM, Camussi G, Serra AM, Curti F, Lonnemann G: Removal of cytokines and activated complement components in an experimental model of continuous plasma filtration coupled with sorbent adsorption. Nephrol Dial Transplant 1998;13:1458–1464.
6 De Vriese AS, Vanholder RC, Pascual M, Lameire NH, Colardyn FA: Can inflammatory cytokines be removed efficiently by continuous renal replacement therapies? Intens Care Med 1999;25:903–910.
7 Mariano F, Tetta C, Guida GE, Triolo G, Camussi G: Hemofiltration reduces the priming activity on neutrophil chemiluminescence in septic patients. Kidney Int 2001;60:1598–1605.
8 Lonnemann G, Bechstein M, Linnenweber S, Burg M, Koch KM: Tumor necrosis factor-alpha during continuous high-flux hemodialysis in sepsis with acute renal failure. Kidney Int 1999; 56(suppl 72):S84–S87.
9 Grootendorst AF, van Bommel EFH, van der Hoven B, van Leengoed LAM, van Osta ALM: High volume hemofiltration improves right ventricular function of endotoxin-induced shock in the pig. Intens Care Med 1992;18:235–240.
10 Cole L, Bellomo R, Journois D, Davenport P, Baldwin I, Tipping P: High-volume hemofiltration in human septic shock. Intensive Care Med 2001;27:978–986.
11 Tetta C, Gianotti L, Cavaillon JM, Wratten ML, Fini M, Braga M, Bisagni P, Giavaresi G, Bolzani R, Giardino R: Coupled plasma filtration-adsorption in a rabbit model of endotoxic shock. Crit Care Med 2000;28:1526–1533.
12 Ronco C, Brendolan A, Lonnemann G, Bellomo R, Piccinni P, Digito A, Dan M, Irone M, LaGreca G, Inguaggiato P, Maggiore U, De Nitti C, Wratten ML, Tetta C: A randomized crossover study on couplet plasma filtration with adsorption in septic shock. Crit Care Med 2002; in press.
13 Cavaillon JM, Munoz C, Fitting C, Misset B, Carlet J: Circulating cytokines: The tip of the iceberg? Circ Shock 1992;38:145–152.

Ciro Tetta, MD, Clinical and Laboratory Research Department,
Bellco Spa, Via Camurana 1, Mirandola (Italy)
Tel. +39 0 535 29241, Fax +39 0 535 29282, E-Mail ciro.tetta@bellcospa.it

Ronco C, La Greca G (eds): Hemodialysis Technology.
Contrib Nephrol. Basel, Karger, 2002, vol 137, pp 189–192

Low Flux Dialysis?

Still a Role

N.A. Hoenich

Department of Nephrology, School of Clinical Medical Sciences, Medical School, University of Newcastle, UK

Introduction

Haemodialysis remains the most widely used modality of treatment for end-stage renal disease. The rationale of treatment being based upon the hypothesis that the uraemic syndrome is a consequence of the accumulation of metabolites and toxic solutes that would normally be removed via the human kidney. The treatment also corrects the fluid and electrolyte imbalance arising from renal insufficiency. Although widely used with close to one million patients benefiting from this type of treatment, it is far from ideal in that it supports life but fails to restore the patient to full functional normality and longevity. Early clinical treatments were undertaken predominantly with membranes based upon unmodified cellulose whose ultrafiltration capacity was low (<5 ml/h/mmHg). Blood and dialysate flow rates were 250 and 500 ml/min, respectively, and treatment was applied three times weekly and lasted between 4 and 6 h. This type of treatment removed low-molecular-weight metabolites across the membrane by diffusion, but the membranes used offered little or no capability for the removal of 'middle' or large molecular weight compounds. The realisation of this inadequate removal prompted the development of alternate therapies along two parallel paths. The first was high-efficiency dialysis by the use of large surface area dialyser and higher blood and dialysate flow rates. Subsequently, the availability of alternative membrane materials in the form of synthetic membranes as well as modified cellulose materials with higher hydraulic flux, a measure of their ultrafiltration capacity, and an increased permeability to middle weight solutes resulted not only in their clinical application in conventional dialysis (high-flux dialysis) but also in their use with therapies in which the predominant mode of solute transport is convection or solvent drag. In this mode of therapy (haemofiltration) no dialysis fluid is used, large volumes of ultrafiltrate are produced during treatment (20–30 litres) and are replaced by a sterile substitution fluid. Fluid replacement is either before the filter (predilution) or after the filter (postdilution). A hybrid technique combining diffusive and convective solute transport is haemodiafiltration. Both haemofiltration and haemodiafiltration simulate the transport mechanism of the human kidney and offer enhanced removal of middle molecular weight solutes compared to conventional low flux dialysis but and require the use of technologically advanced equipment, further more in haemofiltration removal of small molecular weight solutes is not enhanced and as the membranes used are non selective low molecular weight proteins and amino acids can be lost. The clinical application of these new treatment modalities is growing, but an important question remains as to whether there continues to be a role for the more conservative or traditional treatment by low flux techniques. In discussing this, it is proposed to confine discussions to solute removal and cardiovascular stability, both of which play a critical role in outcome and patient quality of life.

Solute Removal

Although much work has been undertaken on the identification of uraemic toxins, our knowledge of them and their potential clinical effects remains incomplete. Interest in solute removal in the clinical setting focuses largely on small molecular weight solutes but a number of studies have demonstrated that an accumulation of β_2-microglobulin over several years of dialysis therapy with conventional low flux membranes results in soft tissue and bone damage [1]. In contrast, therapies with a convective solute transport component offer the ability to remove β_2-microglobulin. The molecular genesis of dialysis related amyloidosis is incomplete and a number of factors other than removal may also contribute. These include the bioincompatibility of the dialysis procedure and the potential influence of advanced glycation end products (AGEs) [2].

Diffusive transport across membranes is a function of the concentration gradient across the membrane. It is rapid for small molecules but decreases with increasing molecular size. It is also governed by the membrane thickness and porosity. Adequacy of small molecular removal is largely based on the retrospective analysis of the classical NCSDS study [3]. However, there are a number of confounding variables such as patient size [4]. Evidence-based clinical practice guidelines have recommended minimum doses of small molecular removal but evidence from the published literature does not yet support a recommendation for an optimal dose. The currently accepted gold standard for dialysis in respect of patient survival is that of the Tassin group in France [5] who have utilized long slow dialysis using unmodified low flux cellulose membranes. The benefits of this modality of treatment are reflected in outcomes, the control of hypertension, as well as the higher removal of small molecules than currently achieved by rapid short duration treatments. There are strong arguments for the reduction of treatment duration (based on the removal of urea). Patients' quality of life is improved, as they spend less time on treatment. The treatment costs may be reduced, and there is better utilization of dialysis spaces. Set against this is are the poorer outcome of patients dialysed less than three times weekly for 3.5 h compared with those dialysed for 4 h or longer [6].

Cardiovascular Stability

Haemodialysis is associated with considerable cardiovascular instability. Its pathogenesis is multi factorial with the age of the patient being an important factor. It is estimated that 20–30% of the dialysis sessions are associated with hypotension, nausea, vomiting and headache [7]. With the clinical introduction of high flux and high efficiency therapies, there has been a reduction in the treatment times. This has required the use of higher blood flow rates, increased rates of ultrafiltration to attain adequate fluid removal during therapy which has further contributed to this problem.

Intradialytic hypotension has been reported as being lower compared to conventional dialysis when using haemofiltration due to a more physiological response arising from better blood volume preservation particularly in patients with a compromised cardiovascular function. This improvement, however, is not explained by a single factor, changes in sodium balance, or the use of more biocompatible membranes influencing vascular reactivity by the reduction of cytokine release may also play a contributory role [8, 9].

Conclusions

A membrane that mimics the glomerular basement membrane in being hemocompatible, having a high hydraulic permeability and a sieving coefficient yet not leading to albumin loss, remains the ideal membrane for renal replacement therapy. Solute removal by convection is equally effective for all solutes that can pass through the membrane; however for enhanced small solute removal, convection needs to be combined with diffusion as in haemodiafiltration, which has the potential to achieve the highest solute removal over a wide molecular weight spectrum among all forms of dialysis. Ideally the clinical application of such therapy should be daily to reduce the peaks in toxin concentration, acidosis and alkalosis, and preserve cardiovascular stability by ensuring that dry weight is maintained. While such therapies are technically feasible today, their clinical application has not been widespread. This has been largely a result of the higher cost of such therapies and the absence of randomised clinical trials comparing conventional low-flux therapy with these new modalities. Until such demonstration is available, low flux dialysis treatments will continue to be the treatment for a large proportion of patients with end stage renal disease.

References

1 Nangaku M, Miyata T, Kurokawa K: Pathogenesis and management of dialysis-related amyloid bone disease. Am J Med Sci 1999;317:410–415.
2 Raj DS, Choudhury D, Welbourne TC, Levi M: Advanced glycation end products: A nephrologist's perspective. Am J Kidney Dis 2000;35:365–380.
3 Gotch FA, Sargent JA: A mechanistic analysis of the National Cooperative Dialysis Study (NCDS). Kidney Int 1985;28:526–534.
4 Wolfe RA, Ashby VB, Daugirdas JT, Agodoa LY, Jones CA, Port FK: Body size, dose of hemodialysis, and mortality. Am J Kidney Dis 2000;35:80–88.
5 Innes A, Charra B, Burden RP, Morgan AG, Laurent G: The effect of long, slow haemodialysis on patient survival. Nephrol Dial Transplant 1999;14:919–922.
6 Port FK, Orzol SM, Held PJ, Wolfe RA: Trends in treatment and survival for hemodialysis patients in the United States. Am J Kidney Dis 1998;32(suppl 4):S34–S38.
7 Daugirdas JT: Pathophysiology of dialysis hypotension: An update. Am J Kidney Dis 2001;38 (suppl 4):S11–S17.
8 Santoro A, Mancini E, Zucchelli P: The impact of haemofiltration on the systemic cardiovascular response. Nephrol Dial Transplant 2000;15(suppl 2):49–54.
9 van der Sande FM, Kooman JP, Leunissen KML: Strategies for improving hemodynamic stability in cardiac-compromised dialysis patients. Am J Kidney Dis 2000;35:E19.

N.A. Hoenich, Department of Nephrology, School of Clinical Medical Sciences,
Medical School, University of Newcastle, Framlington Place,
Newcastle upon Tyne, NE 2 4 HH (UK)
Tel. +44 191 222 6998, Fax +44 191 222 0723, E-Mail nicholas.hoenich@ncl.ac.uk

Ronco C, La Greca G (eds): Hemodialysis Technology.
Contrib Nephrol. Basel, Karger, 2002, vol 137, pp 193–200

High-Flux Hemodialysis and Hemodiafiltration

Impact on Outcome

Francesco Locatelli, Pietro Pozzoni, Celestina Manzoni, Salvatore Di Filippo

Department of Nephrology and Dialysis, A. Manzoni Hospital, Lecco, Italy

A number of complications or symptoms related to the dialytic treatment have been attributed not only to the intermittent and/or insufficient depuration of uremic toxins and to the dialysate composition but also to the type of dialytic treatment (diffusive or convective) and the type of dialytic membrane used. High-flux hemodialysis and hemodiafiltration are renal replacement therapies characterized by an important convective elimination of solutes, thanks to the use of synthetic membranes with a high ultrafiltration coefficient (high-flux membranes). While large solutes are claimed to play an important role in the genesis of several aspects of the morbidity associated with chronic hemodialysis, yet it is still to be definitively proved that a more effective removal of such molecules, as performed by high-flux hemodialysis and hemodiafiltration, could have an effective impact on morbidity and mortality of ESRD hemodialysis patients. In this review among the most recent and meaningful highlights on the effects of high-flux hemodialysis and hemodiafiltration on several clinical end-points of uremic patients undergoing regular hemodialytic treatment, we will analyze the most clinically important potential benefits of these two convective treatments in clinical practice.

Cardiovascular Stability

Cardiovascular instability during hemodialytic treatment is still an important clinical problem affecting a large percentage of uremic patients. Although its pathogenesis is multifactorial, an increasing importance is ascribed to some factors such as the progressive increase in the median age of patients beginning hemodialytic therapy and the prolonged survival of hemodialysis patients and at the same time a tendency to a shorter dialysis treatment time with the consequent use of higher blood flow rates, dialyzer surfaces and ultrafiltration rates. Convective treatments using highly permeable synthetic membranes, such as high-flux dialysis and hemodiafiltration, could theoretically be affected by lower intradialytic hypotension rates than conventional low-flux hemodialysis according to a higher increase of peripheral resistances, a lower removal of sodium, the use of biocompatible membranes and a more efficient removal of adrenomedullin, a hypotensive peptide whose plasma concentrations are more elevated in hemodialysis patients compared with healthy persons and negatively correlate with blood pressure levels both pre-HD and post-HD. Several clinical studies were performed in order to evaluate the effects of different membranes or different dialysis treatments on intradialytic cardiovascular stability. The results of these studies as a whole suggest that convective treatments using highly permeable membranes do not seem to affect cardiovascular stability, and in particular intradialytic hypotension rates, in dialysis patients, but these findings are conditioned by the low incidence of this complication in the studied populations; clinical trials involving a larger number of patients and especially sicker populations with a higher prevalence of intradialytic hypotension are needed.

Residual Renal Function

Preservation of residual renal function in hemodialysis patients is very important, since it may indirectly affect the morbidity and mortality of such patients in different ways: patients with a higher residual renal function could have lower dietary restriction, thus leading to a lesser degree of malnutrition; residual renal function preservation allows shorter treatment times, it may guarantee better removal of β_2-microglobulin thus reducing the risk of dialysis-related amyloidosis, and, finally, it can reduce the loss of production of both calcitriol and erythropoietin resulting in possible decreased rates of osteodystrophy and anemia. It was suggested that the use of highly biocompatible membranes could have a positive effect on the rate of decline of renal function in hemodialysis patients, mainly because of a hypothetically less generation of nephrotoxic substances (including less cytokine induction) by the membrane itself, but this has not yet been confirmed; furthermore, it is not clear whether the use of high-flux biocompatible membranes can have an additive positive effect in comparison with low-flux biocompatible membranes. Several studies were performed in order to clarify this issue. Actually, the possible positive effects of high-flux dialysis and hemodiafiltration on the preservation of residual renal function in hemodialysis patients in comparison with conventional low-flux dialysis is still to be demonstrated, mainly because of the small number of studies performed and the rather small size of most of them.

Anemia

Correction of anemia is of paramount importance in hemodialysis patients, given the relationship existing between anemia and cardiovascular disease. It is well known that anemia improves after the start of conventional low-flux hemodialysis; this positive effect is due to the removal of small- and medium-molecular-weight toxic metabolities inhibiting erythropoiesis that accumulate in the serum of uremic patients. Highly permeable membranes could have an additive positive effect on the improvement of anemia because also high-molecular-weight erythroid inhibitors, cleared only by means of highly porous membranes, could accumulate in uremic serum. Locatelli et al. [1] performed a multicenter prospective randomized controlled trial involving 84 hemodialysis patients over a follow-up period of 12 weeks with the aim of testing whether high-flux (BK-F PMMA membrane) hemodialysis improves anemia in hemodialysis patients in comparison to conventional low-flux (cellulose membrane) hemodialysis. The main result of this study was that a significant difference in the increase of blood hemoglobin levels (the primary response variable of the study) over the trial follow-up between the two treatment groups was not found ($p = 0.485$), in contrast with the results of previous studies. The main explanation for this has to be searched in the particularly restricted selection criteria of the study, as only patients with hematocrit levels of less than 30% ($28.3 \pm 2.3\%$) and without other known factors possibly affecting anemia (malnutrition, vitamin B_{12} and folic acid deficiencies, aluminium intoxication, high PTH plasma levels) were admitted. Further, dialysis dose was adequate (mean level of Kt/V 1.3) and did not change during follow-up in the population as a whole or in the two patient groups, allowing to exclude a hypothetic confounding effect of an inadequate dialysis dose. The main conclusion that can be taken from the results of this study is that when patients are well selected and adequately dialyzed the effect of a high-flux membrane is less than might be expected from the results of uncontrolled trials. Wizemann et al. [2] performed a prospective randomized trial on 44 patients in order to compare the effects of on-line hemodiafiltration and conventional low-flux hemodialysis over a period of 24 months. The same membrane material (polysulphone, although at different levels of biocompatibility and permeability) was used and the same dialysis dose (Kt/V = 1.8) was achieved in each group of randomization, so that the possible role of a different membrane biocompatibility or a different dialysis adequacy between the two groups in affecting the results of the study could be excluded. The author's conclusion was that neither hematocrit levels nor weekly erythropoietin doses over the follow-up period significantly differed between the two groups, suggesting that the addition of convection has no further effects on anemia, at least at the high dialysis dose achieved in the study.

Nutritional Aspects

Malnutrition is a common feature in hemodialysis patients and is an important prognostic factor since a strong association has been found between low plasma levels of serum albumin and increased morbidity and mortality. Its pathogenesis is multifactorial, probably involving less calorie intake, dialysis-related hypercatabolic status, and loss of nutritional substances through dialyzers. If replacement therapies using high-flux biocompatible membranes are able to improve the nutritional status of hemodialysis patients is still a matter of discussion. Locatelli et al. [3] did not find any correlation between Kt/V and protein catabolic rate independently of membrane biocompatibility and flux; however, these results could be explained by the fact that the studied patients, given their high levels of Kt/V, probably were in the plateau region of the curvilinear relationship between PCR and Kt/V, where the correlation between dialysis efficiency and nutrition is in any case lost. Locatelli et al. [1], in a prospective randomized trial comparing high-flux (BK-F PMMA membrane) dialysis and conventional low-flux (cellulose membrane) dialysis, found that total protein levels significantly decreased over the follow-up period of 12 weeks only in the experimental group ($p = 0.043$), but these levels were significantly higher than in the conventional group at baseline ($p = 0.04$); furthermore, no differences between the two groups were found in the patterns of other nutritional status indices such as albumin ($p = 0.098$), transferrin ($p = 0.324$), C3 ($p = 0.315$), C4 ($p = 0.845$). Wizemann et al. [2] reported that any of the studied parameters of nutritional status (body weight, skinfold thickness, nPCR, plasma albumin, prealbumin and transferrin concentrations) did not significantly differ throughout the study follow-up (24 months) between patients treated with low-flux hemodialysis and with on-line hemodiafiltration, using polysulphone membranes and the same dialysis dose (Kt/V = 1.8), but it should be underlined that patients of both groups of this study were well nourished, thus the same results will not necessarily apply to malnourished patients.

β_2-Microglobulin Removal

Deposition of β_2-microglobulin in tissues has been proved to be the primary cause of dialysis-related amyloidosis (DRA). Although an insufficient excretion because of the decreased renal function is the main cause, it is likely that other factors could contribute to β_2-microglobulin deposition in dialysis patients, including the type of membrane used. High-flux biocompatible membranes are thought to be able to obtain a higher removal of β_2-microglobulin in comparison with cellulosic membranes mainly because of their higher permeability to β_2-microglobulin, their ability to absorb it and because of less membrane-mediated inflammatory stimulation that could lead to increased β_2-microglobulin synthesis. Wizemann et al. [2] found that while β_2-microglobulin plasma levels did not change significantly in the hemodialysis group (range between 32 and 43 mg/l) over the 24-month follow-up period, they significantly decreased (from similar values to 18 mg/l, $p < 0.01$) in the hemodiafiltration group over the first 6 months of treatment and then stabilized during the remaining 18 months. Schiffl et al. [4] performed a retrospective study involving 89 patients who had been on hemodialysis for at least 10 years and had been treated with only one kind of membrane and divided them according to the characteristics of flux and biocompatibility of the membranes used into three groups (low-flux cellulose, low-flux polysulphone or PMMA, high-flux polysulphone or AN69) in order to evaluate the effects of flux and biocompatibility on DRA. Clinical manifestations of DRA (such as carpal tunnel syndrome, arthropathy and bone cysts) were found to progressively increase from the first to the third group and a logistic regression analysis showed both flux characteristics and biocompatibility of the membranes to be independent determinants of DRA. Locatelli et al. [1] found that both predialysis and postdialysis β_2-microglobulin levels remained constant in the conventional group treated with low-flux hemodialysis, while they significantly decreased in the experimental group treated with high-flux hemodialysis. Nakai et al. [5] performed a large-sized retrospective study, using data from the Japanese dialysis patient registry, on 1,196 patients who were undergoing renal replacement therapy at the end of 1998 and who developed DRA during 1999: the aim of this study was to investigate and compare the effectiveness of different dialytic treatments (conventional hemodialysis, high-flux hemodialysis, off-line hemodiafiltration, on-line hemodiafiltration) on DRA, using a logistic regression approach. Expressing the results in terms of risk of a worse therapeutic effect (putting this risk at 1.0 for conventional hemodialysis), this risk was found to be progressively lower for high-flux hemodialysis (0.489), for off-line hemodiafiltration (0.117) and for on-line hemodiafiltration (0.013), indicating that high-flux hemodialysis and furtherly hemodiafiltration are more effective treatments for DRA in comparison with conventional low-flux hemodialysis.

Morbidity and Mortality

Several studies investigated the effect of different treatment modalities on the morbidity and mortality of hemodialysis patients, as mainly summarized by Locatelli et al. [6]. Chanard's group reported the positive effect of a biocompatible membrane (PAN) on hospitalization index and the number of days in hospital in comparison with cuprophane membrane, but did not find a significant difference in mortality between the two groups. Hornberger and co-workers in a retrospective study comparing 146 patients on standard hemodialysis with 107 patients on high-flux hemodialysis, found a lower relative risk of mortality in the high-flux group (0.24; 95% CI 0.12–0.49). Woods performed a 5-year retrospective analysis of 715 patients, comparing 252 patients exclusively treated with a low-flux polysulphone membrane and 463 patients treated for at least 3 months with a high-flux polysulphone membrane: patients treated with high-flux polysulphone showed significantly lower mortality (21 vs. 36 per 1,000 years; $p < 0.01$), significantly higher survival at 5 years (90 vs. 60%; $p = 0.029$) and a significantly lower standardized mortality ratio (0.13 vs. 0.2; $p = 0.012$), in comparison with patients treated with low-flux polysulphone only, thus suggesting an advantage of high-flux dialysis at least partially independent of biocompatibility. Hakim's group in a large-sized historical prospective study (2,410 patients) using data from the USRDS, found that, after adjusting for dialysis dose, geographic distribution and the presence of co-morbid factors, the relative risk of mortality estimated with a Cox proportional hazards model in patients dialyzed with modified cellulose or synthetic membrane was at least 20% less than that of patients treated with unsubstituted cellulose membranes. Locatelli et al. [1] did not find significant differences either in mortality or in the number of hospital admissions per year, or in the number of days per year spent in hospital, among the low-flux and high-flux treatment groups, but the study was not designed to tell a difference in mortality and morbidity. Koda et al. [7] found that the switch from a conventional dialysis to a high-flux dialysis led to a reduction in the relative risk of mortality to 0.613 ($p < 0.05$), suggesting that larger molecule removal by a high-flux membrane is an important factor in prolonging the survival of dialysis patients. In a recent large retrospective study using data from the USRDS, Leypoldt et al. [8] showed a 5% reduction in mortality (after correction for case mix, co-morbidities and urea Kt/V) in patients treated with membranes increasing the removal of vitamin B_{12}, assumed to be a middle molecule marker, by 10%. Locatelli et al. [9], in a large historical prospective study performed in 6,440 patients who started renal replacement therapy between 1983 and 1995, found that the relative risk for mortality, evaluated with a Cox proportional regression hazards model and adjusted for age, gender and comorbidities, was not significantly lower in patients treated with hemodiafiltration or hemofiltration compared with patients treated with standard hemodialysis (RR = 0.9; 95% CI 0.766–1.057; p = 0.19). Wizemann et al. [2] reported no significant differences in mortality and morbidity, calculated as hospital days per 3-month period, between patients treated with low-flux hemodialysis and with on-line hemodiafiltration at any time of the 24-month follow-up period. In a very-large-sized historical prospective study evaluating 12,791 patients who were hemodialyzed from 1994 through 1995 (1- to 2-year follow-up), Port et al. [10] found that the relative risk for mortality among reusing patients, estimated with a bootstrapped Cox proportional regression hazards model and adjusted for demographics, comorbidities, facilities, reuse agent and bleach, was lower with high-flux synthetic membranes in comparison with other types of membranes (synthetic low-flux, substituted cellulose low-flux, cellulose; RR = 0.82; 95% CI 0.72–0.93; p = 0.002) and, among synthetic membranes, it was higher with low-flux than with high-flux membranes (RR = 1.24; 95% CI 1.02–1.52; p = 0.04), thus suggesting that clearance of larger molecules may have a role in improving survival of hemodialysis patients.

Conclusion

The results of the studies aimed at evaluating the effects of biocompatible membranes and, more specifically, of high-flux hemodialysis and hemodiafiltration on several clinical end-points of dialysis patients are conflicting. Only the results of further studies with a large-sized study population and a long follow-up period will be able to better clarify the potential benefits of high-flux hemodialysis and hemodiafiltration on morbidity and mortality of patients on chronic renal replacement therapy. Two large randomized controlled clinical trials, aimed at clarifying this important aspect, are now ongoing: the Hemodialysis (HEMO) study [11] and the Membrane Permeability on ESRD Patient Outcome (MPO) study [12]. The HEMO study is a prospective randomized study that begun in 1995 and should conclude at the end of 2001; in a 2×2 factorial design, it considers patient outcomes in relation to two different dialysis doses (an equilibrated Kt/V of 1.05 or 1.45) and two different dialysis membranes (low or high permeability). The MPO study is also a prospective randomized multicenter trial which started in December 1998 and will conclude by the end of 2005, involving a minimum of 666 patients (incident patients only, unlike the HEMO study), and was specifically designed to investigate the long-term effect of membrane permeability on the clinical outcome of dialysis patients.

References

1 Locatelli F, Andrulli S, Pecchini F, Pedrini L, Agliata S, Lucchi L, Farina M, La Milia V, Grassi C, Borghi M, Redaelli B, Conte F, Ratto G, Cabiddu G, Grossi C, Modenese R: Effect of high-flux dialysis on the anaemia of haemodialysis patients. Nephrol Dial Transplant 2000;15:1399–1409.

2 Wizemann V, Lotz C, Techert F, Uthoff S: On-line hemodiafiltration versus low-flux haemodialysis: A prospective randomized study. Nephrol Dial Transplant 2000;15:43–48.

3 Locatelli F, Mastrangelo F, Redaelli B, Ronco C, Marcelli D, La Greca G, Orlandini G: Effects of different membranes and dialysis technologies on patient treatment tolerance and nutritional parameters. Kidney Int 1996;50:1293–1302.

4 Schiffl H, Fisher R, Lang SM, Mangel E: Clinical manifestations of AB-amyloidosis: Effects of biocompatibility and flux. Nephrol Dial Transplant 2000;16:840–845.

5 Nakai S, Iseki K, Tabei K, Kubo K, Masakane I, Fushimi K, Kikuchi K, Shinzato T, Sanaka T, Akiba T: Outcomes of hemodiafiltration based on japanese dialysis patient registry. Am J Kidney Dis 2001;(suppl 38):212–216.

6 Locatelli F, Manzoni C: Treatment modalities in comparison: When do clinical differences emerge? Nephrol Dial Transplant 2000;(suppl 15):29–35.

7 Koda Y, Nishi S, Miyazaki S, Haginoshita S, Sakurabayashi T, Suzuki M, Sakai S, Yuasa Y, Hirasawa Y, Nishi T: Switch from conventional to high-flux membrane reduces the risk of carpal tunnel syndrome and mortality of hemodialysis patients. Kidney Int 1997;52:1096–1101.

8 Leypoldt JK, Cheung AK, Carrol CE, et al: Effect of dialysis membranes and middle molecule removal on chronic hemodialysis patient survival. Am J Kidney Dis 1999;33:349–355.

9 Locatelli F, Marcelli D, Conte F, Limido A, Malberti A, Spotti D for the Registro Lombardo Dialisi e Trapianto: Comparison of mortality in ESRD patients on convective and diffusive extracorporeal treatments. Kidney Int 1999;55:286–293.

10 Port FK, Wolfe RA, Hulbert-Shearon TE, Daugirdas JT, Agodoa LY, Jones C, Orzol SM, Held PJ: Mortality risk by hemodialyzer reuse practice and dialyzer membrane characteristics: results from the USRDS dialysis morbidity and mortality study. Am J Kidney Dis 2001;37:276–286.

11 Eknoyan G, Levey AS, Beck GJ, Agodoa LY, Daugirdas JT, Kusek JW, Levin NW, Schulman G: The Haemodialysis (HEMO) Study: Rationale for selection of interventions. Semin Dial 1996;9:24–33.

12 Locatelli F, Hannedouche T, Jacobson S, La Greca G, Loureiro A, Martin-Malo A, Papadimitriou M, Vanholder R: The effect of membrane permeability on ESRD: Design of prospective randomised multicentre trial. J Nephrol 1999;12:85–88.

Prof. F. Locatelli, Divisione di Nefrologia e Dialisi,
Ospedale A. Manzoni, Via dell'Eremo 9/11 I–23900 Lecco (Italy)
Tel. +39 0341 489850, Fax +39 0341 489860, E-Mail nefrologia@ospedale.lecco.it

Ronco C, La Greca G (eds): Hemodialysis Technology.
Contrib Nephrol. Basel, Karger, 2002, vol 137, pp 201–211

On-Line Hemodiafiltration

Gold Standard or Top Therapy?

Jutta Passlick-Deetjen, Robert Pohlmeier

Fresenius Medical Care, Bad Homburg, Germany

Hemodiafiltration (HDF) combines the excellent low-molecular-weight clearances as achieved in hemodialysis (HD) by diffusive solute transport and the high clearances for the larger uremic toxins, the so-called middle molecules, as achieved with hemofiltration (HF) by convective solute transport. Resulting from this advantageous combination, HDF is superior to both HD and HF with respect to the removal of uremic toxins [1].

The cost for the required sterile substitution fluid, which was obtained usually in ready-to-use bags, was an important reason for the only slowly increasing number of HDF treatments. Each of these bags weighed ca. 5 kg, which also made a great deal of work for the dialysis personnel. Furthermore, the connections of multiple bags and tubing segments often led to relatively complicated technical set-ups. These disadvantages limit in practice the amount of substitution volume used in conventional HDF and, consequently, the potential of HDF to achieve high convective clearance is only partially used in conventional HDF. The development of on-line HDF made the substitution fluid clearly less expensive and simplified the set-up of the dialysis monitor. Thus, compared to a high-quality HD treatment, the advantageous removal characteristics of HDF can be realised with on-line HDF technology at little additional cost.

Technique and Safety

The principal flow diagram of an on-line HDF circuit is shown in figure 1 using thc Fresenius Medical Care ONLINE*plus*™ treatment system as an example. This system uses two specifically designed ultrafilters for cold sterilisation of the dialysis fluid which can be used for up to 100 on-line HDF treatments. The complete dialysis fluid, which has been prepared by the proportioning system,

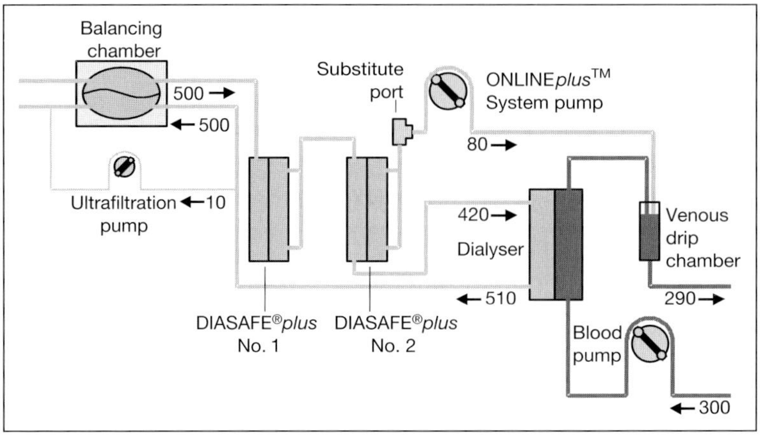

Fig. 1. Schematic depiction of the ONLINE*plus*™ system. The numbers at the arrows indicate flow rate in ml/min during an exemplary operating condition. The fluid balancing system on the left side determines the net fluid removal, in the example 10 ml/min. After the DIASAFE®*plus* No. 1 the dialysis fluid is ultrapure. The DIASAFE®*plus* No. 2 filters a part of the ultrapure dialysis fluid a second time and yields substitution fluid. This substitution fluid is pumped into the extracorporeal circuit in the postdilution mode as shown, alternatively the infusion in the predilution mode is also possible (not shown).

is filtered by the first ultrafilter. Under normal circumstances, the dialysis fluid after this first filtration process has a quality which fulfils the criteria of an infusion fluid, i.e. no detectable bacteria and an endotoxin concentration below 0.25 IU/ml [2]. As first-failure safety is an essential requirement, another ultrafilter is used to filter the infused portion of the ultrafiltered dialysis a second time to protect the patient against a rupture of the first ultrafilter during the treatment. To make the safety concept complete, the integrity of both ultrafilters is checked automatically before an on-line HDF treatment can begin. The safety of this on-line HDF system has been successfully shown [3]. During a 3-month study period of on-line HDF treatments, the microbiological quality of the dialysis fluid after the first and second filtration stages was not different from autoclaved isotonic saline solution. For the LPS-stimulated IL-1Ra production in vitro, no influence of the on-line HDF treatment was detected, neither between pre- and post-treatment blood samples nor between before and at the end of the 3-month on-line HDF treatment period. This demonstrates that these on-line HDF treatments did not cause an activation of the immune system. Other technical solutions for on-line HDF have a different safety concept, e.g. two multiple use ultrafilters are used, one of which is filtering the incoming water and the other one is filtering the ready-to-use dialysis fluid. As prior to each treatment no integrity test of these filters is performed, a third, disposable, ultrafilter is required, on which the safety of the substitution fluid relies and which is a costly disposable.

Principally, the substitution fluid can be infused in the postdilution mode, i.e. after the blood has passed through the dialyser (fig. 1), in the predilution mode, i.e. before the blood enters the dialyser, or combined. Postdilution HDF increases the clearance compared to HD for both small and large uremic toxins. A limitation with postdilution HDF is the intermittent hemoconcentration between the dialyser and the venous drip chamber. A total ultrafiltration rate (i.e. the sum of the substitution flow and the net ultrafiltration) of 30% of the blood flow, e.g., causes an intermittent increase in hematocrit from 35% to 50%. With increasing hematocrit, blood viscosity also increases, which results in an increase in transmembrane pressure and possibly a higher frequency of clotting. Therefore, the total ultrafiltration rate in postdilution on-line HDF should not exceed ca. 30% of the blood flow. The disadvantage of predilution HDF is the dilution of the uremic toxins. As a rule of thumb, comparable clearances of larger uremic toxins like β_2-microglobulin (β_2m, molecular weight 11.8 kD) are achieved with a substitution fluid flow of 30% and 100% of the blood flow in post- and in predilution on-line HDF, respectively. However, it must be noted that the dilutional effect of predilution always causes a drop in clearance of small uremic toxins below that of a comparable HD treatment (identical blood flow, same dialyser, same total dialysis fluid flow) [4]. The combined use of the pre- and postdilution modes was suggested to optimise on-line HDF therapy as the total substitution volume can be increased above the limit set by hemoconcentration in the postdilution mode with only a limited dilution of the uremic toxins [5]. However, the additional technical complexity of this approach has so far only been realised in experimental set-ups.

Comparison of HD and HDF

Zehnder et al. [6] compared high-flux HD and on-line HDF (ca. 24 liters substitution volume) intra-individually using the same 1.6 m^2 high-flux dialyser for both treatment modalities. They repeated the study analogously with a 2.4 m^2 high-flux dialyser. Concerning removal of urea and creatinine no statistically significant differences became apparent between high-flux HD and on-line HDF. In contrast, for phosphate (PO_4) they found a statistically significant increase of the clearance and of the mass removed per treatment. The latter rose by ca. 25% when the treatment was changed from high-flux HD to on-line HDF, thus contributing appreciably to the complicated therapy of hyperphosphatemia. The β_2m reduction ratio increased with the treatment change from high-flux HD to on-line

HDF from 64.1 ± 8.6 to 77.7 ± 8.2% and from 75.0 ± 5.1 to 82.9 ± 8.5% for the 1.6 m^2 and the 2.4 m^2 dialysers, respectively. Unfortunately, each treatment condition was only kept stable for 1 week, thus long-term effects on the pretreatment concentrations of PO_4 and β_2m cannot be compared.

Using a prospective, randomised design, Wizemann et al. [7] compared low-flux HD and on-line HDF over a time period of 2 years, the latter with a substitution volume of 60 liters per treatment in the postdilution mode, which is about the maximum feasible with today's technology. In order to remove possible confounding factors, Kt/V urea for both groups was matched at a high level (1.8) to exclude effects of increased removal of small uremic toxins. For the same reason and as on-line HDF is always performed with ultrapure dialysis fluid, low-flux HD was also performed with ultrapure dialysis fluid. Wizemann et al. [7] demonstrated a statistically significant drop by ca. 40% of the pretreatment β_2m concentration with on-line HDF down to 18 mg/l. It took approximately 9 months after the start of on-line HDF before this effect was apparently complete and a new steady state was established. With low-flux HD, the pretreatment β_2m concentration did not change significantly. PO_4 was reported not to evolve differently for both groups with the values near the upper limit of normal with a nPCR of 1.7–2.1 g/kg/day at the end of the study.

Ward et al. [8] compared prospectively and randomly patients on high-flux HD and on-line-HDF. The single-pool Kt/V_{urea} was 1.58 with on-line HDF (total ultrafiltration volume 21 liters) and 1.39 with high-flux HD (total ultrafiltration volume 2.9 liters). The reduction ratio for β_2m was 73% and 58% with on-line HDF and high-flux HD, respectively. However, both treatment modalities showed a similar small decrease of the pretreatment β_2m concentration. The removal of complement factor D (molecular weight 23.5 kD), a uremic toxin, which enhances the activity of the alternative way of complement activation, was also investigated. With on-line HDF treatment and high-flux HD, a reduction ratio of 33 ± 6 and −2 ± 8%, respectively, was found. However, during the 1-year observation period the reduction of the pretreatment concentration of complement factor D was statistically significantly higher (21%) with on-line HDF vs. 11% with high-flux HD.

Dose-Dependent Effects of On-Line HDF

A few studies investigated the effect of HDF treatments performed with different amounts of substitution fluid. Lornoy et al. [9, 10] showed that with increasing substitution fluid flow in postdilution on-line HDF linear increases of both, β_2m clearance and β_2m reduction ratio result. The effect of on-line HDF became statistically significant in comparison with high-flux HD as the substitution fluid flow exceeded ca. 40 ml/min or the substitution volume ca. 10 liters per treatment. Thus, to achieve clearly improved removal of β_2m compared to high-flux HD, the 10-liters substitution volume typically used in conventional HDF with substitution fluid from ready-to-use bags is not sufficient. Maduell et al. [11] demonstrated improved clinical results after a switch of the patients from conventional HDF to on-line HDF with 4.0 and 22.5 liters substitution fluid in the postdilution mode per treatment, respectively. An increase of both urea and β_2m clearance was documented. After the switch, there was a statistically significant increase in patients' hematocrit despite a parallel and also statistically significant reduction of the erythropoietin (EPO) dose. In addition, blood pressure control was improved with the higher substitution volume, as shown by statistically significant reductions of both the number of hypertensive patients and the number of patients on anti-hypertensive medication. A statistically significant increase of the dry weight was considered to be an indicator of an improved nutritional status. Grillo et al. [12] confirmed the improved response to EPO. Lin et al. [13] compared four patient groups, which received none, one, two, or three on-line HDF treatments per week and the remainder high-flux HD treatments, such that all patients received in total three treatments per week. The higher efficacy for small uremic toxins of on-line HDF resulted in lower pretreatment urea and creatinine concentrations. Furthermore, the incidence of symptomatic hypotension dropped steadily and statistically significantly as the frequency of on-line HDF was increased. This was explained by a higher sodium concentration in the venous return line. The latter is plausible as a small but significant increase of the pretreatment plasma sodium concentration in parallel with an increasing frequency of on-line HDF treatments was found (136.4 ± 2.2 and 138.7 ± 3.0 mmol/l, $p < 0.05$). However, mean pretreatment systolic blood pressures in the four groups of patients with different frequency of on-line HDF were not different. Another possible explanation for the improved cardiovascular stability with on-line HDF may be a slight cooling of the patient by the substitution fluid. Such a cooling effect is well known to be associated with improved cardiovascular stability [14], but measurements on thermal energy balance are not available from the study by Lin et al. [13]. However, van der Sande et al. [15] investigated the relation of temperature effects and cardiovascular stability in HD and conventional HDF. They found, with a constant dialysis fluid temperature of 37.5°C, an improved blood pressure response during conventional HDF (with a substitution fluid at room temperature) compared to HD. A similar improvement of the blood pressure response was found with HD, when the dialysis fluid temperature was reduced to 35.5°C. The authors discussed the improved blood pressure response to be most likely explained by temperature effects, as a decrease of body core temperature causes peripheral vasoconstriction which supports blood pressure stability. In a second study by Lin et al. [16], they used a similar design as in their previous study [13] to investigate the reduction of the pretreatment β_2m concentrations in three groups of patients. The patients of all three groups received three treatments per week, of which were one, two or three on-line HDF treatments and the remaining two, one and none high-flux hemodialysis treatments, respectively. Lin et al. [16] clearly showed a statistically significant increase of the β_2m reduction ratio with increasing substitution volume per session. The pretreatment β_2m concentration was significantly lower when the patients received a higher frequency of on-line HDF treatments. In addition to these results, although performed with conventional HDF, the results of Müller-Steinhardt et al. [17] should not be ignored. They reduced the substitution flow in a stepwise manner using 4-week intervals while keeping the treatment otherwise unchanged. As they expected, a decrease of the β_2m reduction ratios and an increase of the pretreatment β_2m plasma concentrations were revealed, both in a dose-dependent statistically significant relationship with decreasing substitution fluid flow. In addition, the reduction of the substitution fluid flow resulted in alterations of the response of a blood sample to stimulation with LPS: increased concentration of IL-10 and decreased concentrations of IL-1β and IL-6. A return to the higher initial substitution fluid flow reversed this trend after 4 weeks for IL-1β and IL-10, but not for IL-6. In accordance with the authors, 4 weeks after return to the original substitution fluid flow it does not appear, that stable conditions have been reached again, e.g., despite the trend of the pretreatment β_2m concentration to decrease again, this concentration was still significantly higher than at the same treatment conditions at the start of the study, where they had been stable for at least 2 months. Thus, a trend reversal also for IL-6 may have been detected, if the observation period would have been longer. The mRNA concentration of these interleukins showed the same principal pattern, which indicates that not only protein synthesis is influenced by the difference of the substitution fluid flow, but also the transcription of the respective genes. These results show that a higher substitution fluid flow in HDF treatment was associated with a more appropriate immune response to stimulation with LPS.

In conclusion from the above-cited studies, HDF clearly shows effects, which are related to the substitution volume applied per treatment. Therefore and as so far no negative effects of an increased substitution volume have been described, it must be concluded that the substitution volume should be chosen as high as reliably possible. With a typical treatment duration of 4 h and a blood flow of 300–400 ml/min, substitution volumes in postdilution HDF of 20–28 liters are a realistic goal. Substitution volumes in this dimension can only be realised for economic and practical reasons with on-line prepared substitution fluid. Higher substitution volumes in postdilution mode can only be achieved if the processed blood volume is increased, i.e. treatment time and/or blood flow are increased [7].

Alternative Treatment Modalities with Enhanced Convection

Above it was already shown that the convective solute removal with on-line HDF is superior to that with high-flux HD and conventional HDF. The latter is restricted for logistical reasons to relatively low volumes, typically around 10 liters, of substitution volume per treatment, which uses the potential of HDF only partially. Acetate-free biofiltration (AFB) is well described in the literature. The dialysis fluid for AFB is completely free of buffer and the required buffer is supplied by infusion of a bicarbonate containing solution in postdilution mode. Thus, AFB can be considered as a special form of conventional postdilution HDF. With AFB, the substitution volume cannot be easily increased, as such an increase would always mean an automatic increase of the infused bicarbonate, which could lead to alkalosis. Typically with AFB, the substitution volume and consequently the convective solute removal are comparable with conventional HDF and, thus, clearly lower than with on-line HDF. Paired filtration dialysis (PFD) has also been suggested to increase convective solute removal. The convective and the diffusive blood purification are physically separated. In a first step, postdilution hemofiltration is performed with a high-flux dialyser and in a second step hemodialysis is performed with a low-flux dialyser before the blood is returned to the patient. This concept has been designed in an attempt to minimize back-filtration and its possible negative effects. However, different to the concept of ultrapure dialysis fluid, the also important diffusive transfer of small cytokine inducing substances was overlooked. The substitution fluid in PFD is as in conventional HDF supplied in ready-to-use bags with all the related problems of high cost and increased work load of the dialysis personnel as well as the relative to on-line HDF low convective solute removal. Another alternative, conventional HF, i.e. with substitution fluid from ready-to-use bags is a nowadays only rarely used therapy. If a sufficient dose of renal replacement therapy is prescribed, the treatment is quite expensive. In addition, HD therapy has improved markedly during the last decades, such that HF has only little specific advantages nowadays. However, a remaining reason to apply conventional HF is to prevent the spread of highly contagious diseases like Jacob-Creutzfeld disease, as in conventional HF, different to all other set-ups discussed here, all fluids are in contact with disposable material only.

Alternative treatment configurations with increased convective solute removal and without the use of substitution fluid from bags have also been described. Hemodiafiltration with on-line endogenous re-infusion (on-line HFR) was developed based on PFD. The ultrafiltrate from the first (high-flux) dialyser is perfused through an adsorption column and then re-infused into the blood, which is thereafter cleansed in the second (low-flux) dialyser. The re-infused ultrafiltrate, after passage through the adsorption column, still contains some of the ultrafiltered uremic toxins as well as useful substances, e.g. amino acids and vitamins. Whether this is all in all superior to the use of on-line prepared substitution fluid remains at the moment purely speculative. 'Double high-flux dialysis' – two high-flux dialysers in series and an adjusted clamp to limit the dialysis fluid flow between both dialysers – is a possibility to increase internal filtration to such a degree, that a convective solute removal as high as in postdilution on-line HDF can be obtained. Thus, double high-flux dialysis with ultrapure dialysis fluid – to exclude the possible negative effects of backfiltration – is functionally nearly equivalent to postdilution on-line HDF. However, it is more costly as a second high-flux dialyser is required. The so-called 'double chamber on-line HDF' is similarly an approximately functional equivalent of predilution on-line HDF. The ultrapure dialysis fluid (after one stage filtration) is infused into the blood through the high-flux polysulphone membrane of the first dialyser. Thereafter, the blood is cleansed in the second dialyser wherein – in addition to the diffusive blood purification – the required ultrafiltration with the associated convective solute removal takes place. Another modality with enhanced convective solute removal as compared with high-flux HD is push/pull hemodiafiltration (PPHDF), which employs a double chamber piston pump to alternately increase filtration and backfiltration. PPHDF is reported to be functionally close to predilution hemofiltration. All systems for on-line HDF also enable on-line HF both in the post- and in the predilution mode. With postdilution on-line HF it is difficult to achieve sufficient Kt/V_{urea} as recommended in actual guidelines. Therefore, only predilution HF is used in clinical practice. Predilution on-line HF has been compared to high-flux HD while keeping the Kt/V_{urea} constant [18]. In this study, on-line HF is superior to high-flux HD with respect to cardiovascular stability both during treatment and in the inter-treatment interval. This difference was explained to be a consequence of the increased convective removal of uremic toxins associated with on-line HF. This proposed mechanism is plausible as Lin et al. [13] also showed improved cardiovascular stability with increasing convective removal of uremic toxins with on-line HDF in the postdilution mode. As discussed above, the improved cardiovascular stability found in both studies may be partially also explained by differences on the thermal energy balance. A disadvantage of on-line HF is that the potential of a higher small-molecular-weight clearance is not used, which could be easily realised with additional dialysis fluid, i.e. switching the treatment mode to on-line HDF.

Clinical Benefits of On-Line HDF

Summarizing the data above, on-line HDF is superior to other renal replacement therapies in multiple aspects. The excellent clearances for small and large uremic toxins with on-line HDF treatment result in a number of clinical benefits. It is well known that a high Kt/V_{urea} is associated with improved outcome and that such high Kt/V_{urea} values can be easily achieved with on-line HDF. Furthermore, the clinical findings of improved cardiovascular stability [13, 15], reduced EPO requirements [11, 12], and improved immune response with on-line HDF [17] treatment are discussed to be due to the removal of middle molecules with cardiodepressive effects, inhibitory effects on erythropoiesis, or depressive effects on the immune system. Temperature or sodium effects may also explain the improved intradialytic stability with on-line HDF. The clearly proven increased removal of β_2m leads to a reduction of the pretreatment β_2m concentration, which, however, is still above the value found in healthy controls. Nevertheless, β_2m has been shown to be an important constituent of amyloid and therefore it is an important therapeutic goal to reduce the concentration of this uremic toxin as much as possible.

The use of an on-line HDF system automatically is associated with the use of ultrapure dialysis fluid as in all treatment systems the readily mixed dialysis fluid is filtered by one of the used ultrafilters. This has been shown to have important clinical implications by itself [19] and is recommended to enhance the quality of the dialysis treatment in general [20]. Without ultrapure dialysis fluid, a chronic inflammatory state may be induced which has been recognised as an important cardiovascular risk factor. This is even more important as the cardiovascular risk in the ESRD population is markedly elevated as compared with a similar non-ESRD population [21].

By and large, therapies with increased convective solute removal have been shown to have a better outcome. The internal filtration occurring in high-flux HD has been estimated to reach ca. 5–30 ml/min (or 2–8 liters per treatment). Thus, high-flux HD also results in some convective solute removal, which, however, is even less than with conventional HDF. Leypoldt et al. [22] used vitamin B_{12} clearance as a surrogate parameter for middle molecule clearance in HD treatment and showed that a 10% higher vitamin B_{12} clearance reduces the relative risk of mortality significantly to 0.952. Similarly, Port et al. [23] showed that the mortality in low-flux HD was significantly higher than in high-flux HD with a relative mortality risk of 1.24, which they related to the enhanced clearance of larger molecules with high-flux HD. Locatelli et al. [24] analyzed the data of the Dialysis and Transplant Lombardy Registry and found that convective therapies (HF, HDF) compared to diffusive therapies (HD) had a significantly reduced risk for surgical treatment of carpal tunnel syndrome and a trend towards a lower risk of mortality. Even though a prospective comparative study between on-line HDF and low flux/high flux HD with the end-point mortality is missing, it may be assumed that outcome is not worse but even superior.

Summary and Conclusion

In summary, on-line HDF is an extracorporeal blood purification therapy with increased convective removal of uremic toxins as compared to the most frequently used low- or high-flux HD therapy. The clinical advantages of on-line HDF have shown to be dose dependent, which makes on-line HDF superior to other therapies with less convective solute removal. Among the therapies with high convective solute removal, i.e. on-line HDF, on-line HF and double high-flux dialysis, it is difficult to finally decide on the best therapy, as direct comparisons of these therapies are not performed. Theoretical considerations like the relative to on-line HDF lower achievable Kt/V_{urea} with on-line HF, allow to state that on-line HDF is the top therapy now available for patients with ESRD. A gold standard may be defined as something with which everything else is compared if one tries to establish it in the respective field. In order to declare on-line HDF as the gold standard in renal replacement therapy, we need more direct comparisons of on-line HDF with other therapies, including mortality as an outcome parameter. However, based on our current knowledge, it does not seem to be too speculative that high-quality clinical studies will establish on-line HDF in the next years as the new gold standard in renal replacement therapy.

References

1 Wizemann V: Hemodiafiltration – an avenue to shorter dialysis? Contrib Nephrol. Basel, Karger, 1985, vol 44, pp 49–56.

2 Weber C, Groetsch W, Schlotter S, Mitteregger R, Falkenhagen D: Novel online infusate-assisted dialysis system performs microbiologically safely. Artif Organs 2000,24:323–328.

3 Canaud B, Wizemann V, Pizzarelli F, Greenwood R, Schultze G, Weber C, Falkenhagen D: Cellular interleukin-1 receptor antagonist production in patients receiving on-line haemodiafiltration therapy. Nephrol Dial Transplant 2001;16:2181–2187.

4 Wizemann V, Külz M, Techert F, Nederlof B: Efficacy of haemodiafiltration. Nephrol Dial Transplant 2001;16 (suppl 4):27–30.

5 Pedrini LA, de Cristofaro V, Pagliari B, Sama F: Mixed predilution and postdilution online hemodiafiltration compared with the traditional infusion modes. Kidney Int 2000;58:2155–2165.

6 Zehnder C, Gutzwiller JP, Renggli K: Hemodiafiltration – a new treatment option for hyperphosphatemia in hemodialysis patients. Clin Nephrol 1999;52:152–159.

7 Wizemann V, Lotz C, Techert F, Uthoff S: On-line haemodiafiltration versus low-flux haemodialysis. A prospective randomized study. Nephrol Dial Transplant 2000;15(suppl 1):43–48.

8 Ward RA, Schmidt B, Hullin J, Hillebrand GF, Samtleben W: A comparison of on-line hemodiafiltration and high-flux hemodialysis: A prospective clinical study. J Am Soc Nephrol 2000;11:2344–2350.
9 Lornoy W, Becaus I, Billiouw JM, Sierens L, van Malderen P: Remarkable removal of beta-2-microglobulin by on-line hemodiafiltration. Am J Nephrol 1998;18:105–108.
10 Lornoy W, Becaus I, Billiouw JM, Sierens L, van Malderen P, D'Haenens P: On-line haemodiafiltration. Remarkable removal of beta-2-microglobulin: Long-term clinical observations. Nephrol Dial Transpant 2000;15 (suppl 1):49–54.
11 Maduell F, del Pozo C, Garcia H, Sanchez L, Hdez-Jars J, Albero MD, Calvo C, Torregrosa I, Navarro V: Change from conventional haemodiafiltration to on-line haemodiafiltration. Nephrol Dial Transplant 1999;14:1202–1207.
12 Grillo P, Bonforte G, Baragetti I, Scanziani R, Dozio B, Surian M: Haemodiafiltration with substitution of fluid prepared on-line decreases rHuEPO consumption. Nephrol Dial Transplant 1999;14:A207.
13 Lin CL, Huang CC, Chang CT, Wu MS, Hung CC, Chien CC, Yang CW: Clinical Improvement by increased frequency on-line hemodiafiltration. Renal Failure 2001;23:193–206.
14 Maggiore Q, Pizzarelli F, Sisca S, Zoccali C, Parlongo S, Nicolo F, Creazzo G: Blood temperature and vascular stability during hemodialysis and hemofiltration. Trans Am Soc Artif Intern Organs 1982;28:523–527.
15 v. d. Sande FM, Kooman JP, Konings CJ, Leunissen KML: Thermal effects and blood pressure response during postdilution hemodiafiltration and hemodialysis: The effect of amount of replacement fluid and dialysate temperature. J Am Soc Nephrol 2001;12:1916–1920.
16 Lin CL, Yang CW, Chiang CC, Chang CT, Huang CC: Long-term on-line hemodiafiltration reduces predialysis beta-2-microglobulin levels in chronic hemodialysis patients. Blood Purif 2001;19:301–307.
17 Müller-Steinhardt M, Kock N, Härtel C, Kirchner H, Steinhoff J: Production of monokines in patients under polysulphone haemodiafiltration is influenced by the ultrafiltration flow rate. Nephrol Dial Transplant 2001;16:1830–1837.
18 Altieri P, Sorba G, Bolasco P, Asporani E, Ledebo I, Cossu M, Ferrara R, Granadu, Cadinu F, Serra G, Cabiddu G, Sau G, Casu D, Passghe M, Bolasco F, Pistis R, Ghisu T: Predilution haemofiltration – the second Sardinian multicentre study: comparisons between haemofiltration and haemodialysis during identical Kt/V and session times in a long-term cross-over study. Nephrol Dial Transplant 2001;16:1207–1213.
19 Schiffl H, Lang SM, Stratakis D, Fischer R: Effects of ultrapure dialysis fluid on nutritional status and inflammatory parameters. Nephrol Dial Transplant 2001;16:1863–1869.
20 Lonnemann G, Koch KM: Efficacy of ultra-pure dialysate in the therapy and prevention of haemodialysis-associated amyloidosis. Nephrol Dial Transplant 2001;16 (suppl 4):17–22.
21 Locatelli F, Bommer J, London GM, Martin-Malo A, Wanner C, Yaqoob M, Zoccali C: Cardiovascular disease determinants in chronic renal failure: clinical approach and treatment. Nephrol Dial Transplant 2001;16:459–468.
22 Leypoldt JK, Cheung AK, Carroll CE, Stannard DC, Pereira BFG, Agodoa LY, Port FK: Effect of dialysis membranes and middle molecule removal on chronic hemodialysis patient survival. Am J Kidney Dis 1999;33:349–355.
23 Port FK, Wolfe RA, Hulbert-Shearon TE, Daugirdas JT, Agodoa LYC, Jones C, Orzol SM, Held PJ: Mortality risk by hemodialyzer reuse practice and dialyzer membrane characteristics: results from the USRDS dialysis morbidity and mortality study. Am J Kidney Dis 2001;37:276–286.
24 Locatelli F, Marcelli D, Cone F, Limido A, Malberti F, Spotti D: Comparison of mortality in ESRD patients on convective and diffusive extracorporeal treatments. Kidney Int 1999;55:286–293.

Prof. J. Passlick-Deetjen
Fresenius Medical Care Deutschland GmbH
Medicine & Marketing, Else-Kröner-Str. 1
D–61352 Bad Homburg (Germany)
Tel. +49 6172 609 2461, Fax +49 6172 609 2102

Ronco C, La Greca G (eds): Hemodialysis Technology.
Contrib Nephrol. Basel, Karger, 2002, vol 137, pp 212–220

New Options for On-Line Hemodiafiltration

C. Tetta[a], *P.M. Ghezzi*[b], *C. De Nitti*[a], *A. Fiorenzi*[a], *D. Cianciavicchia*[a], *R. Gervasio*[a]

[a] Bellco SpA, Mirandola, and
[b] Nephrology and Dialysis, St. Croce and Carle Hospital, Cuneo, Italy

Hemodialysis insures the survival of more than 900,000 patients with chronic renal failure worldwide. Despite the advances in renal transplantation and organ procurement, the rate of increase of the dialytic population remains steady up to a 6% yearly in the developed world. The picture is, however, incomplete still today. In developing countries, hemodialysis is still not a routine therapy and/or is still based on extensive, uncontrolled reuse. Nevertheless, even in countries where hemodialysis is an established routine practice, both mortality and morbidity are still very high. The major cause is cardiovascular disease which in recent years according to different National Registries has reached true epidemic proportions.

The development of new strategies in hemodialysis must meet today's patients' needs, be applicable in the context of the present cost pressure with the final goal of insuring clinically relevant advantages. On-line techniques were proposed in order to insure ample freedom in prescribing the convective 'dose' of dialysis. Apart from the already existing on-line systems (Fresenius and Gambro), we have recently clinically tested two newly developed techniques: the hemodiafiltration with on-line reinfusion of regenerated ultrafiltrate (HFR on line), and the paired hemodiafiltration (PHF). Both these techniques stem from the original concept of the paired filtration dialysis. In the present editorial, we will try to focus on the technological advances which have led to the formulation of these two new techniques. The following distinction between HFR on line and PHF needs to be made:

HFR on-line combines the possible of advantages derived from the use of regenerated ultrafiltrate as *endogenous* infusion fluid with the use of a double chamber hemodiafiltration which reduces oxidant stress and chronic inflammation (absence of backfiltration).

PHF is a hemodiafiltration system with on-line production of exogenous reinfusion fluid that includes a disposable hemodialyzer as final (second) barrier to bacterial contaminants in the reinfusate. An automatic system checks the fiber integrity during all the session.

HFR On-Line

Inherent to chronic uremia is the accumulation of metabolically active substances that may be responsible for the complex alterations of different biochemical pathways [1]. Schoots et al. [2] described in 1984: 'The discussion of the uremic toxin is probably an oversimplification of the real problem: the entire spectrum of accumulative products may play a role since toxicity can be due to the additive potentialization of specific toxic effects when several components are brought together. The comparison to a puzzle (the uremic puzzle) that presents its total image after it has been completed, seems appropriate here.' Besides the complex scenario of accumulated metabolic products, the uremic syndrome is associated with signs of altered immune response, evidence of oxidative stress and chronic inflammation, and besides being a treatment that removes water, electrolyte, urea and 'uremic toxins' by diffusion and/or convection, hemodialysis should also protect from losses of nutrients and antioxidants as well as from bioincompatibility-related events (cytokine synthesis, complement and kinin generation, erythrocyte fragility). However, convection and diffusion, either alone or in combination, are largely unsatisfactory in removing 'uremic toxins'. Adsorption is a third mechanism that has been applied in extracorporeal therapies. Early studies had shown that 'uremic (chromatographic) peaks' can be efficiently eliminated in haemofiltration with on-line regeneration of the ultrafiltrate, resulting in increased hematocrit and reducing β_2-microglobulin levels (fig. 1) [3].

In hemodiafiltration (HDF), the use of adsorbents could be possible using the double chamber dialyser in paired filtration dialysis (PFD) [4, 5] and the first clinical trial was performed [6].

Originally, the concept of adsorption was applied to the regeneration of dialysate using charcoal-based adsorbents in the search for an easily movable artificial kidney [7]. Subsequently, Shaldon et al. [8] proposed the regeneration of the dialysate via perfusion through the Redy Sorbent Cartridge. However, the need to add aluminum oxide or other aluminum salts to insure stabilization of the urease as well as easy releasibility of microaggregates led to high levels of aluminum with cases of overt aluminum intoxication [9]. The concept of fluid

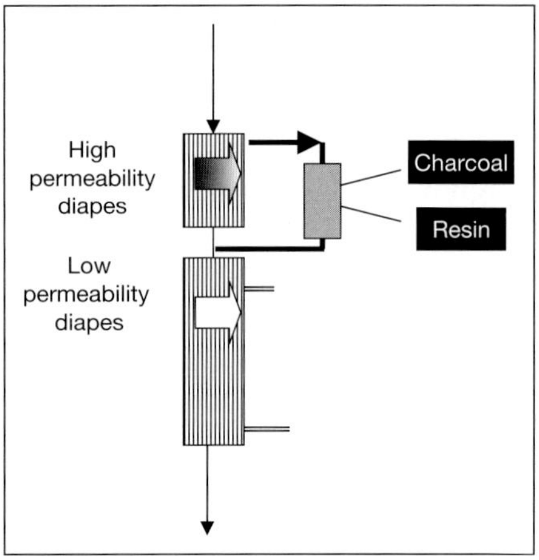

Fig. 1. HFR on-line scheme.

regeneration has been recently revisited in the hemodiabsorption technique where a charcoal-based sorbent mixed with dialysate is recirculated in a closed dialysate circuit [10].

A well-known field for the application of a sorbent has been in the therapy of both chronic renal failure (hemoperfusion in combination with hemodialysis) or in the treatment of acute poisoning [11, 12]. At the time of both benzodiazepine and salicylate accidental or voluntary poisoning, charcoal offered a useful tool for adsorbing the substances directly from the bloodstream because of its high adsorbing capacity and high available surface. However, in extracorporeal therapies, the remarkable characteristics of charcoal for adsorbing a wide range of compounds have been always confronted with the high degree of bioincompatibility. The charcoal in the 'coated' form acquires a much better compatibility in whole blood but greatly diminishes its adsorptive capacities.

As it was stated above, the double chamber technique PFD is the only existing hemodiafiltration (HDF) technique that allows on-line regeneration of the ultrafiltrate. This property relies on the physical separation of convection from diffusion. The solution given by the double hemodialyzer was aimed at improving the clearances of low-molecular-weight substances when this was considered an important goal in dialysis efficiency. As a matter of fact, several other issues such as the absence of backfiltration, the availability of pure ultrafiltrate for biosensing and regeneration were considered additional advantages which could not be verified due to the lack of adequate technology. Later, a number of experimental and clinical data have proven the feasibility of the pure ultrafiltrate for urea biosensing [13, 14]. In the context of the regeneration of the ultrafiltrate, it was initially shown that the ultrafiltrate (patient's own plasma water) could be passed through the sorbent cartridge. The first advantage of the regeneration of the ultrafiltrate that became immediately apparent was that adsorbents may be used in the 'uncoated' form, a remarkable advantage over the 'coated' one that is mandatory when adsorbents be used in whole blood. More recently, beside charcoal, synthetic adsorbents have become available in different extracorporeal therapies: stationary matrixes now encompass ion-exchange [10], or hydrophobic resins [15]. Recently, we examined different uncoated stationary matrixes, charcoals and synthetic resins, to establish their adsorptive capacities in relation to low- (urea, creatinine) and high-molecular-weight (β_2-microglobulin, myoglobin) compounds in in vitro conditions (steady state and flow through) using isotonic solutions or uremic ultrafiltrate. Trace metal, particle release analyses and scanning electron microscopy of different adsorbents were performed. Dynamic flow distribution studies were made using technetium-99 and analyzing the different regions of interest by a single head γ-camera. We showed that adsorbents may differ greatly as to their adsorptive capacity depending on the flow rate, the nature, total mass of the compounds to be removed from the ultrafiltrate. These studies suggested a methodological approach for screening stationary matrixes for possible application in hemodialysis [16].

The second PFD chamber is made of a low-permeability membrane to insure diffusion and patient's weight loss. The low-permeability diffusive membrane eliminates the risk of backfiltration. Backfiltration of dialysate occurs using high-permeability membranes in high-flux hemodialysis and HDF [17]. The transmembrane passage of bacterial pyrogens contaminating the dialysate may lead to monocyte activation and cytokine production, thus representing a mechanism capable of triggering systemic inflammation [reviewed in 18]. To avoid such a low level of biocompatibility, two approaches have been suggested and proved to be effective: the use of ultrapure dialysate and the adoption of techniques that abrogate backfiltration.

A recent long-term, prospective, cross-over study in patients on PFD showed a significant reduction in the generation of both interleukin-1 (IL-1) and IL-1 receptor antagonist (IL-1Ra) in patients treated with PFD versus patients on conventional HDF [19]. The reduced cytokine production in PFD has been related to the absence of backfiltration, a major driving force in the stimulation of monocytes from contaminated dialysate [20]. The same multicenter study [19] also showed significantly higher plasma levels of C-reactive protein and IL-6 in patients on conventional HDF than in PFD [21]. In a prospective, long-term clinical survey on 302 hemodialysis patients, the highest values of C-reactive protein and IL-6 were shown in patients on conventional HDF, but not in PFD [22]. In addition, reinfusion, albeit partial, of hydrosoluble vitamins and amino acids, as occurs in HFR on-line [unpubl. results] could theoretically ameliorate the nutritional status. Hydrophilic vitamins such as vitamin C

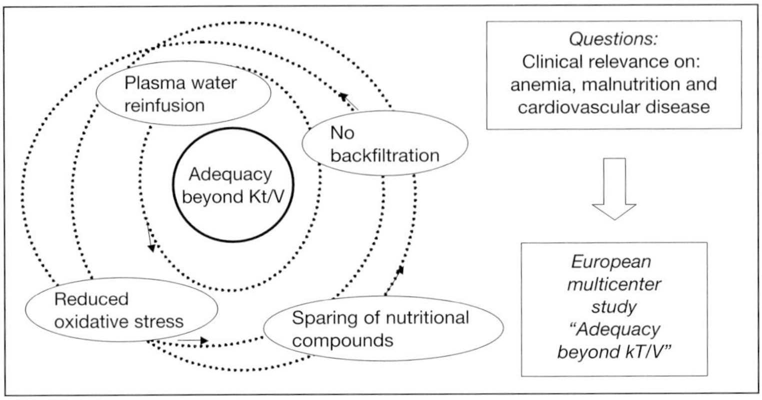

Fig. 2. Rationale of HFR on-line.

are lost during HDF [Cristol and Canaud, pers. commun.]. This loss may further worsen the oxidant/antioxidant unbalance that is known to occur in chronically uremic patients in hemodialysis [23]. Hemodialysis may trigger the formation of radical oxygen species in bioincompatibility-associated phenomena: namely $O_2°$-, its metabolites (H_2O_2 and .OH) and hydroperoxides released from arachidonic acid [24]. Several antioxidant defenses are altered in hemodialysis patients as exemplified by a reduction in the activity of Cu/Zn superoxide dismutase in erythrocytes and glutathione peroxidase [25]. Finally, the vitamin C depletion further aggravates the state of enhanced oxidation of vitamin E [26, 27]. Figure 2 summarizes the various pathophysiologic aspects related to the endogenous reinfusion of the regenerated ultrafiltrate in HFR on-line. Preliminary clinical evidence suggests the possibility for a reduced oxidative stress in patients treated with double-chamber hemodiafiltration [28]. A Multicenter European Collaborative Study is presently ongoing as has been recently published concerning methodology and its main outcomes [29].

PHF

Convective therapies have been shown to improve treatment tolerance and enhance middle molecule removal when compared to standard hemodialysis. However, the high cost of these procedures is a limiting factor for their widespread applicability in any chronic dialysis setting, particularly in this era of limited health care funding. Technogical advances now permit on-line production of substitution fluid, thereby significantly reducing the costs associated with convective treatments.

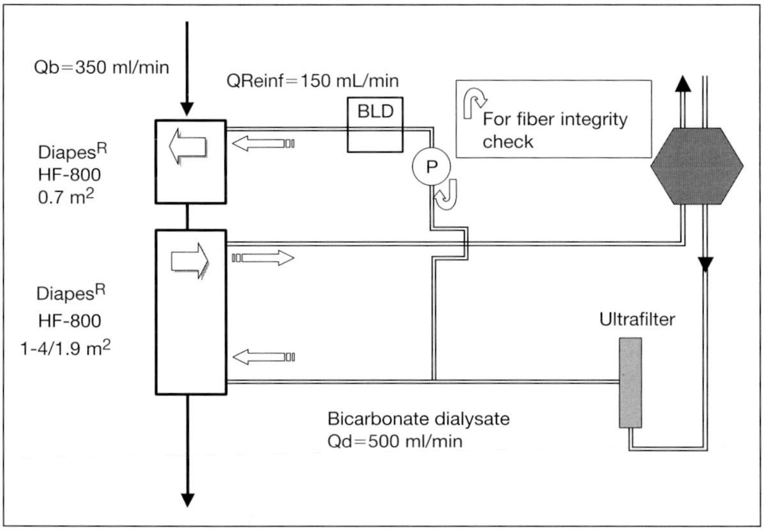

Fig. 3. PHF scheme.

Several clinical studies published so far assessed optimal clinical outcomes and safety of on-line procedures in the long-term [30–33]. Recently, Pizzarelli and co-workers [34, 35] published data showing that on-line fluids have the same, possibly less, cytokine-inducing capability than commercially produced reinfusion fluids. Some monitors specifically conceived for on-line convective treatments have been recently introduced to the market. They fully comply with the regulations for medical devices. Sterility and apirogenicity of infusion fluid is obtained by cold filtration of dialysate and is guaranteed by pretreatment assessment of ultrafilter fiber integrity by pressure test and/or redundancy of dialysate ultrafilters. Notwithstanding the reassuring evidence, many nephrologists are still concerned about the impossibility to check in real time the sterility and apirogenicity of the on-line-produced reinfusion fluid.

Pizzarelli et al. [36] presented preliminary clinical and biological data of PHF, a new on-line treatment. This technique is performed with a double chamber hemodialyzer (fig. 3). Dialysis fluid is filtered through the hollow-fibre ultrafilter (ForClean) embodied in the Bellco Formula 2000 monitor. The ultrafilter is used in the ultrafiltration mode and has been validated for its capacity to retain *Limulus amoebocyte* lysate-positive bacterial products [37]. A definite amount of the ultrafiltered dialysis fluid is continuously collected by the infusion pump and completely backfiltered into the patient's bloodstream in the first chamber of the dialyser (0.7 m^2 high-flux polyethersulfone membrane, Diapes® HF-800, Bellco). The remaining dialysis fluid flows into the dialysate compartment of the second chamber of the hemodialyser (1.9 m^2 high flux polyethersulfone membrane, Diapes HF-800), allowing for mixed convection-diffusion at a controlled flow of 500 ml/min. In this section, the fluid-balancing system of the monitor allows a compensatory convective removal of the back-filtered fluid plus the amount corresponding to the programmed weight loss. Thus, hemodiafiltration takes place in the second chamber, while reinfusion of ultrafiltered dialysate is allowed in the first one. As stated above, reinfusion in the first chamber is performed in a backfiltration mode using a new high-permeability polyethersufone membrane (Diapes HF-800) that has been shown to provide an efficient barrier to pyrogens [38].

Reinfusion rate may be up to 10 liters/h. The PHF system has been evaluated over 6 months with the production of more than 9,900 liters of ultrapure reinfusate according to the French regulation for on-line systems (DGS/DH/AFSSAPS 311 of 07/06/2000). The PHF system is equipped with a newly developed on-line dialyser fiber integrity check. By simply reversing the reinfusion pump, the ultrafiltrate from the patient's blood unmixed with the reinfusate is obtained and the presence of blood analyzed by a blood leak detector. In both in vitro and in vivo experiments, the device showed a great sensitivity even with a minimal dialyser damage (one leaking fiber). At variance with standard treatments, in which the blood leak detector is a slow-working low-sensitive device, the on-line fiber integrity device operates in a fast and high sensitivity fashion since the blood leaking from the dialyser is undiluted. The fiber integrity check can be performed at regular intervals or at any time during treatment. It takes no more than 1–2 min without interference with dialysis efficiency. The PHF system has been recently implemented with automatic procedures for full auto-priming and saline bolus injection. The auto-priming procedure is obtained by backfiltration of the dialysate through the two sections and may allow a better degassing of the whole hemodialyzer.

In conclusion, new options in on-line treatments are now available. Future studies should also clarify clinical indications in the context of absolute safety and better physiology for the treatment of chronic renal failure.

References

1 Vanholder R, De Smet R, Vogeleere P, et al: The uraemic syndrome; in Jacobs C, Kjellstrand CM, Koch KM, Winchester JF (eds): Replacement of Renal Function by Dialysis, ed 4. Amsterdam, Kluwer Academic Publishers, 1996, pp 1–33.

2 Ringoir S, Schoots A, Vanholder R: Uremic toxins. Kidney Int 1988;33(suppl 24):S4–S9.

3 Cerulli N, Politi L, D'Angelo AR, Scandurra R: A purification method by uncoated charcoal. Adv Exp Med Biol 1987;223:193–196.

4 Ghezzi PM, Frigato G, Fantini GF, et al: Theoretical model and first clinical results of paired filtration dialysis. Life Support Syst 1983;(suppl 1):271–275.

5 Ghezzi PM, Gervasio R, Tessore V, et al: Hemodiafiltration without replacement fluid. ASAIO J 1992;38:61–65.
6 De Francisco ALM, Botella J, Escallada R, et al: Hemodiafiltration with sorbent-regenerated ultrafiltrate as replacement fluid: A multicenter study. Nephrol Dial Transplant 1997;12:528–534.
7 Dunea G, Kolff WJ: Clinical experience with the Yatzidis charcoal artificial kidney. Trans Am Soc Artif Intern Organs 1965;2:178–182.
8 Shaldon S, Beau MC, Carlet G, et al: Sorbent regeneration of ultrafiltrate as a long-term treatment of end-stage renal failure. Artif Organs 1978;2:343–347.
9 Pierides AM, Frohnert PP: Aluminum related dialysis osteomalacia and dementia after prolonged use of the Redy cartridge (abstract). ASAIO J 1981;10:53.
10 Ash SR: Hemodiabsorption in treatment of acute hepatic failure and chronic cirrhosis with ascites. Artif Organs 1994;18:355–362.
11 Yatzidis H: The use of ion exchange resins and charcoal in acute barbiturate poisoning; in Mathew H (ed): Acute Barbiturate Poisoning. Amsterdam, Excerpta Medica, 1971, pp 223–232.
12 Yatzidis H, Yulis G, Digenis P: Hemocarboperfusion-hemodialysis treatment in terminal renal failure. Kidney Int 1976;10:S312–S314.
13 Arrigo G, Tetta C, Santoro A, Ghezzi P, Ronco C, Colasanti G, La Greca G, Zucchelli P, D'Amico G: Continuous urea monitoring in hemodialysis: A model approach to forecast dialytic performance. Results of a multicenter study. J Nephrol 2001;14:481–487.
14 Santoro A, Tetta C, Mandolfo S, Arrigo S, Berti M, Colasanti G, D'Amico G, Imbasciati E, Mazzocchi C, Pacini G, Spongano M, Thomaseth K, Wratten ML, Zucchelli P: On-line urea kinetics in hemodiafiltration. Nephrol Dial Transplant 1996;11:1084–1092.
15 Tetta C, Cavaillon JM, Schultze M, Ronco C, Ghezzi PM, Camussi G, Serra AM, Curti F, Lonnemann G: Removal of cytokines and activated complement components in an experimental model of continuous plasmafiltration coupled with sorbent adsorption. Nephrol Dial Transplant 1998;13:1458–1464.
16 De Nitti C, Giordano R, Castellano G, Podio V, Sereni L, Ghezzi PM, Ronco C, Brendolan A, Inguaggiato P, Tonelli M, La Greca G, Tetta C: Choosing new adsorbents for endogenous ultrapure infusion fluid: Performances, safety and flow distribution. Int J Artif Organs 2001; 24:765–776.
17 Ronco C, Brendolan A, Feriani M, Milan M, Conz P, Lupi A, Berto P, Bettini M, La Greca G: A new scintigraphic method to characterize ultrafiltration in hollow fiber dialyzers. Kidney Int 1992;41:1383–1393.
18 Botella J, La Greca G, Klinkmann H, Zucchelli P (eds): Chronic Inflammation in Haemodialysis. Basel, Karger, 2000.
19 Panichi V, De Pietro S, Andreini B, Migliori M, Tessore V, Taccola D, Rindi P, Palla R, Tetta C: Cytokine production in haemodiafiltration: A multicentre study. Nephrol Dial Transplant 1998;13:1737–1744.
20 Schindler R, Serovka F, Frei U: Transport mechanisms of cytokine-inducing substances through hemodialyzers (abstract A1159). J Am Soc Nephrol 1997;8:252A.
21 Panichi V, Tetta C, Rindi P, Palla R, Lonnemann G: Plasma C-reactive protein is linked to back-filtration associated interleukin-6 production. ASAIO J 1998;44:M415–M417.
22 Panichi V, Migliori M, De Pietro S, Metelli MP, Taccola D, Perez R, Palla R, Rindi P, Cristofani R, Tetta C: Plasma C-reactive protein in hemodialysis patients: a cross-sectional, longitudinal clinical survey. Blood Purif 2000;18:30–36.
23 Cristol JP, Canaud B, Rabesandratana H, et al: Enhancement of reactive oxygen species production and cell surface markers expression during hemodialysis. Nephrol Dial Transplant 1994;9:389–394.
24 Tetta C, Biasioli S, Schiavon R, Inguaggiato P, David S, Panichi V, Wratten ML: An overview of hemodialysis and oxidative stress. Blood Purif 1999;17:64–72.
25 Takahashi K, Newburger PE, Cohen HJ: Glutathione peroxidase protein absence in selenium deficiency and correlation with enzymatic activity. J Clin Invest 1986;77:1402–1404.
26 Sullivan JF, Eisenstein AB: Ascorbic acid depletion in patients undergoing hemodialysis. Am J Clin Nutr 1970;23:1339–1346.
27 Descombes E, Hanck AB, Fellay G: Water soluble vitamins in chronic hemodialysis patients and need for supplementation. Kidney Int 1993;43:19–28.

28 Biasioli S, Schiavon R, Petrosino L, Cavallini L, De Fanti E, Zambello A, Borin D, Targa L: Do different dialytic techniques have different atherosclerotic and antioxidant activities? ASAIO J 2001;47:516–521.
29 Cerulli N, La Greca G, Laville M, et al: The effect of hemodiafiltration with on-line endogenous reinfusion (on-line HFR) on anemia: Design of a European, open, randomised, multicentre trial. J Nephrol 2000;13:34–42.
30 Canaud B, Bosc JY, Leray-Moragues H, Stef F, Argiles A, Leblanc M, Mion C: On-line haemodiafiltration: safety and efficacy in long-term clinical practice. Nephrol Dial Transplant 2000; 15(suppl 1):60–67.
31 Canaud B, Bosc JY, Leray-Moragues H, Morena M, Stec F: Microbiologic purity of dialysate: Rationale and technical aspects. Blood Purif 2000;18:200–213.
32 Altieri P, Sorba GB, Bolasco PG, Bostrom M, Asproni E, Ferrara R: On-line predilution hemofiltration versus ultrapure high-flux hemodialysis: A multicenter prospective study in 23 patients. Blood Purif 1997;15:169–181.
33 Maduell F, del Pozo C, Garzia H, Sanchez L, Hdez-Iaras J, Alber MD, Calvo C, Torregrosa I, Navarro V: Change from conventional haemodiafiltration to on-line haemodiafiltration. Nephrol Dial Transplant 1999;14:1202–1207.
34 Pizzarelli F, Cerrai T, Dattolo P, Tetta C, Maggiore Q: Convective treatments with on-line production of replacement fluid: A clinical experience lasting 6 years. Nephrol Dial Transplant 1998;13: 363–369.
35 Pizzarelli F, Maggiore Q: Clinical perspectives of on-line haemodiafiltration. Nephrol Dial Transplant 1998;13(S5):34–37.
36 Pizzarelli F, Tetta C, Cerrai T, Maggiore Q: Double chamber on-line hemodiafiltration: A novel technique with intra-treatment monitoring of dialysate ultrafilter integrity. Blood Purif 2000;15: 237–241.
37 Cappelli G, Inguaggiato P, Perrone S, Gervasio R, Tetta C, Scialoja MG, Albertazzi A: Retention of limulus amoebocyte lysate reactive bacterial products via polysulfone dialysers is affected by the type of disinfectant. ASAIO J 1998;44:M587–M591.
38 Lonnemann G, Sereni L, Lemke HD, Tetta C: Pyrogen retention by highly permeable synthetic membranes during in vitro dialysis. Artif Organs 2001;25:951–960.

Ciro Tetta, MD, Clinical and Laboratory Research Department,
Bellco SpA, Via Camurana 1, I–41037 Mirandola (Italy)
Tel. +39 0535 29241/5, Fax +39 0535 29282, E-Mail ciro.tetta@bellcospa.it

Ronco C, La Greca G (eds): Hemodialysis Technology.
Contrib Nephrol. Basel, Karger, 2002, vol 137, pp 221–226

On-Line Hemofiltration

Old Concept – New Approach

Ingrid Ledebo

Gambro Corporate Research, Lund, Sweden

Original Concept of On-Line Hemofiltration

The difference in solute clearance pattern between convection on one hand and diffusion, as practiced in standard hemodialysis (HD), stimulated Henderson et al. [1] to start clinical experiments with a new therapy initially referred to as hemodiafiltration. At the time retention of medium-sized solutes (0.3–6 kD) played a leading role in the patho-physiological hypothesis for uremia and these solutes are poorly cleared by diffusion-based blood purification. The first clinical experience of hemofiltration (HF) confirmed the removal of solutes over a broad molecular weight spectrum and at rates comparable to the human kidney. For further development beyond that of an investigative tool, the authors pointed out the need for techniques to generate large volumes of sterile, pyrogen-free substitution solution. Three years later, Henderson et al. [2] showed that processing of high-quality dialysis fluid through ultrafilters to retain bacteria and pyrogens could be used as a method for continuous preparation of the substitution solution required for HF. On-line hemofiltration was born.

The technical development required to take on-line HF from bench to bedside for routine clinical use took place mainly during the 1980s and resulted in a number of innovations: highly permeable membranes with desirable sieving properties made from biocompatible, synthetic polymers; fluid balancing systems that control high volume ultrafiltration and accurately match it with reinfusion; hygienic design and maintenance techniques for complex fluid pathways preventing the formation of biofilm; and ultrafilters providing multi-log retention of bacterial products of varying molecular size for effective cold sterilization of fluids.

Development of Modern Hemodialysis

Although triggered by efforts to provide equipment for on-line HF, the technical development was not reserved for this therapy, but has been well integrated in the development of all dialysis equipment. Today, state-of-the-art HD operates with dialyzers with the same type of open membrane as HF. Ultrafiltration control has been a feature of all modern HD machines for well over a decade. The combination of highly permeable membranes and volume control sets the scene for automatic replacement of excess fluid removal by backfiltration of dialysis fluid, which therefore must be of high microbiological quality. To provide so-called ultrapure dialysis fluid, the same type of ultrafilters and similar hygienic measures as for on-line systems are used for the fluid flow-path. HD has thus become similar to HF in many respects, however, with the exception that solutes are still transported from blood mainly by diffusion in HD and only by convection in HF.

New Approach to Hemofiltration

In the early days, the observed clinical benefits of HF over HD were often ascribed to the use of more biocompatible membranes, linear and more accurate volume control and superior fluid quality. Today, these differences no longer exist, but there are still reports of improved treatment tolerance and better overall management of blood pressure in patients treated with HF [3–5]. As a consequence, these patients often experience better quality of life compared to being treated with standard dialysis therapies. What are presently the differences between HF and HD treatment that could explain these clinical benefits?

Prescription, Delivery and Quantification of Therapy

From a practical point of view it is as simple to set up and run a HF treatment as a HD treatment. Often the same machine can be used, the concentrate components for the dialysis fluid may be the same and the filter is of the same type. Because higher flow rates across the membrane are required for convective transport, the optimal surface area for HF is larger than for HD. The machine set-up varies because of the different fluids used; for HD the dialysis fluid flow is connected counter-currently to the blood flow; for HF the infusion solution is mixed with the blood before or after it enters the filter, predilution or postdilution, and there is no dialysis fluid, only a drain line for the filtrate.

The treatment parameters are also similar. For both therapies the blood flow is of major importance and should be optimised with regard to the vascular access of the patient. The weight loss is also patient related. Once the filter is selected and the blood flow rate is set, the dose of dialysis in HD is determined by the treatment time. In HF, the total volume of ultrafiltrate determines the amount of convective solute transport and thus the dose of dialysis. With present targets for adequate dialysis similar treatment times are often achieved [4, 5].

In order to quantify the dose in HD the removal of a marker solute must be measured either by sampling the blood before and after the treatment or by collection of dialysate and direct measurement. Urea has become the marker solute of choice, originally because it was believed to be a uremic toxin, secondly because it is a good marker of protein metabolism, thirdly and presently because we have generated so much data connecting urea removal to various outcome parameters that we would loose the empirical ground for all dialysis prescription if we abandoned it. If we select another marker solute in HD the values cannot simply be calculated or deduced from the values for urea, but new measurements need to be made. Quantification in HF is simpler because convective transport is directly related to molecular size via the sieving coefficient. The total volume of ultrafiltrate, corrected for the degree of dilution in predilution mode, is the total clearance of all solutes that are completely sieved by the membrane. Thus, we only need to know the volume of ultrafiltrate, and in relevant cases the degree of dilution, to have information about the clearance of a whole range of solutes [6].

Solute Removal

In HD, solutes are removed from blood in relation to their molecular weight irrespective of the choice of membrane. The clearance of small solutes is high but the transport rate across the membrane falls rapidly when the weight and size of the molecules increase. In HF, the pore size of the membrane determines the range of solutes removed because all solutes that can pass through the pores of the membrane are cleared at an equal rate. This has always been and still is the main difference between HF and HD and the main argument for HF. Because the standards for dialysis adequacy are based on experience gained with HD, small solute clearance has become a goal in itself. When dialysis therapy has been upgraded to provide greater overall blood purification, this has usually been expressed as a higher clearance goal for small solutes, which has not always been possible to achieve with HF. However, the implementation of predilution rather than postdilution has made it possible to reach realistic targets for small solute clearance also in HF [6].

Every year a number of solutes are added to the list of potential uremic toxins, some of them closely associated with inflammatory and cardiovascular complications in ESRD patients [7]. Most of these solutes are of a size that makes them poorly removed by HD but effectively cleared from circulating blood by HF. The impact of convective therapies on a large molecule such as β_2-microglobulin (β_2m) has been addressed in retrospective studies based on registry data from Europe and Japan [8, 9]. They show that complications from accumulation and deposition of β_2m are increasingly delayed by therapies that promote the removal of the molecule from blood, even though plasma levels are not normalized.

Hemodynamic Stability

Loss of fluid from the vascular space normally elicits an increase in peripheral resistance that preserves the blood pressure. This physiological mechanism is also the response to fluid removal during HF, while its absence during HD often leads to hypotensive episodes and other symptoms of intolerance. A number of investigators have documented the stabilising effect on blood pressure by HF, whether conducted in postdilution or predilution mode [3, 10]. In addition to this acute effect, a long-term progressively stabilizing action of HF was noted in two recent prospective studies, conducted in Sardinia [4, 5]. Each study included around 20 stable dialysis patients, treated in cross-over design with HD and HF under similar conditions – membrane, fluid quality and treatment time were unchanged – and in the second study even the urea clearance was kept constant. Both studies show a significant difference in the frequency of symptoms during as well as between the dialysis sessions, all to the advantage of HF. These data are confirmed by observations from Bologna where a group of 9 unstable patients with severe comorbidities were transferred from HD to HF because of treatment intolerance [11]. This resulted in a significantly reduced number of symptomatic sessions and premature interruptions of treatment.

Mechanism for Hemodynamic Stability

Only a few of the originally proposed mechanisms for the observed hemodynamic stability of HF remain when the comparison is made with modern HD. The difference in solute transport is a fact and if there were a large vasoactive molecule, the function of which was to destabilize the capillary wall, its removal might bring about the effect we see in HF. A candidate for this could be calcitonin gene-related peptide [12].

Since the early days, sodium retention has been proposed to contribute to the preservation of vascular volume and stability in HF. Ultrafiltration of blood creates protein polarisation on the membrane and sodium ions are held back through the Donnan effect. Such sodium retention should be less in predilution HF, but this was not confirmed by recent measurements [13]. If sodium retention were the main mechanism behind the cardiovascular stability in HF, one would expect HD with correspondingly elevated sodium levels to produce a similar result, but this has not been shown to be the case [14]. Furthermore, one would expect to see an effect of sodium retention on plasma sodium levels, but no observations of such phenomena have been reported among patients chronically treated with HF.

A third proposed mechanism is based on the cooling and thus stabilizing effect induced by the absence of temperated dialysis fluid in HF. It has been shown that the use of heated infusion solution which increases the temperature of blood abolishes the increase of peripheral resistance in HF [10]. However, if this were the major mechanism providing hemodynamic stability it should be possible to mimic the effect by performing HD with cold dialysate. Although cold HD is known to confer a certain vascular stability, the effect is of short duration and probably has little impact on overall blood pressure control. The evasive nature of the mechanism behind the hemodynamic stability of HF therapy leads us to conclude that it is most likely of multifactorial origin.

Conclusion

Convective transport across membranes with sieving properties that mimic those of the glomerular basement membrane results in a solute removal profile that is closer to that of the human kidney than any diffusion-based therapy can provide. Thus, HF is the renal therapy that most closely approaches the function of the human kidney [15]. To make the therapy even more physiological, we need to adapt the duration and the frequency of treatment towards a more continuous schedule. However, also in its present application HF deserves to be utilized to a greater extent than is presently practised, because it fulfils two important requirements that we may be missing with standard dialysis therapy. HF clears blood from solutes of a wider molecular weight spectrum, including many recently identified uremic toxins that may be associated with severe complications and are discriminated against by standard HD. Furthermore, HF seems to provide better protection of the cardiovascular system against the fluctuations in extracellular volume unavoidable for renal failure patients. These features are desirable characteristics of an ideal dialysis therapy for our aging, often diabetic, dialysis population with severe cardiovascular comorbidity.

References

1 Henderson LW, Colton CK, Ford CA: Kinetics of hemodiafiltration. II. Clinical characterization of a new blood cleansing modality. J Clin Lab Med 1975;85:372–391/J Am Soc Nephrol 1997;8: 494–508.

2 Henderson LW, Sanfelippo ML, Beans E: On line preparation of sterile pyrogen-free electrolyte solution. Trans Am Soc Artif Intern Organs 1978;XXIV:465–467.

3 Fox SD, Henderson LW: Cardiovascular response during hemodialysis and hemofiltration: Thermal, membrane, and catecholamine influences. Blood Purif 1993;11:224–236.

4 Altieri P, Sorba GB, Bolasco PG, Bostrom M, Asproni E, Ferrara R, Bolasco F, Cossu M, Cadinu F, Cabiddu GF, Casu D, Ganadu M, Passaghe M, Pinna M: On-line predilution hemofiltration versus ultrapure high-flux hemodialysis: A multicenter prospective study in 23 patients. Blood Purif 1997;15:169–181.

5 Altieri P, Sorba G, Bolasco P, Asproni E, Ledebo I, Cossu M, Ferrara R, Ganadu M, Cadinu F, Serra G, Cabiddu G, Sau G, Casu D, Passaghe M, Bolasco F, Pistis R, Ghisu T: Predilution hemofiltration – the second Sardinian multicenter study: Comparisons between hemofiltration and hemodialysis during identical Kt/V and session times in a long-term cross-over study. Nephrol Dial Transplant 2001;16:1207–1213.

6 Ledebo I: Predilution hemofiltration: a new technology applied to an old therapy. Int J Artif Organs 1995;18:735–742.

7 Vanholder R, Argilés A, Baurmeister U, Brunet P, Clark W, Cohen G, de Deyn PP, Deppisch R, Descamps-Latscha B, Henle T, Jörres A, Massy ZA, Rodriguez M, Stegmayr B, Stenvinkel P, Wratten ML: Uremic toxicity: Present state of the art. Int J Artif Organs 2001;24:695–725.

8 Locatelli F, Marcelli D, Conte F, Limido A, Malberti F, Spotti D: Comparison of mortality in ESRD patients on convective and diffusive extracorporeal treatments. Kidney Int 1999;55: 286–293.

9 Nakai S, Iseki K, Tabei K, Kubo K, Masakane I, Fushimi K, Kikuchi K, Shinzato T, Sanaka T, Akiba T: Outcomes of hemodiafiltration based on Japanese dialysis patient registry. Am J Kidney Dis 2001;38:S212–S216.

10 van Kuijk WHM, Hillion D, Savoiu C, Leunissen KML: Critical role of the extracorporeal blood temperature in the hemodynamic response during hemofiltration. J Am Soc Nephrol 1997;8: 949–955.

11 Mancini E, Sorice M, Santoro A: Chronic effects of on-line hemofiltration (HF): Monocenter study. J Am Soc Nephrol 2001;12:270 A.

12 Henderson LW: Hemodynamic instability during different forms of dialysis therapy: Do we really know why? Blood Purif 1996;14:395–404.

13 Locatelli F, Di Filippo S, Manzoni C: Removal of small and middle molecules by convective techniques. Nephrol Dial Transplant 2000;15(suppl 2):37–44.

14 de Vries PMJM, Olthof CG, Solf A, Schuenemann B, Oe PL, Quellhorst E, Schneider H, Donker AJM: Fluid balance during hemodialysis and hemofiltration: The effect of dialysate sodium and a variable ultrafiltration rate. Nephrol Dial Transplant 1991;6:257–263.

15 Ledebo I: Does convective dialysis therapy applied daily approach renal blood purification? Kidney Int 2001;59:(suppl 78):286–291.

Ingrid Ledebo, PhD, Gambro Corporate Research,
Box 10101, S–220 10 Lund (Sweden)
Tel +46 46 16 91 76, Fax +46 46 16 96 91, E-Mail ingrid.ledebo@gambro.com

Ronco C, La Greca G (eds): Hemodialysis Technology.
Contrib Nephrol. Basel, Karger, 2002, vol 137, pp 227–232

The Ideal Hemodialysis Machine

Hans-Dietrich Polaschegg

Medical Devices Consultant, Köstenberg, Austria

The ideal dialysis machine does not exist and will never exist, simply because the term 'ideal' is not well defined. The 'medical ideal' machine would automatically adjust treatment parameters according to the need of the patient. This, however, would require a clear understanding of the dialysis physiology and clear goals for control parameters. Although sensors have been developed allowing balancing of electrolytes and energy and measuring blood volume changes, appropriate control algorithms are missing, possibly with the exception of thermal energy balancing. I therefore abstain from defining the 'medical ideal' machine that would require too many 'may' and 'might'.

For this investigation I define 'ideal' as realization of the utilitarian philosophers' *ideal* of 'the greatest good for the greatest number'.

Even so, I am unable to define a single 'ideal' machine good for all purposes. Rather the definition must be adapted to the environment in which the dialysis machine is used.

The 'greatest good for the greatest number' must include confirmed medical requirements, e.g., minimum dialysis doses, accuracy of controlled values, but also costs because the cost of dialysis prevents treatment of most of the world's population.

Systems Approach

The dialysis machine cannot be discussed isolated from the rest. It is part of an assembly consisting of the water treatment system, the dialysate concentrate supply, the dialysis machine, the extracorporeal circuit, the dialyzer and the data network. Its operation is related to processes. The most important ones being control of treatment, disinfection, waste management and maintenance.

A dialysis machine can only be optimized for a given environment. While dialysis machines are well standardized, water treatment and concentrate supply is not. A dialysis machine adaptable for every possible environment is not 'ideal' because it is too costly to manufacture and to operate because of many redundant components. In this paper I will therefore attempt to sketch the ideal dialysis system rather than the 'ideal machine'.

The GENIUS™ System

For medium-sized dialysis units, the GENIUS™ developed by the late Dr. Tersteegen appears close to ideal. It has the lowest number of components of any dialysis system on the marked, does not require elaborate water and electrical installation of the treatment rooms and can run on batteries for hours. It is a simple batch type dialysis machine. Some features that are regarded as drawbacks, e.g. fixed ratios of dialysate to blood flow, maximum blood flows of 300 ml/min were specifically chosen by Dr. Tersteegen and can easily be changed without changing the principle of operation. With Dr. Tersteegen's patents expiring in ~3 years competition may reduce the market prices for the system and make it more popular. For a description of the machine and the clinical applications see Kleophas et al. [1]. The batch system does not allow 'sodium profiles' which need not be regarded as drawback anyway but it allows individualization of the dialysate composition in a way not possible with conventional systems, e.g. addition of amino acids or vitamins.

Conventional Dialysis Units

Conventional dialysis units may still be preferable for the existing organizational structures. In the past such units were often operated with central dialysate delivery machines and bed side monitors. Criticisms of such systems were the lack of individual dialysate adjustment, bacterial contamination and the hazard of catastrophic failure in case of a chemical disinfection malfunction. Despite the lack of individualization of dialysate excellent and even superior patient survival rates have been reported from clinics using such systems as, e.g. Tassin in France [2]. Also, central delivery systems have been used widely in Japan and are still in use there. Today's technology makes it possible to design such systems without the drawbacks mentioned above.

State-of-the-art individual dialysis delivery systems reduce water pressure of the RO water to a level that can be handled by the hydraulic components of the machine. The machines heat and degas water, mix dialysate from two solid

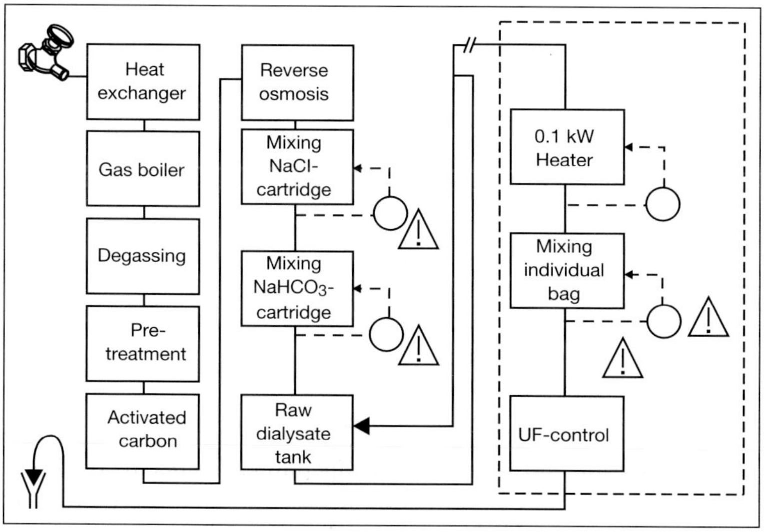

Fig. 1. Dialysis system with centralized heating, degassing and mixing of basic dialysate. Individual adjustment of dialysate composition and temperature is done at the bedside station.

and one liquid concentrate and provide for disinfection of the dialysate fluid path. Functional drawbacks of such systems are: separate disinfection of water treatment and dialysis machines with the connection between water distribution and individual machines often not disinfected at all; handling of concentrates and disinfectants, and waste of concentrates.

Technical drawbacks are an enormous waste of energy, complicated machine hydraulics and increased maintenance costs.

It is obvious that some functions as, e.g. degassing of water, can be done centrally without affecting the clinical usefulness of the dialysis machine. But also heating up to 35°C and mixing of a base dialysate containing, e.g. 134 mmol/l of Na and 30 mmol/l of bicarbonate can be done centrally. Also, automatic heat disinfection of the complete system can be easily carried out. Such a system is sketched in figure 1.

The following components of a dialysis machine would become redundant: The pressure reduction valve, heat exchanger, head tank, high-power heater, NaCl mixing, $NaHCO_3$ mixing and the disinfection system. The high-power heater would be replaced by a low-power heater allowing the machine to be designed as class II equipment.

Centrally, a high efficiency heat exchanger made from copper or a copper alloy can be used for heat recovery. Heat exchangers from copper are by far more cost efficient compared with stainless steal heat exchangers and would reduce fouling by bacteria. Next, heating can be done by a gas boiler alternatively hot water from a central boiler can be used. Effective degassing can be done by a combination of heat and reduced pressure. The quality of the material of all components upstream of the RO unit is uncritical which means that mostly conventional components used for hot water piping can be used.

Estimate of Potential Cost Savings from Heating Energy

Mean electrical heating power can be calculated by equation 1:

$$P_{heater}[kW] = (T_d - T_{in}) * Q_D * c_p * (1 - R) \qquad (1)$$

with T_d and T_{in} the dialysate and water input temperatures, respectively, [K] or [°C], Q_D. Dialysate flow [liters/s], c_p...specific heat of water [kJ/kg·K] and R ... recovery rate of the heat exchanger.

For $T_d = 37°C$, $T_{in} = 10°C$, $Q_D = 500\,ml/min$, $c_p = 4.18$ and $R = 0$ (no heat exchanger) we get:

$$P_{heater} = 0.94\ kW.$$

A dialysis machine running two 4- to 5-hour shifts a day will run ~4,000 h per year that means that each machine consumes ~3,760 kWh of electricity per year for heating. Heat exchangers as used in some dialysis machines recover approx. 30–50% of this energy.

The following example uses oil and electricity prices for an Austrian household 2001:

Electricity cost per kWh ~0.13 €.

Oil heating cost per kWh are ~0.039€ (heat of combustion for 1 liter of oil extra light ~10.2 kWh, 90% boiler efficiency).

We can now calculate the cost for dialysate heating per year (per dialysis station). With central heating, the individual temperature adjustment, an increase of 2°C maximal will still be done by electrical heating.

Depending on the comparison used (with/without heat exchanger) the cost saving ranges from ~97 to 411 € per machine and year (table 1). In the USA, where the price difference between electricity and natural gas is higher, the cost savings may be more. Also, the savings do not take potential cost savings by using environmental sources, e.g. solar collectors into account.

Most suppliers of electricity charge a basic fee depending on installed power in addition to the delivered electricity. This basic fee will be considerably reduced because the installed electrical power will be reduced by ~80%.

Table 1. Cost of dialysate heating (EURO) per dialysis machine and year

	Conventional	Central (oil, gas)	Bedside (electricity)	Central (sum)
Without heat exchanger	488.80	135.78	36.21	171.99
With optimized heat exchanger	268.84	40.73	36.21	76.94

Reduced Complexity of Bedside Stations

As an example, the flow diagram of the Fresenius 4008 from 1998 was checked. From 83 hydraulic components listed (pumps, valves, chambers, connectors) 43 could be eliminated if degassing, dialysate mixing, heating and disinfection is centralized as described above.

Reduction of the complexity of the dialysis machine will not only reduce the initial cost of the hydraulic system but also the cost and power consumption of the electronics required for operation of the hydraulic components. The machine described as example dissipates approx. 500 W to the environment. In countries where air conditioning is required this energy loss must be removed by air conditioning, usually with an efficiency of 50% or less. This means that savings of 200 W in the dialysis machine will result in reduced energy consumption for air conditioning of 400 W or power savings of 600 W total per machine. These savings are in the same order of magnitude as the savings for dialysate heating.

Reduced Concentrate Consumption

Powder cartridges are usually designed for 6 h of dialysis operation. The residues remaining after shorter treatments are usually discarded. The residues in a central supply system are much lower. Also, the volume of solid waste will be reduced.

Discussion

The basic idea of the system proposed has been described by Murisasco et al. [3]. With today's technology and knowledge this system can be further simplified. Technical development of such a system is comparably simple. Any change of the infrastructure of dialysis units, however, involves many people who must be educated and trained, and the necessary modifications can only be introduced gradually. It requires long-term thinking for introducing such a system. A country or an organization intending to develop a dialysis program for 10,000 people will require ~2,500 dialysis machines. With estimated cost savings for system investment of 25% or 5,000€ per dialysis station the initial cost savings would be 12.5 Mio€, enough for covering the costs of development. For existing systems, step-wise adaption is possible by, e.g. starting with central heating.

References

1 Kleophas W, Haastert B, Backus G, Hilgers P, Westhoff A, van Endert G: Long-term experience with an ultrapure individual dialysis fluid with a batch type machine. Nephrol Dial Transplant 1998;13:3118–25.

2 Charra B, Calemard E, Laurent G: Importance of treatment time and blood pressure control in achieving long-term survival on dialysis. Am J Nephrol 1996;16:35–44.

3 Ragon A, Reynier JP, Murisasco A, Elsen R, Leblond G: Dialysate sodium control during modeling in hemodialysis. Artif Organs 1985;9:63–65.

Dr. Hans-Dietrich Polaschegg
Oberdorf 92, A–9231 Köstenberg (Austria)
Tel. +43 4274 4045, Fax +43 4274 4096, E-Mail pg@compuserve.com

Ronco C, La Greca G (eds): Hemodialysis Technology.
Contrib Nephrol. Basel, Karger, 2002, vol 137, pp 233–244

Blood Volume Monitoring Systems and Biofeedback

Antonio Santoro, Elena Mancini

Malpighi Nephrology and Dialysis Department, Policlinico S. Orsola-Malpighi, Bologna, Italy

Dialysis treatment involves fluid removal from the circulating blood with a view to returning the patient's hydration status to normal levels. The consequent changes in blood volume (BV) strongly affect the patient's intradialytic well-being, and probably his/her interdialytic one, too. The preservation of BV and an adequate cardiovascular response to the BV reduction are the patient's main weapons for maintaining a certain hemodynamic stability [1, 2].

The sequence of the events addressed to maintaining blood pressure (BP) stability can be schematically depicted in this way [3]. Initially, ultrafiltration (UF) induces a progressive BV reduction, the magnitude of which is the result of a balancing between the ultrafiltration rate (UFR) and the vascular refilling rate (VRR). The compensation for impending hypovolemia is then based on: (1) the progressive hemoconcentration, which recalls water from the extravascular (interstitial and cellular) to the vascular space, and (2) the activation of the sympathetic nervous system, which induces peripheral vasoconstriction and a heart rate increase.

All of these compensatory reactions are blunted in older patients, having a high degree of comorbidity, especially the cardiovascular pathology, or in the hypotension-prone patients, in whom there is a reduced tolerance to fluid withdrawal and a high incidence of acute intradialysis hypotension (IDH) episodes, for a variety of reasons that are not always absolutely clear.

Preventive measures for reducing the incidence of IDH first of all include an accurate definition of dry body weight, its regular updating, the avoidance of ultrashort aggressive ultrafiltration, morning and fast dialysis, the avoidance of any drug potentially reducing BP, bicarbonate as a buffer, and an adequate sodium concentration in dialysate. Alternative dialysis techniques, such as hemofiltration which is based on a purely convective solute removal, must also be taken into account [4].

Hemodynamic Monitoring

The physicians' attention to the problem of intradialytic cardiovascular instability has increased greatly over the last decade for a number of reasons: its clinical impact may be extremely dangerous, above all in patients with a high degree of vasculopathy; its negative repercussions in terms of rehabilitation are evident, but there is also a high price to be paid in terms of dialysis efficiency. The need to control the physiological parameters related to BP preservation has thus grown stronger and stronger [5]. Technological research has tried to satisfy this need, by realizing a number of devices aimed at a noninvasive, continuous, on-line monitoring of the different parameters, both of a hemodynamic and of a biochemical kind [6].

The main aim of the continuous monitoring of the physiological variables involved in the genesis of the cardiovascular instability is a better hemodynamic surveillance, making it possible to analyze some of the adaptive responses to the UF-induced body fluid reduction and to deepen our understanding of the pathogenetic aspects of IDH. Next, some systems for continuous hemodynamic monitoring can be implemented in the dialysis instrumentation with a view to preventing the onset of acute events, such as hypotension and arrhythmias.

Ideally, all of the variables involved in maintaining blood pressure during dialysis warrant continuous measurement (BV, heart rate, stroke volume, peripheral resistances, blood temperature). However, due to the crucial role of hypovolemia in the genesis of dialysis hypotension, most of the research has inevitably been devoted to the realization of BV monitoring systems.

BV Monitoring

In the past, the only method to measure BV was of a radiopharmacological kind, with the use of dilution techniques [7, 8]. The advantage was the availability of an absolute measurement. Substances like albumin, chromium or technetium are, however, limited by their radioactivity, on the one hand, and by the need for long equilibration times, on the other, thus turning out to be impracticable for a repeated routine use. Methods measuring the relative BV changes, rather than their absolute values, have proved much more suited to the dialysis needs for instant information and repeatability.

Underlying most of the indirect methods described over the last few years is the mass concentration principle: if the mass of a certain substance does not undergo variations during hemodialysis (HD) treatment then its variations are exclusively due to the volume of the solution in which the substance is dissolved.

The relationship that allows for the calculation of the BV change after any time interval (t) can be calculated with a mathematical formula which takes into account the variations of the concentrations of the substance (x) in time:

$$BV_t(\%) = \frac{BV_t - BV_0}{BV_0} = \frac{Cx,_0}{Cx,_t}$$

Red blood cells (hematocrit), hemoglobin, plasma proteins and blood density are all variables to which the mass concentration principle can be applied for a continuous measurement of the relative changes of BV during dialysis.

The traditional hematocrit (Hmt) measure by means of the Wintrobe tube was one of the first immediate methods for obtaining information on the BV trends by way of a straightforward mathematical calculation:

$$BV\ (\%) = (Hmt_0/Hmt_t) - 1.$$

Stiller's group [9], as early as 1980, discussed the need for a continuous intradialytic measurement of BV and suggested the use of the physical principles governing light transmission of through blood to derive a measurement of the hemoglobin concentration and thus the relative changes in BV. In 1986, Maeda's group [10] described a system, suitable for hemofiltration, which, starting with the measure of the electrical resistance of blood and ultrafiltrate, could evaluate volemia variations. In 1988 De Vries et al. [11] described a much more straightforward system for the conductivity measurement of Hmt. However, one drawback of the conductivity measurement of Hmt is the possible interference with the measure of the variations in the electrolytes, the anticoagulant substances and the plasma proteins [12]. Moreover, Hmt may not vary as a result of the hemoconcentration but owing to changes in the mean corpuscular volume, as in HD with a sodium dialysate concentration higher or lower than the patient's plasma sodium one. Schneditz et al. [13] described an ultrasonographic measurement of BV exploiting the reflection properties of the sound waves by the plasma proteins. Intradialytic variations in the plasma protein mass consequent to a transcapillary escape and/or a reentry with the lymphatic circulation can, however, invalidate the measures obtained with the serum protein evaluation.

A number of years ago we tested an optical absorbance device, running with the physical principle of the transmission of light through blood [14],

Table 1. Factors affecting vascular refilling dynamics in dialysis

Related to the patient	Related to the dialysis procedure
Tissue hydration state	UFR/UF volume
Predialysis plasma volume	Dialysate osmolality
Plasma osmolality	Dialysate buffer
Plasma oncotic pressure	Dialysate temperature
Transcapillary hydrostatic/oncotic pressure gradient	Dialysate membrane
Venous compliance	
Pre- to post-capillary sphincter tonus ratio	
Regional blood flow distribution	
Vasoactive substances (ANP, nitric oxide, CGRP, NPY)	
Eating	
Body position	

capable of providing a continuous measurement of the hemoglobin concentration, from which the relative variations of BV could be calculated:

$$\Delta\%\ BV = (Hb_0/Hb_t - 1) \cdot 100$$

where Hb_0 and Hb_t are the basal (0) Hb concentration and the one measured at any time (t) during dialysis.

Today, this optical device is completely integrated into the dialysis machine which provides a continuous graphic display of the curve of the BV reduction [15]. Repeated observations on the very same patient and on different groups of patients have shown that there is an extreme variability in the BV profiles, from one patient to the next, and even in the very same patient, not just related to the entity of the UFR [3, 5, 16, 17].

This is largely due to the main patient-dependent variable affecting BV, i.e. the VRR. Indeed, at any time during dialysis, the instantaneous BV change is the result of the continuous balancing between the UFR, negatively affecting the BV, and the VRR, instead aimed at BV preservation. A number of factors, both of a dialysis nature and patient-related, may generate a different VRR behavior (table 1) and consequently a more or less acute variation in BV [17–19]. Among these, the patient's hydration state, closely related to his/her clinically defined 'dry body weight', is of paramount importance [20, 21].

Moreover, the variability of BV changes is also related to the patient's BV state prior to the start of treatment. This may vary from a state of expansion to a relative contraction, depending on the quantity, the times of accumulation and the fluid distribution modality into the different body water compartments. With a radiolabelled isotopic technique aimed at the absolute measurement of

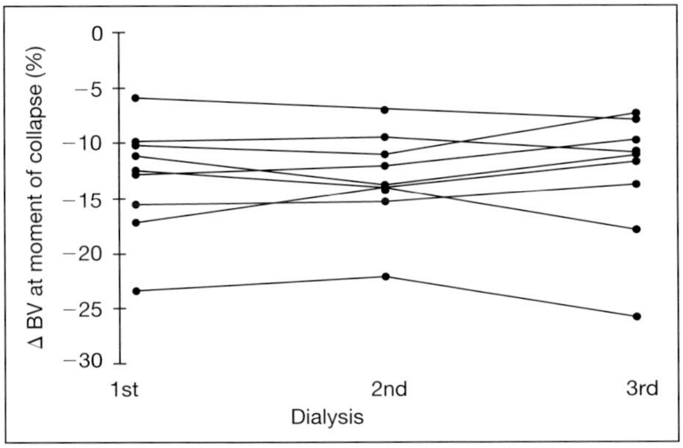

Fig. 1. Reductions in BV detected at the onset of arterial hypotension in 9 hypotension-prone patients at three different hemodialysis sessions.

BV before the dialysis sessions, we observed that patients with higher values of predialysis BV showed a smaller BV reduction normalized for the UF (ΔBV/UF) when compared to that of the patients with the lowest predialysis blood volumes.

On the whole, intradialytic BV monitoring is useful in providing information on individual vascular refilling dynamics, the individual patient's characteristics concerning the hypotension episodes and the individual critical BV for blood pressure stability [18].

Considering the latter aspect in particular, in our experience there does not seem to exist a general hypovolemia threshold level to be considered critical for the hypotension onset, since a collapse can appear in a wide range of BV reductions (5–20%). However, this may not be true for the individual patient. Steuer et al. [22] have shown that the appearance of symptoms such as hypotension, muscular cramps, or dizziness is correlated with the reaching of a clearly identified Hmt threshold with a standard deviation of only 1.4%. Even in our experience, we have found a certain consistency in the volemic reductions at the time of the collapse in the individual patient (fig. 1). It can be hypothesized that, at least in the short-medium run, each patient maintains his/her own critical level of BV reduction; beyond that, the mechanisms counteracting hypovolemia are no longer effective.

The validity of this hypothesis has paved the way for new prospects in the use of continuous volemia monitoring systems and automatic volemia modelling control during the dialysis session. But it is necessary to stress that the detection of an individual level of critical hypovolemia is not enough to rectify the problem of dialysis hypotension: any changes in the variables affecting vascular

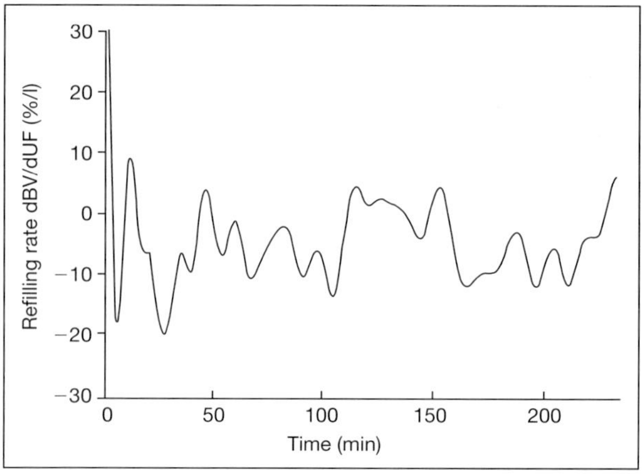

Fig. 2. Variability of plasma refilling rate expressed as change in BV per liter of ultrafiltrate (dBV/dUF): wide and acute variations throughout the dialysis session in spite of a constant UFR.

refilling regulation, serum osmolarity, electrolyte and protein concentrations, changes in body position and/or eating during dialysis and drugs, can always unpredictably modify the 'critical BV level', which should always be regularly controlled and updated.

Moreover, the continuous BV monitoring device could be implemented in a multivalent hemodynamic monitoring system, with a view to realizing a statistical model, operating on-line during HD, predicting the onset of a critical hemodynamic condition with an acute blood pressure drop. The practical realization of an on-line alarm system is, however, hindered by the fact that these models can only be used in patients repeatedly studied before [5]. Indeed, the coefficients and the constants relating BV and other hemodynamic variables to BP need to be repeatedly evaluated before an alarm system can be devised. This fact makes the widespread use of such a system in an unselected patient population impossible.

However, BV monitoring alone cannot take account of all the variables that unpredictably interfere with vascular refilling [17, 23], which vary erratically throughout dialysis (fig. 2). Hence, the relationship between the UFR and BV cannot be linear; actually, continuous monitoring proves that it changes not only from patient to patient but it is also variable during the dialysis session. So it is unlikely that BV changes can be instantaneously predicted from mathematical models. Only an adaptive control method can overcome the variabilities in vascular refilling dynamics, and guide the BV intradialytic trends along a preset trajectory (biofeedback systems).

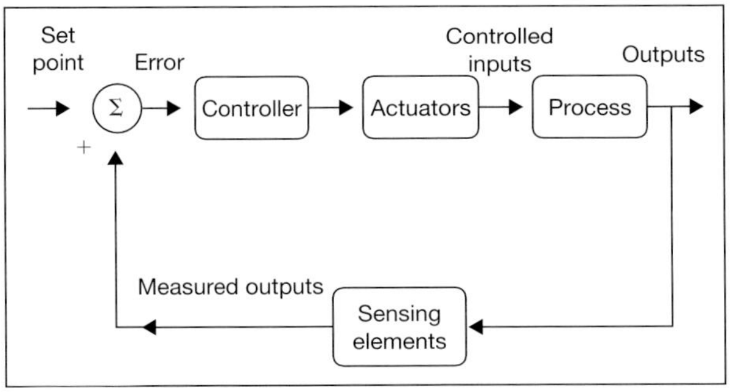

Fig. 3. Components and the relationships of the program in a feedback control system.

The Biofeedback Control

The idea of an automatic BV feedback control system during dialysis re-proposes what already exists in nature. In physiology, the term biofeedback is synonymous with a servo-system, which controls a biological process, such as muscular coordination and metabolism. A classic example is that of body temperature regulation, which is kept constant independently of the outside temperature. Deep and skin thermoreceptors continuously measure core and surface temperature and send this information to the hypothalamic integrated control centers. From here the orders are transmitted that modify the activity of the effectors, the skin blood flow first of all, the sweat rate and shivering, all of which contribute to keeping the body core temperature constant, in spite of any great or small changes in the outside temperature. Learning from nature, bioengineering has codified the basic components of a biofeedback system: the plant, the sensors, the actuators and the controller (fig. 3). The plant is the biological process that we need to control, while the sensors are the devices used for measuring the output variables. These are the variables measured and compared to the inputs, i.e. the reference value for the output. The controller is the mathematical model that continuously sets the measured output variable against the reference input and modifies the actuators in order to reduce any discrepancies.

Mathematically speaking, the formulation of a control problem requires three kinds of information: the behavior of the system (plant), the aim of the control, and the environment (noise): all three of these items of information must be specified in a mathematically accurate way. Yet in practice there are a number of conceptual, physical and technological difficulties to be overcome. In particular, in some circumstances, the behavior of what is to be controlled may be nonlinear and time-varying depending on the turbulence from the environment, and there may also be an interaction between the actuators and the controlled variable. In these cases, more sophisticated control systems are needed, which must be capable of identifying the behavior of the process, i.e. finding out the mathematical relationship linking the input and the output variables, and continuously update these data while the control is on. These complex systems are called adaptive controllers. The intradialytic BV control system described here belongs to this category.

The Biofeedback Control of BV

Having built up a large body of knowledge on BV monitoring, and starting from the same basal instrumentation (an optical device), several years ago we developed and tested a BV control system capable of forcing the patient's spontaneous BV changes along a desired preset trajectory (BV tracking). In the first version, the system could control BV via UFR modulation alone [24], but it was not always capable of guaranteeing the desired volemia trends together with the target of the total planned body weight loss (BWL): in nearly 30% of the sessions these goals turned out to be incompatible within the predefined treatment times [24]. A second effector, dialysate conductivity (DC), was then introduced. The increase or decrease of dialysate sodium concentration, via a variation of the extracellular fluid osmolarity, can in fact promote a two-directional water movement between the extra- and intravascular compartments, consequently varying the BV behavior [25–28]. Moreover, apart from BV preservation, 'boluses' of high sodium dialysate with a consequent temporary increase in plasma sodium allow the autonomic nervous system to make better compensatory adjustments to hypovolemia-induced BP reduction, namely an increase in the systemic vascular resistances.

The BV tracking system does not analyze the numerous factors affecting vascular refilling, which are treated here as if they were a 'black box', and only input (the BV changes, controlled variable) and output variables (UFR and DC, control variables) are necessary. In actual fact, the systems on-line also measure: (1) the difference between the instant actual BWL and that predicted by the model at that moment, and (2) the difference between the actual and predicted equivalent conductivity (the conductivity value which, in standard dialysis, produces the same sodium balance as in the BV-controlled dialysis). The system then turns out be a multi-input/multi-output closed loop system, with 3 controlled variables: the BV changes, the BWL and the equivalent conductivity, and 2 control variables, the UFR and DC (fig. 4) [29].

The two control variables are modified according to a mathematical model, so that the actually obtained BV profile, and consequently the BWL and EC, come as close as possible to the preset desired profiles.

The core of the system is an adaptive controller, which, at any time during dialysis, after the measurement of the spontaneous BV variations, the actual

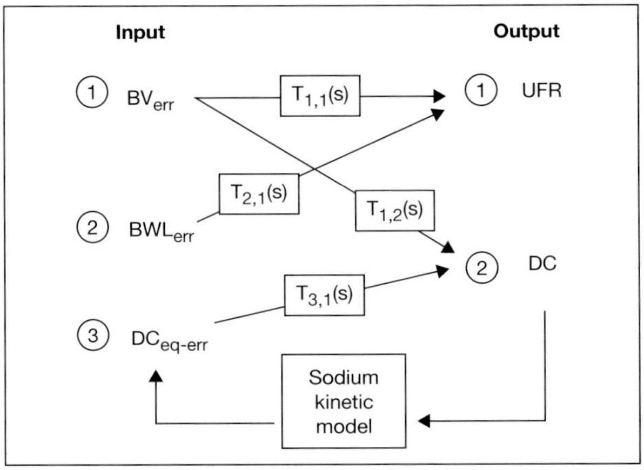

Fig. 4. Structure of the multi-input/multi-output (MIMO) controller. During the dialysis session it manages three kinds of error (differences between the prescription and the actual results obtained): BV errors, BWL errors and equivalent conductivity (DC_{eq}) errors. On the basis of the estimated errors, the controller modifies the instantaneous values of the effectors, the UFR and the dialysate conductivity.

total BWL and the actual EC, calculates: the mathematical coefficients that link the controlled variables to the control variables, the instantaneous errors in the actual BV trajectory compared to the ideal one, and the resulting new values of the control variables (UFR and DC) able to offset the error in the BV trajectory, also taking into account the desired BWL and EC.

A kinetic two-compartment sodium model actually operates together with the automatic model, as described by Pedrini et al. [30], which continuously calculates the theoretical systemic concentration of the patient's plasma sodium. This kinetic model, which considers the systemic sodium concentration as a function of time, has been validated by comparing computer simulation results with experimental data and allows for a continuous control of the sodium balance [29].

Aiming at the same time at three different targets (the BV change, the BWL and the desired EC), the adaptive controller adopts a strategy which makes it possible to obtain the best compromise among the errors in the three targets for that individual patient in that single session. The continuous and combined correction of each error throughout the session leads to an equilibrium point at the end of dialysis, which must match the initial choices made in terms of BV, BWL and EQ [29].

The largest clinical validation of BV tracking is represented by a multicenter protocol involving 10 Italian nephrology units (Bologna Malpighi,

Chieti, Gorizia, Leno, Lodi, Martina Franca, Novara, Milano San Carlo, Ostia and Trieste). In this study [31], carried out in 36 patients with a high degree of cardiovascular comorbidity and suffering from frequent dialysis-induced hypotensive episodes, cardiocirculatory stability during dialysis was compared in two different treatments: conventional dialysis (A treatment) and dialysis with BV tracking (B treatment). Each patient served as his/her own control, and was randomly assigned either to a sequence A-B-A-B or B-A-B-A, with each period lasting 4 weeks. At the end of the study, a 30% reduction in the dialysis hypotension incidence resulted in dialysis with the BV tracking system. The effect was particularly evident in patients with the highest number of hypotensive events in conventional dialysis (in these patients the reduction of hypotension was by as much as 65%). The results concerning the hemodynamic treatment tolerance were reinforced by the observation of a 10% overall reduction in interdialysis symptoms (thirst, cramps, fatigue). Body weight gain, predialysis blood pressure, and Kt/V did not differ between the two treatments.

Confirmation of our results comes from Basile et al. [32], who also compared conventional bicarbonate dialysis with biofeedback-equipped dialysis in 19 HD patients over the short-medium term. They found a reduction in both acute hypotension and muscle cramps and a significant difference in postdialysis asthenia. The residual BV %/Δ extracellular fluid volume % ratio (measured by a bioimpedance technique) was significantly higher during HD with biofeedback, suggesting a better capacity of refilling in dialysis with BV control. Once again the BV tracking system proves less 'unphysiological' compared to conventional treatment. The continuous adaptation of both the UFR and DC to the instant vascular refilling capacity preserves more water in the interstitial fluid compartment or reduces the intracellular shift: vascular refilling is in any case optimally safeguarded and enhanced.

Ronco et al. [33], besides observing similar results in terms of hypotension prevention, reported also better values of equilibrated Kt/V in BV-controlled HD, with a striking reduction in postdialysis percentage urea rebound (6.4 ± 2.3 vs. $14.2 \pm 2.7\%$, in BV controlled and standard HD, respectively). Hence, the better hemodynamic stability obtained thanks to the biofeedback reflects positively in terms of HD efficacy: it reduces solute compartmentalization and favors a better blood flow distribution within the body. As a consequence, the amount of urea accessible to the dialyzer is greater, as is the amount of urea actually removed.

In conclusion, our clinical experience confirms that the intradialytic BV control proves to be particularly useful in improving the tolerance to treatment in (1) patients with hypovolemic hypotension with an identifiable critical BV threshold; in these circumstances the cause-and-effect relationship between hypovolemia and hypotension may be broken, preventing the achievement of critical volemia, and (2) patients with an instability or inefficacy of the vascular refilling dynamics (diabetic patients above all, but also patients with severe malnutrition or dehydration); in this case, the system guarantees the continuous adaptation of water withdrawal to the instant capacity of the vascular refilling, forcing fluid removal when refilling is efficient and instead smoothing ultrafiltration and increasing plasma osmolarity, via dialysate conductivity, in the periods of acute BV decrease indicating refilling insufficiency.

This instrumentation is at present the most advanced application of the systems for monitoring BV. Nevertheless, it should not be considered a static system. By definition, integrated control systems have an open architecture, and new devices, to measure, or even to control variables other than BV, should be freely integrated if and when required. Blood temperature and solute clearance are two examples of parameters which could be monitored and controlled, together with BV, by a unique complex system. Researchers have already oriented their technological research in that direction.

References

1 Zucchelli P, Santoro A: Dialysis-induced hypotension: A fresh look at pathophysiology. Blood Purif 1993;11:85–98.
2 Daugirdas JT: Dialysis hypotension: A hemodynamic analysis. Kidney Int 1991;39:233–346.
3 Leunissen KML, Noordzig JC, Van Hoff JP: Pathophysiology aspects of plasma volume preservation during dialysis and ultrafiltration, in Klinkman H, Smeby IC (eds): Terminal Renal Failure: Therapeutic Problems, Possibilities and Potentials. Contrib Nephrol. Basel, Karger, 1990, vol 78, pp 201–211.
4 Santoro A, Mancini E, Zucchelli P: The impact of hemofiltration on the systemic cardiovascular response. Nephrol Dial Transplant 2000;15(suppl 2):49–54.
5 Santoro A: On-line monitoring. Nephrol Dial Transplant 1995;10:615–618.
6 Santoro A, Mancini E, Spongano M, Di Giovannantonio C, et al: The continuous monitoring of dialysis adequacy parameters. Issues Nephrosci 5.94. Milano, Wichtig Editore, 1995, pp 69–88.
7 International Committee for Standardisation in Haematology: Recommended methods for measurement of red cell and plasma volume. J Nucl Med 1980;21:793–800.
8 Santoro A, Mancini E, Paolini F, Zucchelli P: Blood volume monitoring and control. Nephrol Dial Transplant 1996;11(suppl 2):42–47.
9 Schallenberg U, Stiller S, Mann H: A new method of continuous hemoglobinometric measurement of blood volume during hemodialysis. Life Support Syst 1987;5:293–305.
10 Maeda K, Shinzato T, Yoshida F, et al: Newly developed circulating blood volume monitoring system and its clinical application for measuring changes in blood volume during hemofiltration. Artif Organs 1986;10:452–459.
11 De Vries PMJM, Kouw PM, Mejer JH: Changes in blood parameters during hemodialysis as determined by conductivity measurements. ASAIO Trans 1988;34:623–626.
12 Steuer RR, Harris DH, Conis JM: A new optical technique for monitoring hematocrit and circulating blood volume: Its application in renal dialysis. Dial Transplant 1993;22/5:260–265.
13 Schneditz D, Pogglitsch H, Horina J, Binswanger U: A blood protein monitor for the continuous measurement of blood volume changes during hemodialysis. Kidney Int 1990;38:342–346.
14 Mancini E, Santoro A, Spongano M, Paolini F, et al: Continuous on-line optical absorbance recording of blood volume changes during hemodialysis. Artif Organs 1993;17:691–694.

15 Paolini F, Mancini E, Bosetto A, Santoro A: Hemoscan™: A dialysis machine-integrated blood volume monitoring. Int J Artif Organs 1995;18:487–494.
16 Kimura G, Van Stone JC, Baven J: Model prediction of plasma volume change induced by hemodialysis. J Lab Clin Med 1984;104:932–938.
17 Schneditz D, Roob J, Osvald M, Pogglitsch H, et al: Nature and rate of vascular refilling during hemodialysis and ultrafiltration. Kidney Int 1992;42:1425–1433.
18 Santoro A, Mancini E: Clinical significance of intradialytic blood volume monitoring. Int J Artif Organs 1997;20:1–6.
19 Ilimura O, Tabei L, Nagashima H, Asano K: A study on regulating factors of plasma refilling during hemodialysis. Nephron 1996;74:19–25.
20 Koomans HA, Geers AB, Meers EJD: Plasma volume recovery after ultrafiltration in patients with chronic renal failure. Kidney Int 1984;26:848–854.
21 Wizeman V, Leibinger A, Mueller K, Nilson A: Influence of hydration state on plasma volume changes during ultrafiltration. Artif Organs 1995;19:416–419.
22 Steuer RR, Leypolt JK, Cheung AK: Hematocrit as an indicator of blood volume and predictor of intradialytic morbid events. ASAIO J 1994;40:M691–M696.
23 Keshaviah PR, Ilstrup KM, Shapiro FL: Dynamics of vascular refilling. Prog Artif Organs 1983; 2:506–510.
24 Santoro A, Rossi M, Paolini F, Mancini E, et al: Parameter estimator and adaptive controller in regulating intradialytic blood volume trends, in Blood Purification in Perspective: New Insight and Future Trends. ICAOT Press, 1992, vol 2, p 74.
25 Santoro A, Mancini E, Paolini F, Zucchelli P: Automatic control of blood volume trends during hemodialysis. ASAIO J 1994;40:M419–M422.
26 Fleming SJ, Wilkinson JS, Greenwood RN, Aldridge C, et al: Effect of dialysate composition on intercompartmental fluid shift. Kidney Int 1987;32:267–273.
27 Swartz RD, Somermeyer MG, Hsu CH: Preservation of plasma volume during hemodialysis depends on dialysate osmolality. Am J Nephrol 1982;2:189–194.
28 Kouw PM, Olthof CG, Gruteke P, de Vries PMJM: Influence of high and low sodium dialysis on blood volume preservation. Nephrol Dial Transplant 1991;6:876–880.
29 Santoro A, Mancini E, Paolini F, Cavicchioli G, et al: Blood volume regulation during hemodialysis. Am J Kidney Dis 1998;32:739–748.
30 Pedrini L, Ponti R, Faran P, Cozzi G, et al: Sodium modelling in hemodiafiltration. Kidney Int 1991;40:525–532.
31 Santoro A, Mancini E: Effects of automatic blood volume control on the cardiovascular stability of hypotension-prone hemodialysis patients. J Am Soc Nephrol 1998;9:1364.
32 Basile C, Giordano R, Vernaglione L, Montanaro A, et al: Efficacy and safety of hemodialysis treatment with the Hemocontrol biofeedback system: A prospective medium-term study. Nephrol Dial Transplant 2001;16:328–334.
33 Ronco C, Brendolan A, Milan M, Rodeghiero MP, et al: Impact of biofeedback-induced cardiovascular stability on hemodialysis tolerance and efficiency. Kidney Int 2000;58:800–808.

Dr. Antonio Santoro, U.O. Nefrologia e Dialisi Malpighi,
Policlinico S. Orsola-Malpighi, Via P. Palagi 9, I–40138 Bologna (Italy)
Tel. +39 051 6362430, Fax +39 051 6362511, E-Mail santoro@orsola-malpighi.med.unibo.it

Ronco C, La Greca G (eds): Hemodialysis Technology.
Contrib Nephrol. Basel, Karger, 2002, vol 137, pp 245–253

Blood Temperature Monitor: A Novel Tool in the Management of Dialysis-Induced Hypotension

Frank M. van der Sande, Jeroen P. Kooman, Karel M.L. Leunissen

Department of Nephrology, University Hospital Maastricht, The Netherlands

Intradialytic hypotension continues to be a leading problem, especially in the elderly and cardiovascular compromised patient. This predominance can be explained by the fact that structural abnormalities of the heart and blood vessels increase the sensitivity of the patient to changes in fluid status. Intradialytic hypotension does not only cause discomfort, but also increases mortality, according to recent data in which a low postdialytic blood pressure was associated with a significantly increased risk for mortality [1]. Therefore, prevention of intradialytic hypotension, especially in the elderly and vulnerable patient, remains an important challenge for the dialysis physician.

The pathogenesis of hemodialysis hypotension is multifactorial, but generally results from a disturbance in any of the three major factors implicated in the maintenance of hemodynamic stability during hemodialysis: first, the refilling of blood volume from the interstitial to the intravascular compartment, so-called blood volume preservation; secondly, the constriction of the resistance vessels such as small arteries and arterioles, leading to an increase in systemic vascular resistance; thirdly, the maintenance of cardiac output, which occurs through an increase in myocardial contractility, heart rate, and constriction of the capacitance vessels such as venules and veins, leading to centralisation of blood volume. In this respect, an intact cardiovascular system is of major importance in preserving hemodynamic stability [2]. There are very strong arguments for an important role of temperature in the pathogenesis of the impaired vascular response during dialysis. New devices, such as the blood temperature monitor, enabled us to study the effects of different dialysate temperatures, but also the effect of different treatment modalities on core temperature and extracorporeal heat gain or loss on intradialytic hypotension [3–5].

Vascular Response and Temperature

An impaired vascular response is implicated in the pathogenesis of intradialytic hypotension. Isolated ultrafiltration and hemofiltration have been shown to improve hemodynamic stability, which is due to a larger increase in vascular resistance, as compared to hemodialysis combined with ultrafiltration [6, 7]. Factors like changes in osmolality and ionized calcium do not appear to be responsible for this phenomenon [8–10]. It has also been suggested that the production of cytokines, such as interleukin-1 and tumor necrosis factor-α during dialysis, leads to an increased production of inducible nitric synthetase in smooth muscle, which attenuates the vasoconstrictor response during hemodialysis [11]. However, in several studies no effect at all of ultrapure dialysate, or the use of biocompatible and bioincompatible membranes on vascular reactivity was observed [12, 13]. In addition, the time required for nitric oxide production is in disagreement with the fact that differences in vascular reactivity between isolated ultrafiltration and hemodialysis are present as early as 15–30 min into the dialysis run [14, 15].

It is likely that the energy balance between the patient and the extracorporeal circuit plays an important role in the pathogenesis of the impaired vascular response during dialysis, as the hemodynamic reaction appears to differ between dialysis with standard (37–38°C) versus cool (35–36°C) temperature of the dialysate. Both the blood pressure response and vascular reactivity is improved with the use of cool dialysate, whereas the blood returning from the extracorporeal circuit to the patient is also much cooler during isolated ultrafiltration and hemofiltration compared with 'standard' dialysis [16, 17]. Interestingly, the differences in vascular reactivity between hemodialysis and hemofiltration disappear largely when both treatment modalities were matched for blood temperature in the venous blood lines [18].

Temperature of the Dialysate and Intradialytic Hypotension

Since the early 1980s the effects of different dialysate temperatures on hemodynamic stability have been investigated [6, 19–23]. Most authors who studied the relation between the dialysate temperature and cardiovascular stability during hemodialysis found an improvement in hemodynamic stability when dialysate temperature was lowered to about 35.0°C [24, 25]. A better increase in total peripheral resistance [6, 26, 27] and myocardial contractility [28] in association with higher levels of plasma noradrenaline [24, 27] is probably responsible for these observations.

Baldamus et al. [29] observed an increase in systemic vascular resistance during the first 2 h of dialysis treatment, after which it tended to decrease. We observed only minor changes in forearm vascular resistance and decrease in venous tone during standard temperature dialysis, in contrast to isolated ultrafiltration and cold temperature dialysis, during which the vascular response was more pronounced [14, 17, 18]. During isolated ultrafiltration in the absence of dialysate and infusate blood cools during extracorporeal circulation. Maggiore et al. [30] found a difference of 2.0°C in blood temperature between the arterial and venous in isolated ultrafiltration. More recent studies showed the same results [31, 32].

During standard temperature dialysis (37–38°C) core temperature increases, which suggest an effect of the dialysis treatment on the regulation of core temperature [33–35]. The pathophysiologic mechanism behind the increase in core temperature during standard dialysis remains speculative. It was hypothesised by Gotch et al. [36] that this phenomenon was caused by initial peripheral vasoconstriction resulting in a reduction in surface heat loss, leading to an increase in core temperature. An increase in core temperature causes vasodilatation and might thus interfere with the normal vascular response to a decrease in blood volume [18]. During cold temperature dialysis (35.5°C) core temperature remained unchanged as has been shown in several studies [37–39]. Moreover, the relation between predialytic core temperature and the change in core temperature during dialysis, as shown in one of our studies [40], might provide an explanation for the findings of Fine and Penner [35] that cold temperature dialysis is most effective in patients with a low predialytic core temperature, because in these patients during standard temperature dialysis, the increase in core temperature is more distinct (fig. 1). Although often a standard dialysate temperature of 37.5–38.0°C is chosen based on the erroneous belief that this temperature is physiological, most patients have subnormal predialysis core temperatures of less than 36.5°C [32, 37–39]. Moreover, small changes in core temperature during hemodialysis have a great impact on intradialytic hemodynamic stability, as shown by several studies.

Heat Gain or Loss and Energy Transfer Rate in the Management of Hypotension

Although the effect of dialysate temperature on hemodynamics is well recognised, information on the energy transfer rate between the patient and extracorporeal system is scarce. As mentioned above, it has been observed that core temperature increases with the use of standard dialysate temperature.

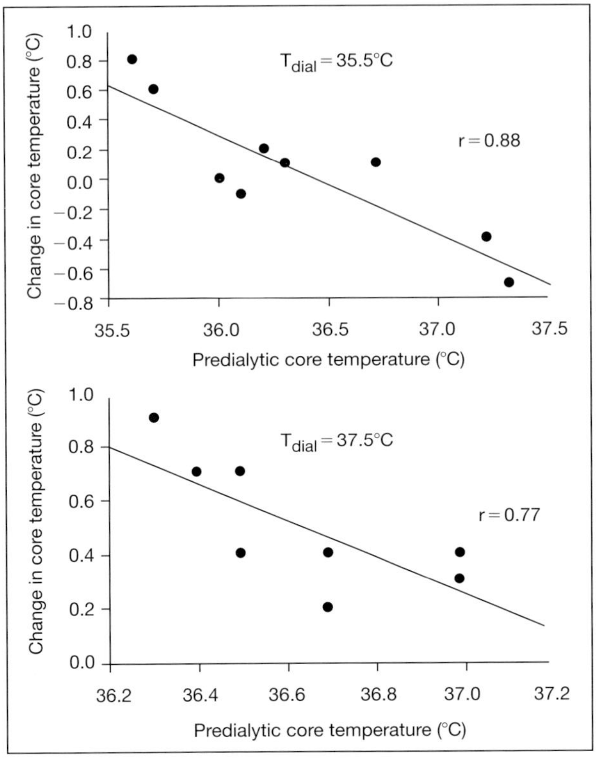

Fig. 1. Relation between predialytic core temperature and change in core temperature.

However, whether this is caused by heat load from the extracorporeal system or an effect of the dialysis procedure on core temperature regulation is not known. Moreover, there is little detailed information on the difference in energy balance between standard and cold temperature dialysate.

In a study by Schneditz et al. [41] arterial blood temperatures increased with mild extracorporeal cooling, whereas arterial blood temperature slightly decreased when heat flux was more negative (heat loss from the patient to the extracorporeal system). Moreover, the results of this study showed that during cold temperature dialysis energy flow rates were more negative the higher the arterial blood temperature and the higher the blood flow rate. On the other hand, during standard temperature dialysis energy flow rates were less negative and became even positive when arterial blood temperature was lower and blood flow rates higher. In a recent study the energy transfer rate between the extracorporeal circuit and patient, as well as the blood pressure response, during hemodialysis with the use of cold and standard temperature dialysate

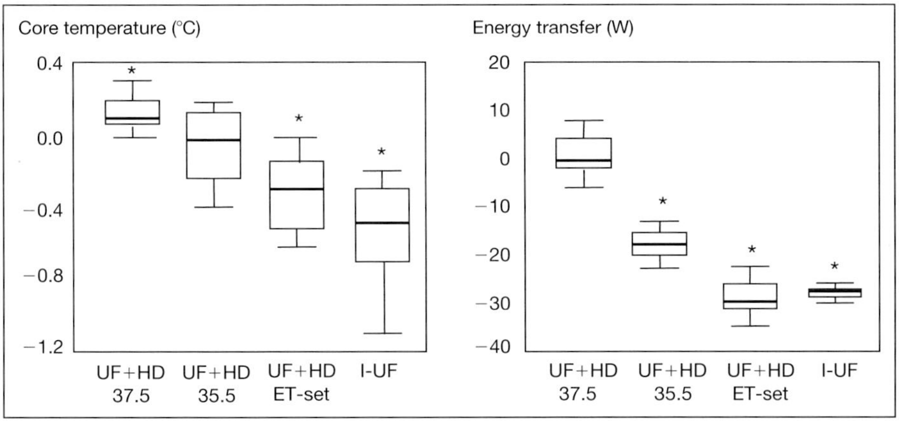

Fig. 2. Changes in core temperature and energy transfer.

was assessed [42]. Core temperature increased during standard temperature dialysis despite a small negative energy balance from the patient to the extracorporeal circuit, which might be explained by the thermal effects of hemodialysis as discussed above. However, during cold temperature dialysis, energy loss was much more pronounced, whereas core temperature remained stable, and even increased in some patients with a low predialytic core temperature. Core temperature generally remains stable during cool dialysis and decreases during isolated ultrafiltration due to pronounced energy loss from the patient to the extracorporeal circuit [31]. Thermal factors may therefore be of great importance in this respect. However, until recently, it is not known to what extent differences in extracorporeal energy transfer or changes in core temperature are responsible for the divergent vascular response between isolated ultrafiltration and hemodialysis. In a more recent study, the effect of isolated ultrafiltration, standard temperature hemodialysis, cold temperature hemodialysis, and hemodialysis matched for the same extracorporeal energy transfer rate as found during isolated ultrafiltration on changes in core temperature and vascular reactivity was investigated [32]. Core temperature decreased significantly during isolated ultrafiltration and hemodialysis matched for the extracorporeal energy transfer rate, remained unchanged during cold temperature hemodialysis, and increased significantly during standard temperature hemodialysis (fig. 2). Vascular reactivity increased significantly during the first three treatment sessions, but not during the latter (fig. 3). So when isolated ultrafiltration and hemodialysis are matched for the extracorporeal energy transfer rate, all differences in vascular response disappear, showing that differences in extracorporeal energy transfer rate are the single most important factor for the

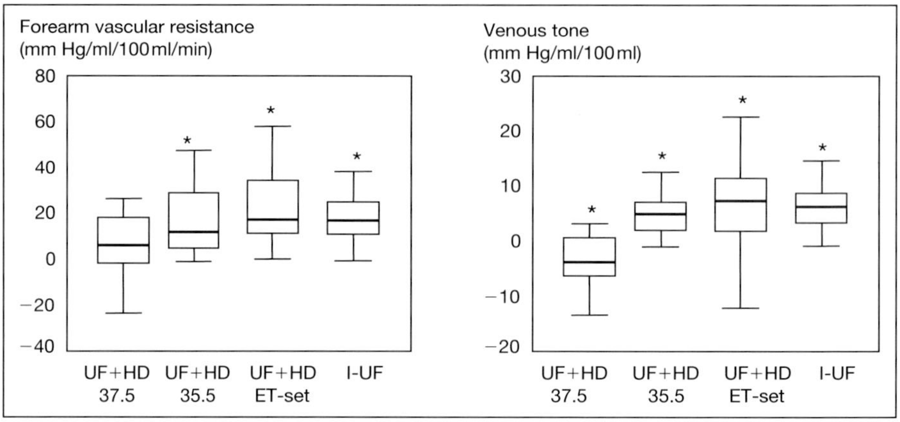

Fig. 3. Changes in forearm vascular resistance and venous tone.

observed difference in vascular response between isolated ultrafiltration and hemodialysis. In contrast to standard temperature hemodialysis vascular reactivity was improved when the increase in core temperature was prevented during cold temperature and appeared to increase more when core temperature was lowered. Finally, in another study it was concluded that in order to prevent an increase in core temperature approximately 6% of energy expenditure must be removed through the extracorporeal circulation for each percent of ultrafiltration-induced body weight change [42].

The disadvantage is that a negative energy balance and a decrease in core temperature are uncomfortable for the patient. It is sufficient, however, to only prevent the increase in core temperature during dialysis sessions [32, 43], which is not associated with complaints of shivering.

In hemofiltration, heat transfer from the substitution fluid to the blood compensates extracorporeal blood cooling. However, depending upon the infusate temperature and as a result of the relatively large extracorporeal circuit and a low infusate temperature this compensation is only partial. During hemodiafiltration with a relatively low exchange volume of 1 liter/h, extracorporeal blood temperature increased significantly, whereas on the other hand extracorporeal blood temperature remained unchanged during hemodiafiltration with an exchange volume of 2.5 liters/h [44].

Conclusion

Although the fact that decreasing the dialysate temperature improves hemodynamic stability during dialysis, the influence of this parameter seems to be widely underestimated. New techniques enable the clinician to measure and model core temperature and energy transfer continuously during dialysis. They may be of great help in the prevention of intradialytic hypotension.

Improving hemodynamic stability during dialysis is of main importance. This can be achieved with relatively simple maneuvers, such as a standard dialysate temperature of 35.5°C, which led to a stable core temperature and improvement of vascular reactivity. Decreasing the core temperature by adjusting the energy transfer over the extracorporeal system might have an additional, but minor, beneficial effect on vascular reactivity.

By using the blood temperature monitor, it is possible to automatically adjust the dialysate temperature according to the individually chosen profile of the patient. Such an approach may be of great clinical importance in preventing hemodialysis-associated hypotension.

References

1 Zager PG, Nikolic J, Brown RH, et al: 'U' curve association of blood pressure and mortality in hemodialysis patients. Kidney Int 1998;54:561–569.

2 Leunissen KML, Kooman JP, van Kuijk W, Luik AJ, van der Sande F, van Hooff JP: Preventing haemodynamic instability in patients at risk for intra-dialytic hypotension. Nephrol Dial Transplant 1996;11:S11–S15.

3 Provenzano R, Sawaya B, Frinak S, Polaschegg H, Roy T, Zasuwa G, Dumler F, Levin NW: The effect of cooled dialysate on thermal energy balance in hemodialysis patients. Trans Am Soc Artif Intern Organs 1988;17:515–518.

4 Krämer M, Steil H, Polaschegg HD: Optimization of a sensor head for blood temperature measurement during haemodialysis. Proc Annu Int Conf IEEE-EMBS 1992;14:1610–1611.

5 Krämer M, Polaschegg HD: Control of blood temperature and thermal energy balance during hemodialysis. Proc Annu Int Conf IEEE-EMB 1992;S14:2299–2300.

6 Maggiore Q, Pizzarelli F, Sisca S, Zocalli C, Parlongo S, Nicolo F, Creazzo G: Blood temperature monitor and vascular stability during haemodialysis and hemofiltration. Trans Am Soc Artif Intern Organs 1982;28:523–527.

7 Fox SD, Henderson LW: Cardiovascular response during hemodialysis and hemofiltration: Thermal, membrane, and cathecholamine influences. Blood Purif 1993;11:224–236.

8 van Kuijk WHM, Wirtz JJM, Grave W, de Heer F, Menheere PPCA, van Hooff JP, Leunissen KML: Vascular reactivity during combined ultrafiltration-haemodialysis: Influence of dialysate sodium. Nephrol Dial Transplant 1996;11:323–328.

9 van Kuijk WHM, Mulder AW, Peels CH, Harff GH, Leunissen KML: Influence of changes in ionized calcium on cardiovascular reactivity during haemodialysis. Clin Nephrol 1997;47:190–196.

10 van der Sande FM, Cheriex EC, van Kuijk WHM, Leunissen KML: Effect of dialysate calcium concentrations on intradialytic blood pressure course in cardiac-compromised patients. Am J Kid Dis 1998;32:125–131.

11 Henderson LW, Koch KM, Dinarello CA, Shaldon S: Hemodialysis hypotension: The interleukin-1 hypothesis. Blood Purif 1993;1:3–8.

12 Bergamo Collaborative Dialysis Study Group: Acute intradialytic well-being; Results of a clinical trial comparing polysulfone with cuprophane. Kidney Int 1991;40:714–719.

13 van Kuijk WA, Buurman WA, Gerlag PG, Leunissen KM: Vascular reactivity during combined ultrafiltration-hemodialysis: Influence of dialysis derived contaminants. J Am Soc Nephrol 1996;7:2664–2669.

14 Kooman JP, Gladziwa U, Bocker G, van Bortel LMAB, van Hooff JP, Leunissen KML: Role of the venous system in hemodynamics during ultrafiltration and bicarbonate dialysis. Kidney Int 1992;42:718–726.
15 Converse RL, Jacobson TN, Jost CM, Toto RD, Jost CM, Cosentino F, Fouad-Tarazi F, Victor RG: Sympathetic overactivity in patients with chronic renal failure. N Engl J Med 1992;327: 1912–1918.
16 Coli U, Landini S, Lucatello S, Fracasso A, Morachiello P, Righetto F, Scanferla F, Onesti G, Bazzato G: Cold as cardiovascular stabilizing function in hemodialysis: hemodynamic evaluation. Trans Am Soc Artif Int Org 1983;29:71–75.
17 van Kuijk WH, Hillion D, Savoiu C, Leunissen KM: Critical role of the extracorporeal blood temperature in the hemodynamic response during hemofiltration. J Am Soc Nephrol 1997;8:949–955.
18 van Kuijk WH, Luik AJ, de Leeuw PW, van Hooff JP, Nieman FH, Habets HM, Leunissen KM: Vascular reactivity during hemodialysis and isolated ultrafiltration: thermal influences. Nephrol Dial Transplant 1995;16:1852–1858.
19 Daugirdas JT: Dialysis hypotension: A haemodynamic analysis. Kidney Int 1991;39:233–246.
20 Coli U, Landini S, Locatello S, Fracasso A, Morachiello P, Righetto F, Scanferla F, Onesti G, Bazzato G: Cold as cardiovasular stabilizing factor in haemodialysis: Haemodynamic evaluation. Trans Am Soc Artif Intern Organs 1983;29:71–75.
21 Mahida BH, Dumler F, Zasuwa G, Flieg G, Levin NW: Effect of cooled dialysate on serum catecholamines and blood pressure stability. Trans Am Soc Artif Intern Organs 1983;29:384–389.
22 Sherman RA, Faustino EF, Bernholc AS, Eisinger RP: Effect of variations in dialysate temperature on blood pressure during haemodialysis. Am J Kidney Dis 1984;4:66–68.
23 Levy FL, Grayburn PA, Foulks CJ, Brickner ME, Henrich WL: Improved left ventricular contractility with cool temperature haemodialysis. Kidney Int 1994;41:961–965.
24 Lindholm T, Thysell H, Yamamoto Y, Forsberg B, Gullberg CA: Temperature and vascular stability in hemodialysis. Nephron 1985;39:130–133.
25 Marcen R, Quereda C, Orofino L, Lamas S, Teruel JL, Matesanz R, Ortuna J: Hemodialysis with low-temperature dialysate: A long-term experience. Nephron 1988;49:29–32.
26 Bazzato G, Coli U, Landini S, Lucatello S, Fracasso A, Morachiello P, Righetto F, Scanferla F: Temperature monitoring in dialysis-induced hypotension. Kidney Int 1985;28:S161–S165.
27 Jost CMT, Agarwal R, Khair-El-Din T, Grayburn PA, Victor RG, Henrich WL: Effects of cooler temperature dialysate on hemodynamic stability in 'problem' dialysis patients. Kidney Int 1993;44:606–612.
28 Levy FL, Grayburn PA, Foulks CJ, Brickner ME, Henrich WL: Improved left ventricular contractility with cool temperature haemodialysis. Kidney Int 1994;41:961–965.
29 Baldamus CA, Ernst W, Frei UW, Koch KM: Sympathetic and hemodynamic response to volume removal during different forms of renal replacement therapy. Nephron 1982;31:324–332.
30 Maggiore Q, Pizzarelli F, Zocalli C, Sisca S, Nicolo F: Influence of blood temperature on vascular stability during hemodialysis and isolated ultrafiltration. Int J Artif Organs 1985;8:175–178.
31 Keijman JMG, van der Sande FM, Kooman JP, Leunissen KML: Thermal energy balance and body temperature: Comparison between isolated ultrafiltration and haemodialysis at different dialysate temperatures. Nephrol Dial Transplant 1999;14:2196–2200.
32 van der Sande FM, Gladziwa U, Kooman JP, Bocker G, Leunissen KML: Energy transfer is the single most important factor for the difference in vascular response between isolated ultrafiltration and hemodialysis. J Am Soc Nephrol 2000;11:1512–1517.
33 Kluger M, Turnbull A, Cranston W, Wing A, Gross M, Rothenburg B: Endogenous cryogen excreted by the kidneys. Am J Physiol 1981;241:R271–R276.
34 Davenport A, Davison A, Will E: Membrane biocompatibility: Effects on cardiovascular stability in patients on hemofiltration. Kdiney Int 1993;43:S230–S234.
35 Fine A, Penner B: The protective effect of cool temperature dialysate is dependent on patients' predialysis temperature. Am J Kidney Dis 1996;28:262–265.
36 Gotch FA, Keen ML, Yarian SR: An analysis of thermal regulation in hemodialysis with one and three compartment models. Trans Am Soc Artif Intern Organs 1989;35:622–624.
37 Swartz RD, Fitzgerald F, Budd M: Body temperature in patients undergoing hemodialysis. Kidney Int 1979;16:1954.

38 Swartz RD, Fitzgerald FT, Kalousdian S, Budd M: Hypothermia in the uremic patient. Dial Transplant 1983;12:584–590.
39 Jones PG, Kaufman CA, Port FK, Kluger MJ: Fever in uremia: Production of leucocyte pyrogen by chronic dialysis patients. Am J Kidney Dis 1985;6:241–244.
40 van der Sande FM, Kooman JP, Burema JH, Hameleers P, Kerkhofs AM, Barendregt JM, Leunissen KM: Effect of dialysate temperature on energy balance during hemodialysis: Quantification of extracorporeal energy transfer. Am J Kidney Dis 1999;33:1115–1121.
41 Schneditz D, Martin K, Krämer M, Kenner T, Skrabal F: Effect of controlled extracorporeal blood cooling on ultrafiltration-induced blood volume changes during hemodialysis. J Am Soc Nephrol 1997;8:956–964.
42 Rosales LM, Schneditz D, Morris AT, Rahmati S, Levin NW: Isothermic Hemodialysis and Ultrafiltration. Am J Kidney Dis 2000;36:353–361.
43 Maggiore Q: Multicentre randomized study on the effect of thermal balance on vascular stability in hemodialysis patients. J Am Soc Nephrol 1999;10:219A.
44 van der Sande FM, Konings S, Kooman JP, Leunissen KML: Thermal effects and blood pressure response during hemodiafiltration and hemodialysis. J Am Soc Nephrol 2001;12:1916–1920.

F.M. van der Sande, MD, PhD, Department of Internal Medicine and Nephrology,
University Hospital Maastricht, P. Debeyelaan 25, PO Box 5800
NL–6202 AZ Maastricht (The Netherlands)
Tel. +31 43 3875007, Fax +31 43 3875006, E-Mail fvs@sint.azm.nl

Ronco C, La Greca G (eds): Hemodialysis Technology.
Contrib Nephrol. Basel, Karger, 2002, vol 137, pp 254–259

Optimization of Convection on Hemodiafiltration by Transmembrane Pressure Monitoring and Biofeedback

Luciano A. Pedrini, Vincenzo De Cristofaro, Bruno Pagliari, Maria Filippini, Pio Ruggiero

Nephrology and Dialysis Unit, Ospedale di Sondrio, Italy

The use of synthetic membranes has been shown to reduce both the morbidity (amyloidosis, cardiovascular disease and lipid derangement) and the mortality of chronic dialysis patients [1, 2]. Increasing evidence suggests that this reduction may be associated with the enhanced removal of toxic middle-molecular solutes which is promoted by high flux membranes, in addition to the recognized effects related to their high biocompatibility [3, 4]. To take full advantage of high flux membranes, they should be used in hemodiafiltration (HDF), and ultrafiltration (UF) should be forced in order to obtain a substantial improvement and widening of the molecular spectrum of the uremic compounds removed by convection [5]. On-line production of substitution fluid from the dialysate can supply an indefinite amount of sterile infusion at low cost. However, in order to operate safely at the very high UF flow rates needed to optimize the efficiency of the technique, knowledge of the dialyzer machine performance in terms of its hydraulic permeability and UF control system is essential. The complex interactions between the system and the patient must also be taken into account.

Hydraulic Permeability

The water permeability of a dialyzer is defined clinically as the ultrafiltration coefficient of the dialyzer (K_{UF} D, ml/h/mm Hg). K_{UF} D is usually calculated in an experimental setting, in which bovine blood at a defined hematocrit

(Hct, 28–30%) and total protein concentration (~6 g/dl) is ultrafiltered at different transmembrane pressures (TMP). For high flux membranes, the obtained UF flow rate is linearly related to TMP up to certain TMP values (200–300 mm Hg), and the slope of the linear regression defines the K_{UF} D value [6]. At higher TMP values, principally due to the main effect of plasma protein concentration polarization on the membrane surface, the relationship becomes curvilinear and eventually reaches a plateau, at which point TMP increments do not further increase the flux rate [6]. In vitro, K_{UF} D largely depends on the membrane size and characteristics (mainly their pore radius) and on the dialyzer geometry, while the level of the plateau is a function of the blood flow rate (Qb).

Even if these standard requirements for K_{UF} D determination are satisfied (and this is not always the case), setting the UF rate during HDF only on the basis of an in vitro K_{UF} D value may be misleading for several reasons. Basal Qb, Hct and protein concentration vary widely between patients, while in any one patient these parameters can vary greatly throughout the session. Protein concentration, which progressively increases with body weight loss, contributes to a thickening of the secondary layer and so limits the hydraulic permeability of the membrane. At the same time, it exerts an increasing oncotic pressure that resists UF [6]. High UF rates exacerbate this phenomenon by increasing polarization on the blood side of the membrane, while low Qb acts in the same way, by reducing the shear rate that stirs the protein layer. Even at constant Qb, K_{UF} D decreases as the session progresses, and increasingly higher and unpredictable TPM gradients are often necessary to maintain the programmed UF.

Ultrafiltration Control Systems

Dialysis machines incorporate UF control systems (fluximetric or volumetric) which set the hydrostatic pressure necessary to drive the planned water flux across the membrane. In clinical practice, the infusion volume of an HDF session is set arbitrarily, based on individual judgement. If the maximum TMP value set by the operator is reached, the infusion rate (Q_S) either scales down automatically and dilutes in time (Gambro system) or must be reset manually (Fresenius system). In both systems the recorded and displayed TMP is calculated as the difference in the pressure values as read by two transducers placed on the blood and dialysate outlet lines. In this way, it is only weakly related to the mean pressure acting across the membrane and is not at all representative of the pressure regimens occurring along the dialyzer [7].

The present technology of HDF machines does not allow the precise calculation of the infusion volume able to maximize solute removal by convection, nor does it allow the control of the complex biophysical events occurring at the capillary wall during the sessions and the consequences may be unpredictable. On one hand, critical hemoconcentration may result in total or partial clotting of the dialyzer, and beyond certain TMP or UF values protein denaturation and red cell damage may also occur [6]. On the other hand, if a too low TMP is adopted as a result of caution, reduced convective flux limits the efficiency of the technique. Predilution HDF ensures better rheologic conditions and the possibility of higher infusion and UF rates, but this advantage may be offset by dilution of the solute concentration available for diffusion and convection, with a consequent reduction of the cumulative transfer.

Biofeedback Module for TMP Control

Probably due to the scarce diffusion of HDF, there have been few studies on this subject over the last few years, after a report of the past, which established an empirical limit for UF at a filtration fraction (FF) of 0.5 [6]. Indeed, a model has only recently been proposed to monitor K_{UF} D on-line [8].

A new biofeedback mechanism for the automatic control of the UF rate through TMP has been developed in our unit on the basis of some observations. (1) At a given Qb the maximal efficiency in convective removal of small and medium molecular weight solutes occurs at the highest FF [9, 10]. (2) The highest achievable FF is often unpredictable, due to patient-related variable factors which have not yet been fully elucidated. (3) At any given Qb, TMP is exponentially related to FF, and the slope of the curve is a function of K_{UF} D [10]. (4) Above a certain level of TMP the system becomes unstable and sudden dangerous peaks are likely to occur due to small changes in blood flow or viscosity, venous pressure, or for technical reasons. A small reduction in the UF rate restores safer and stable TMP values, but the relation between UF rate and TMP has to be reset to a lower level, due to an irreversible loss of hydraulic membrane permeability (fig. 1).

In our system, using a prototype device adapted from a 4008 Fresenius monitor (Fresenius, FMC, Bad Homburg, Germany), instantaneous inlet and outlet blood and dialysate pressures of the dialyzer (Pbi, Pbo, Pdi, Pdo, mm Hg) are recorded continuously by means of four pressure transducers. Data are elaborated using computer software and the mean TMP along the dialyzer calculated using the equation:

$$TMPm = (Pbi + Pbo)/2 - (Pdi + Pdo)/2 - \pi$$

where π = oncotic pressure of plasma (in mm Hg).

Six hundred TMPm values are recorded per minute and then filtered, buffered and averaged for each minute. Instantaneous changes in plasma water

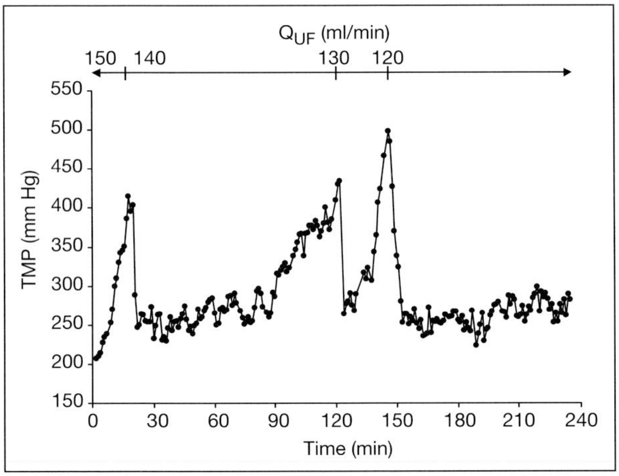

Fig. 1. Example of TMP behavior during on-line postdilution HDF at the highest UF rates and FF.

flow rate (Q_{pw}) are calculated from on-line values for effective Qb and Hct is monitored with devices integrated into the system, and using a default value for protein concentration.

Defining FF as the ratio Q_{UF}/Q_{pw}, the initial rate of substitution fluid infusion (Q_S) is set automatically in order to obtain an FF of 0.5, taking into account the desired session length (t, min) and body weight loss (ΔBW, kg). The automatic volume control system sets TMPm in order to obtain an initial $Q_{UF} = Q_S + \Delta BW$. The integrated software of the device is programmed in order to maintain TMPm within a strict range (250–300 mm Hg) by regulating the infusion pump speed: Q_S is increased by 5 ml/min at intervals of 1 min when TMPm falls below the minimum value of the set pressure range and, vice versa, Q_S is reduced by the same amount if TMPm reaches its maximum value. The biofeedback does not interfere with the planned weight loss. Whatever the Qb, Hct or protein concentration, the highest FF compatible with the actual K_{UF} D is maintained throughout the treatment.

The biofeedback was validated in 20 patients on renal replacement therapy, each of whom underwent one session of post-HDF with a high flux 2.1 m^2 polysulfone hemodiafilter (HDF 100, Fresenius, FMC). The mean effective Qb was 373 ± 57 ml/min, Hct 33.4 ± 2.2%, total proteins 6.6 ± 0.3 g/dl, and treatment time 227 ± 18 min. The device algorithm, after setting the initial Q_S to 110 ml/min (Q_{UF} = 120 ml/min, FF = 0.51), caused repeated increases of Q_S in steps of 5 ml/min in the following 10 min until TMPm stabilized within the planned range at Q_{UF} of 150 ml/min and at an FF of 0.64 (fig. 2). Subsequently, Q_{UF} was

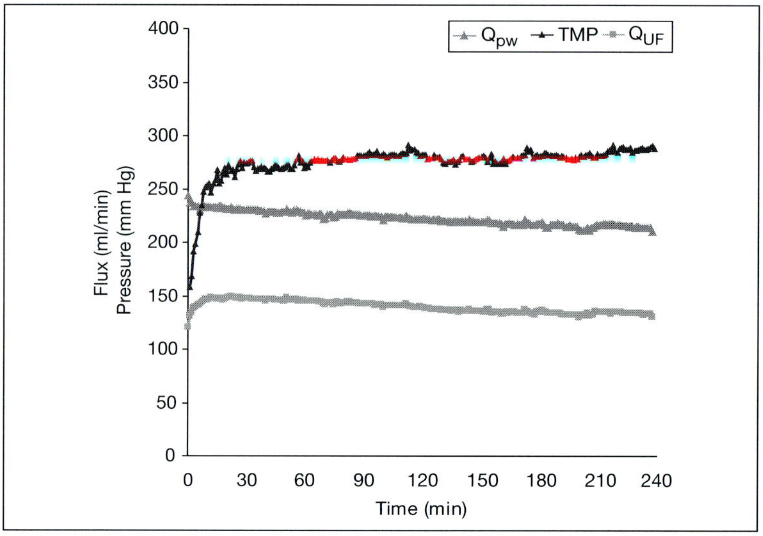

Fig. 2. Optimization of the UF rate with the biofeedback control of TMP (explanation in the text).

reset to a lower value whenever TMPm rose to its upper level, due to a progressive reduction of Q_{pw} (hemoconcentration) and the hydraulic permeability of the dialyzer membrane (the mean K_{UF} D decreased from 57 to 32 ml/h/mm Hg from the start to the end of the sessions). The final recorded Q_{UF} was 130 ml/min (FF = 0.63), and the mean amount of substitution fluid infusion averaged 30.5 ± 5.6 liters per session. The system operated automatically, without any intervention by the operators. No clinical or technical adverse effects (filter clotting or membrane damage) were observed in any experimental session.

To summarize, biofeedback allows the TMP to be set and profiled from parameters recorded on-line by the machine. It automatically adjusts the infusion rate at the maximum FF taking into account the blood flow conditions, the hydraulic permeability of the dialyzer, and their complex interactions. The device helps to fully exploit the convective mechanism of solute removal while safely optimizing the depurative capacity of HDF.

References

1 Hakim RM: Influence of high-flux biocompatible membrane on carpal tunnel syndrome and mortality. Am J Kidney Dis 1998;32:338–340.

2 Woods HF, Nandakumar M: Improved outcome for haemodialysis patients treated with high-flux membranes. Nephrol Dial Transplant 2000;15(suppl 1):36–42.

3 Leypoldt JK, Cheung AK, Carroll CE, Stannard DC, Pereira BJ, Agodoa LY, Port FK: Effect of dialysis membranes and middle molecule removal on chronic hemodialysis patient survival. Am J Kidney Dis 1999;33:349–355.
4 Port FK, Wolfe RA, Hulbert-Shearon TE, Daugirdas JT, Agodoa LY, Jones C, Orzol SM, Held PJ: Mortality risk by hemodialyzer reuse practice and dialyzer membrane characteristics: Results from the usrds dialysis morbidity and mortality study. Am J Kidney Dis 2001;37:276–286.
5 Ward RA, Schmidt B, Hullin J, Hillebrand GF, Samtleben W: A comparison of on-line hemodiafiltration and high-flux hemodialysis: A prospective clinical study. J Am Soc Nephrol 2000; 11:2344–2350.
6 Henderson LW: Biophysics of ultrafiltration and hemofiltration; in Maher JF (ed): Replacement of Renal Function by Dialysis. Dordrecht, Kluwer Academic, 1989, pp 300–326.
7 Ronco C: Backfiltration in clinical dialysis: Nature of the phenomenon, mechanisms and possible solutions. Int J Artif Organs 1990;13:11–21.
8 Vaussenat F, Bosc JY, LeBlanc M, Canaud B: Data acquisition system for dialysis machines. A model for membrane hydraulic permeability. ASAIO J 1997;43:910–915.
9 Lornoy W, Becaus I, Billiouw JM, Sierens L, Van Malderen P: Remarkable removal of beta-2-microglobulin by on-line hemodiafiltration. Am J Nephrol 1998;18:105–108.
10 Pedrini LA, De CV, Pagliari B, Sama F: Mixed predilution and postdilution online hemodiafiltration compared with the traditional infusion modes. Kidney Int 2000;58:2155–2165.

Luciano A. Pedrini
Piazza Mascheroni, 8, I–24129 Bergamo (Italy)
Tel. +39 0338 5719480, Fax +39 035 237277, E-Mail la.pedrini@katamail.com

Ronco C, La Greca G (eds): Hemodialysis Technology.
Contrib Nephrol. Basel, Karger, 2002, vol 137, pp 260–267

Potassium Profiling in Acetate-Free Biofiltration

Antonio Santoro[a], *Elena Mancini*[a], *Francesco Fontanazzi*[b], *Francesco Paolini*[b]

[a]Malpighi Nephrology and Dialysis Department, Policlinico S. Orsola-Malpighi, Bologna, and [b]Gambro Dasco, Medolla, Italy

Cardiac arrhythmias are of the most dangerous side effects of hemodialysis (HD) therapy. Electrocardiographic alterations are frequently observed in patients receiving maintenance HD [1]. HD therapy alters the duration and homogeneity of ventricular repolarization: the QT interval results significantly prolonged at the end of the treatment and this prolonging is more evident when complex premature ventricular beats occur [2]. The nonhomogeneity of ventricular repolarization induced by the HD therapy may amount to an important arrhythmia-inducing factors [1].

The mechanisms underlying the ECG alterations are not clearly known nor is their clinical relevance wholly clear. HD has a substantial impact on body fluid composition, tissue hydration and circulatory blood volume. All these factors are known to have considerable effects on the excitability of cardiac cells favoring cardiac arrhythmias and can contribute to the ECG changes observed during HD. Between these factors, the sudden reduction in the plasma potassium concentration as well as the elevation of ionized calcium plasma levels [3] may have a pivotal role in increasing ventricular arrhythmia susceptibility.

One of the aims of the dialysis treatment is to remove the potassium accumulated in the interdialytic period due to the dietary intake. The amount of potassium removed during the dialysis is strictly related to the existing gradient between the serum potassium concentration and the concentration in the dialysate usually set at a constant (lower) value (about 2 mEq/l).

In conventional HD therapy, hyperkalemic patients, who start the treatment with a high plasmatic concentration of potassium (up to 8 mEq/l), are immediately faced with a high concentration gradient between blood and dialysate. This gradient induces high K^+ diffusive fluxes through the filter membrane (dialysis ↔ extracellular), which, in turn, determines high fluxes through the cell membranes (intracellular ↔ extracellular), thus affecting the resting electric membrane potential and, consequently, cell excitability. Since this mechanism also affects the cardiac pacemaker cells, the patient is exposed to the risk of intradialytic cardiac arrhythmias. This phenomenon is much more evident in the case of cardiac diseases and may give rise to a stroke volume reduction which compromises the cardiovascular flow.

The need to combine adequate potassium removal with a limited concentration gradient calls for the introduction of potassium concentration modulation in the dialysate during the dialysis treatment.

The main aim of our study was to assess the possibility of implementing potassium concentration profiling to the dialysate in acetate-free biofiltration in order to modulate the patient's plasma K. The secondary aims of the study were the evaluation of both (1) serum potassium removal and (2) the appearance of cardiac arrhythmias during standard acetate-free biofiltration (AFB_{st}) and during AFB with potassium profiling in the dialysate (AFB_K).

Materials and Methods

Dialysate K^+ concentration profiling was implemented on standard AFB dialysis and was performed using the two dialysate preparation stages available on the Integra machine (Gambro Dasco, Medolla, Italy) in order to modulate the concentrates from two separate bags with equal concentration of all ions (Na^+, Ca^+, Mg^+) except for potassium, which is only present in one bag in a high concentration. It is therefore possible, to obtain a final dialysate liquid with a potassium concentration ranging from a maximum to a minimum value maintaining, at the same time, the concentration of other ions (fig. 1).

In $AFB_{st,}$ the usual prescription was given to the patient. The concentrate bag used was the SAFEBAG 93G, with the following composition: NaCl = 284.31 g/l, KCl = 5.22 g/l, CaCl = 10.29 g/l, $MgCl_2$ = 2.63 g/l, anhydrous glucose = 35 g/l.

In AFB_K, a special two-compartment concentrate bag (SAFEBAG KV 93G), connected to the AF and B connectors on Integra, was used to prepare the dialysate (fig. 1). The composition of the B compartment of the bag was: NaCl = 284.31 g/l, KCl = 19.57 g/l, $CaCl_2$ = 10.29 g/l, $MgCl_2$ = 2.63 g/l, anhydrous glucose = 35 g/l.

The composition of the AF compartment of the bag was: NaCl = 284.31 g/l, KCl = 0 g/l (no potassium), $CaCl_2$ = 10.29 g/l, $MgCl_2$ = 2.63 g/l, anhydrous glucose = 35 g/l.

The Integra machine automatically mixes the concentrates from the two bags in order to prepare a dialysate with a constant concentration (set by the user) of Na^+, Ca^{2+}, Mg^{2+}, and a variable concentration of K^+ according to the exponential profile.

In AFB_K, prescription was delivered according to standard AFB treatment (the same duration, infusion bags, and infusion flow). The dialysate composition (sodium, calcium,

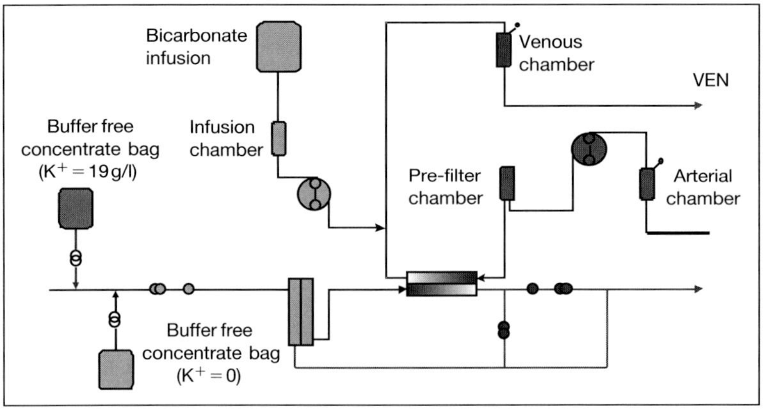

Fig. 1. Schematic representation of AFB_K dialysis. Two concentrate bags are used to prepare a dialysate with a time-varying potassium concentration, while keeping the concentration of the other solutes constant.

magnesium) was the same as in AFB except for potassium. An exponential profile was chosen for the potassium concentration in the dialysate. The initial value of such an exponential was chosen each time as 1 mEq/l below the value of the plasmatic concentration at the start of dialysis, whereas the final value was set at 1.5 mEq/l for all the patients.

Patients

For this study, 15 patients aged between 55 and 75 years old were recruited from the Nephrology and Dialysis Division of Policlinico S. Orsola-Malpighi (Bologna, Italy). Each patient was studied on two different treatments: one during AFB_{st} and one during AFB with potassium profiling (AFB_K). Potassium kinetics was evaluated in the two types of treatment by collecting samples of blood and dialysate (upstream and downstream to the dialyzer). ECG was also recorded throughout the dialytic treatment by means of a 12-derivation Holter. The machine data for each treatment were recorded by means of a PC connected to the machine and using DIALMASTER™ software.

The following patient inclusion criteria had to be satisfied: (1) a chronic renal disease, (2) on dialysis for at least 6 months, (3) undergoing three treatments per week, and (4) on AFB for at least 1 month.

Exclusion criteria were hypokalemic conditions and blood access recirculation greater than 10%. AFB_K dialysis was performed using standard Integra machines (by Hospal Dasco), whose software had been previously upgraded. The following parameters were measured on the collected samples: potassium blood concentration, sodium blood concentration, potassium dialysate concentration (pre- and post-filter), sodium dialysate concentration (pre- and post-filter).

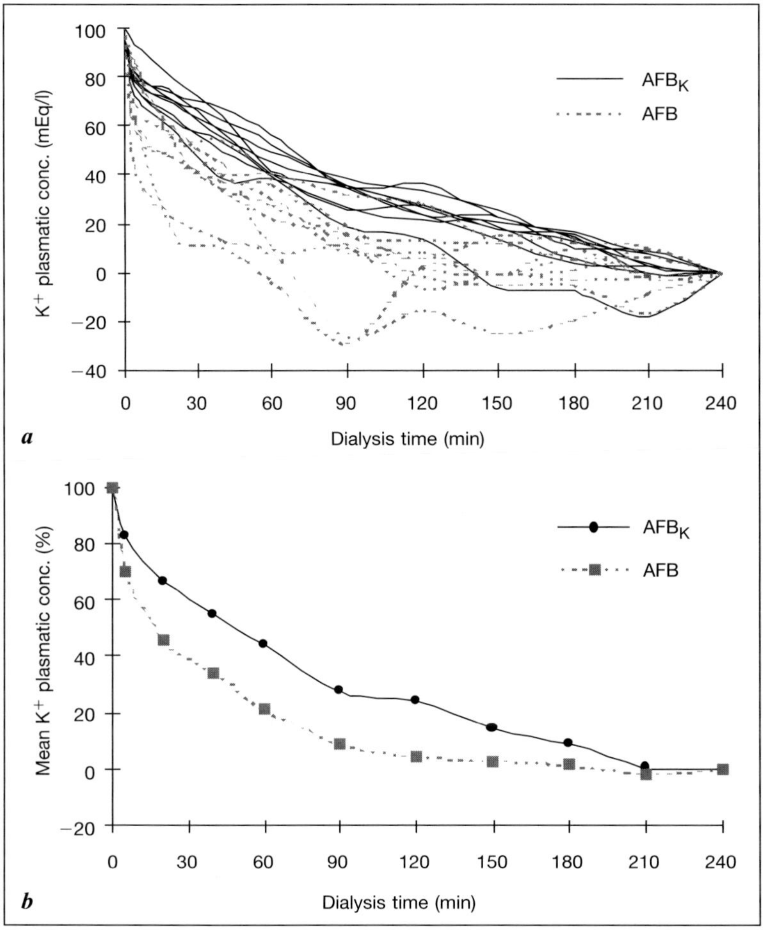

Fig. 2. a Plasmatic potassium concentrations in AFB_{st} and AFB_K expressed as a percentage of the range given by the plasmatic initial (start dialysis) and final (end dialysis) values. ***b*** Mean percentage values of the plasma concentrations.

Results

Figure 2 shows the individual and mean plasma potassium concentrations and the mean plasma potassium concentration during AFB and AFB_K dialysis. The higher concentration gradient existing between the blood and the dialysate in AFB determines a faster decay in the plasmatic potassium concentration in AFB_{st} than in AFB_K (1 mEq/l in the first 30 min in AFB vs. 1 mEq/l in the 1 hour in AFB_K).

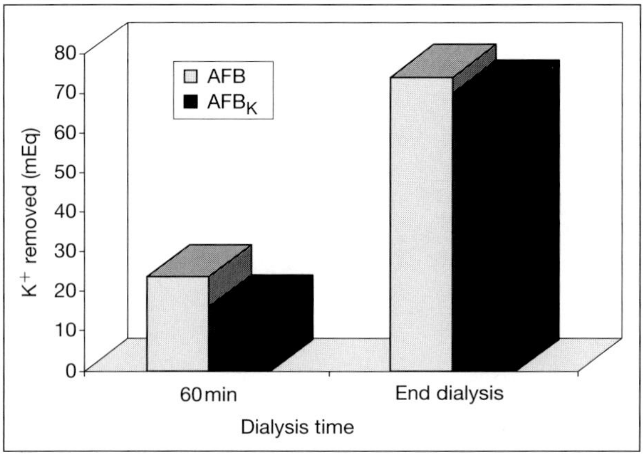

Fig. 3. Potassium mass removed at 1 h from the start of dialysis and at the end of dialysis in AFB_{st} and AFB_K. Potassium removal was significantly different ($p < 0.05$) for the two treatments at 1 h, but then was substantially equivalent by the end of the dialysis.

The quantities of potassium removed in AFB_{st} and AFB_K, to which the risk of cardiac arrhythmias in the dialytic period is related, were evaluated from the measurement of the concentration in the post-filter dialysate, after the solute exchange with the blood. In fact, by knowing the concentration in the pre-filter (prepared by Integra) and in the post-filter dialysate and the effective ultrafiltration flow rate, the potassium mass removed from the patient can be calculated. The two treatments were significantly different at 1 h from the start of dialysis, but not at the end of dialysis (fig. 3). This can be explained by considering that the mean dialysate potassium concentration in AFB_K (about 2 mEq/l) was comparable to the concentration in AFB_{st}.

A reduction in the number of intradialytic cardiac arrhythmias was observed in AFB_K dialysis. Such a phenomenon was more evident in patients for whom the presence of ventricular ectopic beats is pathological (see, for example, patients. 4, 7, 8, 13 in fig. 4). The population of the study also included nonarrhythmic patients, for whom a non-significant change in the number of arrhythmias was observed during the treatment.

Discussion

Our study showed that potassium removal during AFB might also be obtained by means of a dialysate profiling. At the end of the dialysis the amount of potassium removed from the patient is similar in AFB_{st} with a constant

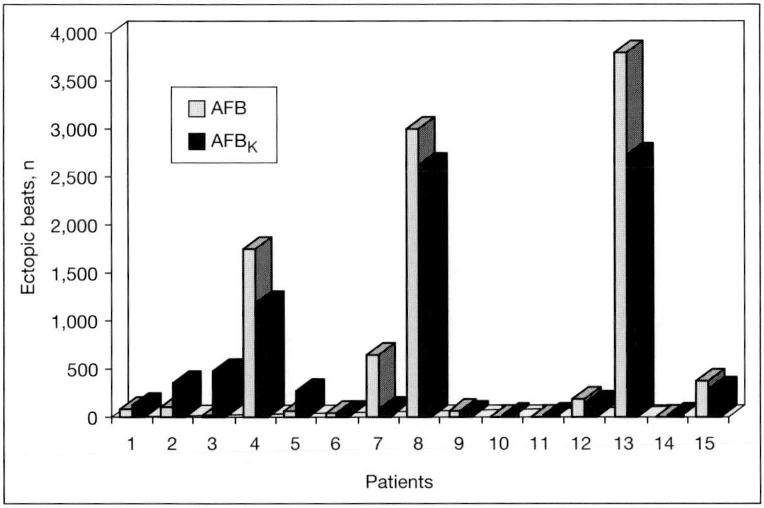

Fig. 4. The effect of AFB_K dialysis on the intradialytic cardiac arrhythmias was evaluated by studying the ECG recorded during each treatment. Arrhythmias were classified depending on their atrial or ventricular nature. In particular, the distributions of the supraventricular premature beat and of the premature ventricular contraction were calculated.

potassium concentration in the dialysate and in the AFB_K with K modulation. On the other hand, in the 1 hour of the treatment the mass of potassium removed was significantly higher in AFB_{st}. The different potassium kinetics can elicit electrocardiographic modifications and a 12-lead Holter recording adequately quantifies the complexity of these abnormalities, particularly as concerns ventricular repolarization. A slower potassium removal rate occurring in AFB_K guarantees a higher cardiac tolerability since it induces a significantly less pronounced alteration in the homogeneity of ventricular repolarization. Cardiac electrophysiology strictly relates to the kinetics of the K ion [4]. In particular, the K concentration gradient across the cell membrane is critical for the repolarization process, being responsible for both the resting and threshold membrane potentials. In fact, cardiac arrhythmias are known to be related to the imbalance of plasma K concentrations and the frequency and severity of arrhythmias increases during HD. The rise in ventricular ectopic activity during HD is correlated with low dialysate K concentrations. Hou et al. [5] observed an increase in ventricular ectopic activity during HD as the dialysate K concentration was reduced from 2 to 1 and 0 mEq/l, demonstrating that a large K removal is a critical arrhythmia-inducing factor. As a confirmation, Redaelli et al. [6] found a 32% reduction in ventricular ectopic beats using a decreasing intra-HD dialysate concentration instead of a constant K concentration of no more than 3 mEq/l. However, using dialysate K concentrations ranging from 1.7 to 3.0 mEq/l, Kyriakidis et al. [7] found that ventricular ectopic activity was unusual. This apparent contradiction in the prevalence of cardiac arrhythmias during HD may be due to the different patient populations examined or differences in cardiovascular therapies. In patients with a high incidence of cardiac diseases, such as congestive cardiomyopathy or left ventricular hypertrophy, as the majority of the patients on dialysis nowadays, dialysis may be more arrhythmia-inducing than in healthy individuals. In these patients, sudden K removal represents a dangerous arrhythmia-inducing side effect.

In the present study, a correlation is observed between the modality of potassium removal, plasma K changes and the appearance of hyperkinetic arrhythmias.

Both AFB treatments have ensured a similar and effective K removal, but because of the lower plasma-dialysate K gradient, AFB_K has produced a smooth trend in the plasma K concentration (fig. 2). The difference was well evident in the first part of treatment (first 2 h), when the continuous reduction in the dialysate K concentration occurring in HDF_K was effective and the K diffusive flux through the dialyzer was limited. In both AFB modalities, the majority of arrhythmic events occurred in the first 2 h, when the plasma K concentration change was larger. Notably, AFB_K treatment had a less destabilizing effect on repolarization compared to AFB_{st}.

Concluding Remarks

This study confirms the considerable impact of dialysis therapy on ECG modifications particularly concerning the arrhythmia onset. At the same time, this study has demonstrated that the profiling of the dialysate K concentration represents a feasible method within the AFB technique. Furthermore, the optimal K profile in AFB_K or the individual patient can be easily realized by adapting the initial potassium dialysate concentration to the patient's plasma potassium. This may reduce the therapy impact on the repolarization homogeneity as well as preventing cardiac arrhythmias.

References

1 Abe S, Yoshizawa M, Nakanishi N, Yazawa T, Yokota K, Honda M, Sloman G: Electrocardiographic abnormalities in patients receiving hemodialysis. Am Heart J 1996;131:1137–1144.

2 Suzuki R, Tsumura K, Inoue T, Kishimoto H, Morii H: QT interval prolongation in the patients receiving maintenance hemodialysis. Clin Nephrol 1998;49:240–244.

3 Nishimura M, Nakanishi T, Yasui A, Tsuji Y, Kunishige H, Hirabayashi M, Takahashi H, Yoshimura M: Serum calcium increases the incidence of arrhythmias during acetate hemodialysis. Am J Kidney Dis 1992;19:149–155.
4 Katz AM: Mechanism of disease. Cardiac ion channels. N Engl J Med 1993;328:1244–1251.
5 Hou S, Mc Elroy PA, Nootens J, Beach M: Safety and efficacy of low potassium dialysate. Am J Kidney Dis 1989;13:137–143.
6 Redaelli B, Locatelli F, Limido D, Andrulli S, Signorini MG, Sforzini S, Bonoldi L, Vincenti A, Cerutti S, Orlandini G: Effect of a new model of hemodialysis potassium removal on the control of ventricular arrhythmias. Kidney Int 1996;50:609–617.
7 Kyriakidis M, Voudielaris S, Kremastinos D, Vyssoulis G, et al: Cardiac arrhythmias in chronic renal failure. Nephron 1984;38:26–29.

Dr. Antonio Santoro, U.O. Nefrologia e Dialisi Malpighi,
Policlinico S. Orsola-Malpighi, Via P. Palagi 9, I–40138 Bologna (Italy)
Tel. +39 051 6362430, Fax +39 051 6362511, E-Mail santoro@orsola-malpighi.med.unibo.it

Ronco C, La Greca G (eds): Hemodialysis Technology.
Contrib Nephrol. Basel, Karger, 2002, vol 137, pp 268–271

On-Line Clearance: Advanced Methodology to Monitor Adequacy of Dialysis at No Cost

Frank A. Gotch

San Francisco, Calif., USA

The Dose of Dialysis

The dose of dialysis is generally defined as the total dialyzer urea clearance (K) provided during each treatment (dialyzer clearance × treatment time or K·t) divided by the urea distribution volume (V). This is the definition of single pool Kt/V (spKt/V) where V is calculated from a variable volume single pool urea kinetic model (UKM) [1]; K is dialyzer urea clearance calculated from a generic dialyzer transport constant (overall permeability area product or KoA) and the prescribed blood and dialysate flows (Qb, Qd) and ultrafiltration rate (Qf); t is the dialysis treatment time. In recent years it has become apparent that the spKt/V parameter may overestimate the dose of dialysis because of the double pool nature of urea distribution in the body and consequent rebound of BUN immediately postdialysis. Thus the delivered dose is thought to be better expressed as the equilibrated Kt/V or eKt/V which reflects the dose calculated from the postdialysis BUN after rebound has occurred. It has been established that eKt/V is a predictable function of spKt/V and the length of dialysis or the treatment time, t, expressed in minutes [2] in accordance with

$$eKt/V = spKt/V[t/(t + 35)] \qquad (1)$$

where 35 is the patient equilibration time for urea as defined by Tattersall et al. [2].

Prescribed and Delivered Dialysis Doses

There may be substantial differences between prescribed and delivered dialysis doses since the prescribed dose is based on a calculated dialyzer clearance with the assumption that Qb and Qd are constant throughout the treatment and there is no dialyzer clotting or access recirculation. There may be significant errors, often unrecognized, in these calculated dialyzer clearances resulting in underdelivery of dialysis. Measurement of the delivered dialysis dose of dialysis is typically done at most monthly from measurements of pre- and post-BUN (Co, Ct). The most rigorous method to measure the delivered dialysis dose has been analysis of Co, Ct with UKM using the recorded treatment parameters (Qb, Qd, Qf, t) and, as described above, a generic KoA for the dialyzer to estimate K and calculate V, spKt/V and eKt/V. All errors in dialysis delivery will be quantified in the calculated value for V which can be compared to the historical mean kinetic V for the patient or a value predicted from anthropometric measurements. With on-line clearance (OLC) the UKM analysis is far simpler and more precise because there is no need to estimate K from all the parameters listed above since the measured mean conductivity clearance can be entered directly into the modeling equations.

The V calculated with UKM provides a quantitative estimate of the delivered dose (since any K·t error appears as an error in V) but the confidence limits on the Kt/V estimation have been very broad, ±25% of the dose (1). Thus, if an eKt/V of 1.05 were prescribed and an eKt/V of 0.85 calculated from kinetic analysis of a set of monthly pre- and post-BUNs, there would likely be no change made in the dialysis prescription since 0.85 is within the ±25% confidence limits of measurement error with UKM. The major reason for these wide confidence limits on dose calculation with UKM is thought to be substantial variance in the time-averaged effective dialyzer urea clearance, K_e, during the treatment compared to the clearance value (K) calculated from the generic dialyzer transport constant and recorded blood and dialysate flows. It is hoped that this variability will be substantially reduced with OLC.

If the low eKt/V is due to ongoing flow errors, clotting or access recirculation resulting in a low K_e, the inadequate level of therapy will likely continue at least for another month until the next pre- and post-BUNs are measured and the patient may have undergone a minimum of 2 months of inadequate dialysis. Morbidity and mortality are highly nonlinear functions of eKt/V [3] and increase sharply as eKt/V falls below 1.0. Thus intervals of therapy with eKt/V $<$ 1.0 might be expected to substantially increase the risk of poor outcome. It is very difficult to assure adequate therapy when the dose is monitored at monthly intervals and confidence limits on each measurements are ±25%.

On-Line Effective Conductivity Clearance (K_{ecn}) and Effective Urea Clearance (K_e)

It has long been known that Na clearance (K_{Na}) is equal to urea clearance (K) and, since NaCl is the major salt in dialysate, it contributes more than 95% of the electrolyte conductivity (Cn) of dialysate. Conductivity can be measured automatically and at no cost with on-line conductivity meters deployed in inlet and outlet dialysate streams and precision of Cn measurement is 10 times greater than precision of Na measurement using ion-selective electrodes.

In view of these relationships the idea of on-line measurement of conductivity dialysance (K_{cn}) was conceived as an automated method for monitoring of K throughout the dialysis [4, 5]. Since there is a negligible Na concentration gradient between blood and dialysate during regular dialysis, it was necessary to devise a method to abruptly change inlet dialysate Cn (ΔCn_{di}) by changing Na proportioning to achieve a dialysate to blood inlet conductivity gradient ($Cn_{di} - Cn_{bi}$). The two methods used have consisted of (1) sequential increase and decrease Cn_{di} over a 5- to 6-min interval [4] or (2) a single step function increase in Cn_{di} over 2–3 min [5]. Both methods result in two simultaneous equations which can be solved for K_{cn} in accordance

$$K_{cn} = \left(\frac{\Delta Cn_{di} - \Delta Cn_{do}}{\Delta Cn_{di} - \Delta Cn_{bi}} \right) (Qd + Qf) \tag{2}$$

where ΔCn_{do} is change in dialysate outlet conductivity and over the short time interval of measurement, Cn_{bi} is assumed to be stable so the term $\Delta Cn_{bi} = 0$ and we can write

$$K_{ecn} = \left(1 - \frac{\Delta Cn_{do}}{\Delta Cn_{di}} \right) (Qd + Qf) \tag{3}$$

In equation (3) K_{ecn} represents the effective conductivity dialysance and will be equal to K_{cn} only when $\Delta Cn_{bi} = 0$. The relationship between K_{ecn} and K_{cn} can be shown by dividing equation (3) by equation (2) to give

$$K_{ecn}/K_{cn} = \left(1 - \frac{\Delta Cn_{bi}}{\Delta Cn_{di}} \right) \tag{4}$$

Note in equation (4) that the ratio $K_{ecn}/K_{cn} < 1$ when there is any change in Cn_{bi}. Effective conductivity clearance is defined as flux divided by the gradient between systemic blood conductivity (Cn_{bs}) and Cn_{di}. It has been shown in the case of access recirculation (R_{ac}) the ratio K_{ecn}/K_{cn} is identical to the ratio K_e/K where K_e is urea flux divided by systemic concentration. With R_{ac}, Cn_{bi} will increase and decrease relative to Cn_{bs} due to salt transfer into and out of the recirculating dialyzer bloodstream during the measurement as Cn_{di} is increased and decreased. Mathematical analysis [5, 6] shows that the effect of recirculation on K_{cn} is exactly the same as the effect on K so K_{ecn} will be equal to K_e and replicate measurements of K_{ecn} over the course of dialysis can be expected to yield a much more accurate value for the true time averaged effective urea clearance provided during the treatment compared to a theoretical value which is calculated from a generic dialyzer KoA and not corrected for clotting, recirculation, flow and time errors.

Clinical Use of OLC

In the new patient UKM with Co, Ct and $K_{ecn} \cdot t$ are required to kinetically determine a unique value for the patient V. After this is determined V can be stored in the delivery system along with software to compute the actually delivered spKt/V and eKt/V every dialysis from the automated measurement of mean $K_{ecn} \cdot t$. Periodically the V should be updated and PCR can be calculated as desired from a predialysis BUN with appropriate software. We believe OLC can result in a substantial improvement in the quality of dialysis therapy. It has the potential to eliminate long intervals of inadequate therapy by virtue of monitoring the delivered dose of dialysis for each treatment and at a level of precision substantially higher than that achieved with urea kinetic modeling and estimated urea clearance.

References

1 Gotch F: Kinetic modeling in hemodialysis; in Nissenson A, Fine R, Gentile D (eds): Clinical Dialysis, ed 3. Norwalk, Appleton & Lange, 1995, pp 156–189.

2 Tattersall J, DeTakats D, Chamney P, Greenwood R, Farrington K: The post-hemodialysis rebound: Predicting its effect on Kt/V. Kidney Int 1996;50:2094–2102.

3 Gotch F, Levin N, Port F, Wolfe R, Uehlinger D. Clinical outcome relative to the dose of dialysis is not what you think: The fallacy of the mean. Am J Kidney Dis 1997;30:1–15.

4 Polsachegg H: Automatic, noninvasive intradialytic clearance measurement. Int J Artif Organs 1993;16:186–191.

5 Petitclerc T, Bene B, Jacobs C, Jaudon M, Goux N: Non-invasive monitoring of effective dialysis dose delivered to the haemodialysis patient. Nephrol Dial Transplant 1995;10:212–216.

6 Gotch F, Buyaki R, Panlilio F, Folden T: Measurement of blood access flow rate during hemodialysis from conductivity dialysance. ASAIO J 1999;45:139–146.

Frank A. Gotch, 144 Belgrave Ave., San Francisco, CA 94117 (USA)
Tel. +1 415 661 6191, Fax +1 415 731 7876, E-Mail frank.gotch@fmcna.com

Ronco C, La Greca G (eds): Hemodialysis Technology.
Contrib Nephrol. Basel, Karger, 2002, vol 137, pp 272–278

Dry Weight Determination

N.W. Levin[a], *T. Folden*[b], *F. Zhu*[a], *C. Ronco*[c]

[a] Renal Research Institute, New York, N.Y.,
[b] Fresenius Medical Care North America, USA;
[c] St. Bortolo Hospital, Vicenza, Italy

Chronic fluid overload in dialysis patients is a two-edged sword: hypertension and cardiac hypertrophy on one edge and intradialytic hypotension, primarily due to high ultrafiltration rates, on the other. The missing factor has been some accurate measure of changes in extracellular fluid (ECF) content as opposed to changes in blood volume. Blood volume change is better related to ultrafiltration than it is to extracellular volume.

Dry weight is a term which generates confusion. It is used every day by nephrologists to prescribe an ultrafiltration goal for dialysis treatments, but in practice this is based on an assessment, and not hard evidence. Factors included in this decision include previous history, patient symptoms, especially dyspnea, the absence or presence of peripheral edema, raised blood pressure and occasionally the clinical assessment of jugular venous pressure. When patients are seen frequently and responses to changes in the above are observed, especially after planned ultrafiltration, an approximation of dry weight might be made, but observations in our dialysis clinics would suggest that this does not happen often. A reasonable question is: How to go about the decision more rationally? One solid fact is the decrease in blood pressure (BP) to the point of intradialytic hypertension observed when dry weight is gradually approached over time. There are strong indications that patients in the US are generally overhydrated and well above their dry weight. In such patients the relative absence of symptoms during ultrafiltration, because plasma volume refilling from an expanded interstitial fluid compartment is rapid, provides little incentive to a busy dialysis unit to reduce dry weight. In addition the ubiquitous presence of hypertension is often not considered to be treatable by systematic reduction in extracellular volume, or short dialysis makes this too difficult. However, accurate measurement of dry weight, when the ECF volume is reduced to that of the healthy

Table 1. Methods to determine dry weight

	Methods	Comments
Trial by gradual sodium depletion	Weight ↑; BP ↑; jugular venous pressure ↑	Effectiveness depends on quality of assessment
Clinical assessment	Reduction in weight and BP; added to by with ↓ in sodium intake	Successful but may not be best in quality of life
Biochemical measurements	BNP, ANP; brain natriuretic peptide; atrial natriuretic peptide	Good population correlation but little use in individual patients; correlates much better with cardiac disease
Blood volume change	Intradialytic refilling rate	Better at indicating overhydration than dry weight
Segmental bioimpedance	Whole body comparison with normal controls; segmental analysis of leg with (1) comparison to normal population and (2) software analysis of resistivity curve during dialysis	Unproved but possibly the most accurate method
Inferior vena caval diameter	Ultrasonic measurement	Requires 1–2 h postdialysis for equilibration

Table 2. Methods to reduce interdialytic weight gain

	Method	Comments
Decreased sodium intake	Dietary counsel	Dependent on compliance and thirst
Equating dialysate sodium to patient's predialysis Na^+	Knowledge of predialysis Na^+ and ability to change dialysate Na^+	Successful in reducing interdialytic weight gain, but more trials needed

population, would appear to be of value to patients. Reliable, practical methods for dry weight assessment might also have a place in other disorders such as acute renal failure and congestive heart failure.

This paper briefly discusses (1) current methods for assessment of dry weight (table 1) and (2) methods for reducing interdialytic weight gain which facilitate reaching dry weight (table 2).

Body Fluid Depletion (Extracellular Mainly)

Charra et al. [1] have virtually had the corner on the market of reduction of body weight by dialysis patients using gradual depletion of ECF during dialyses, through low dialysate sodium concentration, long slow ultrafiltration and encouraging compliance to a low salt diet. Their obvious success in reducing BP by this procedure is well documented. It can be assumed that with this approach patients are at their dry weight. When patients are at their dry weight utilization of antihypertensive drugs is very low. It is noteworthy that over months there is an increase in body weight while BP remains low [2]. These results have accessioned much debate and it is generally conceded that a reduction in ECF volume can only be of benefit. It is not possible in the USA to adopt this approach and routinely dialyze patients for 8 h (except at home). Consequently other methods are necessary which will provide information about the dry weight status of the patient and adapt to the dry weight prescription frequently to gradually get to the desired fluid status.

Clinical Assessment

Interdialytic BP increase is expected to follow salt and water intake, but may only be useful as a measure of overhydration when the patient is close to dry weight. (Current USRDS results relating hypertension to mortality suggest that levels of BP in the higher ranges are not associated with increases in adjusted mortality risk. Absence of large-scale longitudinal studies has made it difficult to differentiate the effect of severe systolic dysfunction in lowering previously high BP to normal levels BP from the effect of the BP level itself on mortality. Overhydration may well be playing a role here).

An increase in jugular venous pressure assessed by careful inspection of the level of pulsation in the internal jugular veins (preferably on the right side) in relation to the sternal angle is a routine sign in cardiology but is rarely used in dialysis patients. Overhydrated patients will usually display this physical sign, which is much more valuable and easier to elicit by a trained individual than the rapid cursory auscultation of the heart and lungs demanded by the state surveyors in the US of many clinicians in the dialysis unit.

The blood levels of ANP, BNP and to a lesser extent GMP have been suggested as indicators of fluid overload. Most of the literature deals with the relationship as a measure of ventricular function and structure in patients with and without cardiac failure. Cataliotti et al. [3] suggested that the levels of these substances predict overall and cardiovascular mortality. Yoshihara et al. [4] found that BNP levels before and after hemodialysis correlated with the degree of fluid removal but these levels also reflected LV function in terms of LV mass and BP.

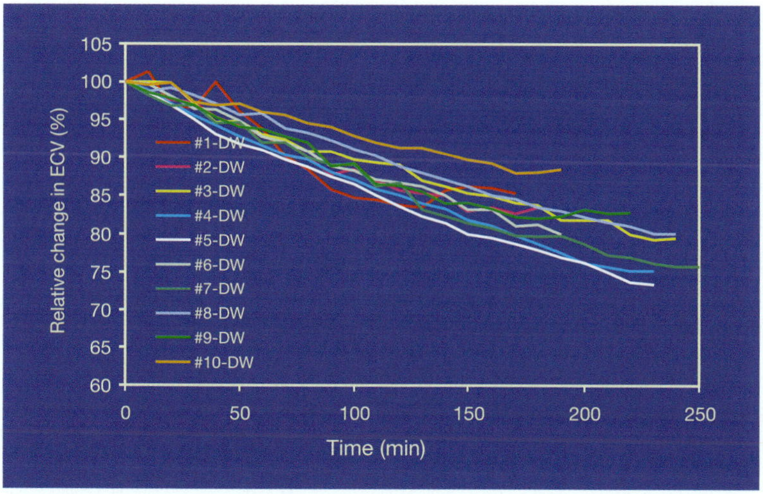

Fig. 1. Patients reaching dry weight. ECV = Extracellular volume.

Zhu et al. [5] explored the relationship between BNP and ANP weight loss and indices of LV function in HD patients with and without coronary artery disease. After HD, reductions in weight did not correlate significantly with plasma ANP and BNP. Baseline levels correlated with LV function (end-diastolic pressure and ejection fraction and pulmonary artery pressure). While many authors have also shown a similar reduction in the plasma concentration of these peptides following dialysis, evidence that a particular change or level indicates dry weight in individual patients is lacking.

Segmental bioimpedance analysis was performed using very low currents (0.8 mA) at a frequency of 5 kHz for ECF measurement. For measurement of dry weight a cuff containing injecting and sensing electrodes is placed around the leg [6].

Using segmental bioimpedance, Shulman et al. [7] demonstrated that plasma water is being removed more from the arm and leg than from the trunk and the movement of water from the leg is more dynamic than elsewhere. We have also chosen the leg for estimation of dry weight because in most individuals, more fluid is present in the leg due to the effects of gravity so that it is unlikely that excess fluid would remain elsewhere if the leg were 'dry'.

Figures 1 and 2 show examples of patients who presumably have and have not reached their dry weight using segmental bioimpedance. The measurement of resistivity is highly sensitive and at the low frequency of 5 kHz externally produced noise is much less of a problem than with higher frequencies when

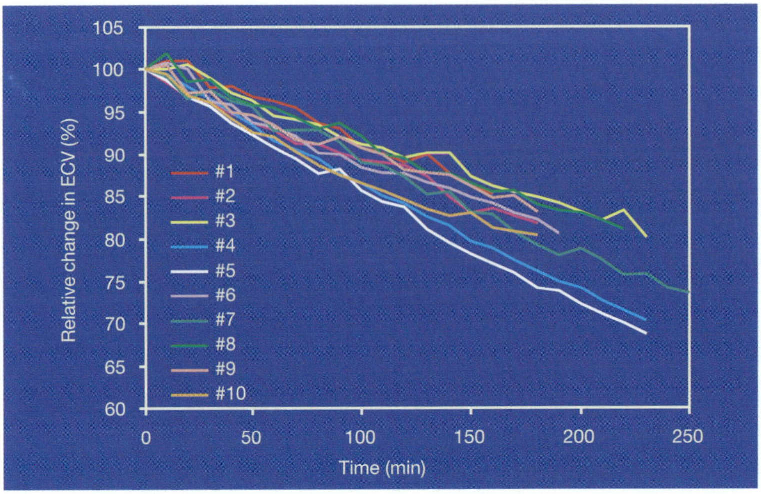

Fig. 2. Patients not reaching the dry weight. ECV = Extracellular volume.

ICF is also measured. Zhu et al. [5] have shown that in patients who have reached dry weight MAP is 5 mm Hg lower than those who have not. Resistivity is in the same range as in a normal population. Further development would permit analysis of the volume curves so that an intervention could be made at the point when the curve flattens out, i.e. ultrafiltration could be manually or automatically controlled.

Interdialytic Weight Gain

The weight gained between the end of one dialysis and the beginning of the next dialysis is clinically important in terms of its effect on the cardiovascular system and particularly the level of BP. Interdialytic fluid intake increases with total nutrient intake [8], thus representing a longitudinal indicator. Being disproportionately related to body size, higher fluid intake may be an influence in the increased death rate of small as opposed to large individuals on dialysis.

What factors determine the relevant fluid intake? The predominant influence is the magnitude of the interdialytic increase in osmolality. There is evidence that osmolality set points are individually constant and that these may be genetically determined. The higher the dialysate sodium the greater is the stimulus to thirst responding to the increase in osmolality. The history of dialysate sodium concentration has been influenced by dialysis prescription and strategies. When dialysis times were very long, dialysate sodium was at the lower end of the normal plasma concentration since fluid removal rates could be low. As dialysis times were reduced, dialysate sodium was increased so as to maintain ECF volume and to prevent decreases in BP and the incidence of vascular cramps. When dialysate sodiums were increased above the patients' set point, thirst increased. Zhu et al. [5] reporting Keen's data have demonstrated a statistically significant correlation between the Na^+ gradient (dialysate minus patient's predialysis Na^+) and interdialytic weight and BP increase. Individualizing management by providing dialysate sodium close to that of the patient reduced interdialytic weight gains and BP increase. The ability to reduce interdialytic fluid gain facilitates the task of getting closer to the dry weight of the patient. The higher the ultrafiltration rate the greater is the danger of hemodynamic disaster especially when dialysis times cannot be prolonged. In order to align dialysate to plasma sodium concentrations one needs to know the plasma sodium at the beginning of the treatment. In theory it would be possible to obtain a series of plasma sodium concentrations from the laboratory and rely on the mean, but the availability of a plasma sodium measurement derived from the on-line clearance (Fresenius Medical Care) is more practical.

The Fresenius 2008H and 2008K hemodialysis machines equipped with on-line clearance (OLC) capability can also determine predialysis serum sodium concentration indirectly from determination of dialyzer efficiency. The treatment begins once blood has been 'sensed' by the machine. At least 2 min after the blood is sensed and pre- and post-conductivity are stable the pre- and postconductivity measurement values are recorded as well as the base conductivity of the delivered dialysate. Fifteen minutes into the treatment the first OLC conductivity clearance test (Kecn0) is performed. This value as well as blood flow rate (Qb), dialysate flow rate (Qd) and ultrafiltration rate are recorded and used to calculate predialysis serum Na by the following equation:

$$\text{Plasma Na} = [\text{Kecn0} \cdot (1 - \text{Qf/Qe}) - \text{Qd}] \cdot [\text{Qd} \cdot (1 - \text{Cond. poststart/Cond. prestart}) + \text{Qf}] \cdot [(\text{base Na Cond./Kecn0}) \cdot (1 - \text{Qf/Qe}) + \text{Qf}]$$

where

$$\text{Qe (plasma flow rate)} = (0.94 + 0.0022 \cdot \text{Hct}) \cdot \text{Qb}$$
$$\text{Qf} = \text{ultrafiltration rate.}$$

The hematocrit (Hct) is manually input to the machine by the clinician. The Fresenius 2008 series machines that include OLC capabilities are manufactured with two independent conductivity probes to be used in the determination of dialysis treatment efficiency, one located in the predialyzer dialysate flow stream and the second in the postdialyzer dialysate stream. These conductivity monitors are sensitive to variations in dialysate conductivity of 0.001 mS/cm^2. Stability of conductivity is defined as the dialysate conductivity reaching steady state with no more than 0.5% variation in the reading.

At the initiation of treatment and after the 2 min of 'blood sensed' the machines automatically record pre- and postconductivity values. Differences in the pre- and postconductivity readings indicate that there is a difference in the blood plasma sodium concentration relative to the fixed initial dialysate conductivity. For example, a patient that has a predialysis plasma sodium of 138 mEq/l is dialyzed against a dialysate sodium of 143 mEq/l. The postconductivity sensor will be higher than the preconductivity indicating that there has been a transfer of sodium from the patient's blood to the dialysate through convection to reach equilibrium. The rate that this equilibrium process occurs is directly dependent on the efficiency (mass transfer) of the hemodialyzer being used. To determine this rate of efficiency an OLC test is performed. Based on the OLC Kecn0 value the plasma sodium concentration in mEq/l is corrected for the rate of convection.

References

1 Charra B, Bergstrom J, Sribner BH: Blood pressure control in dialysis patients: Importance of the lag phenomenon. Am J Kidney Dis 1998;32:720–724.

2 Chazot C, Charra B, Vo Van C, et al: The Janus-faced aspect of 'dry weight'. Nephrol Dial Transplant 1999;14:121–124.

3 Cataliotti A, Malatino LS, Jougasaki M, et al: Circulating natriuretic peptide concentrations in patients with end-stage renal disease: Role of brain natriuretic peptide as a biomarker for ventricular remodeling. Mayo Clin Proc 2001;76:1111–1119.

4 Yoshihara F, Nishikimi T, Sasako Y, et al: Plasma atrial natriuretic peptide concentration inversely correlates with left atrial collagen volume fraction in patients with atrial fibrillation: Plasma ANP as a possible biochemical marker to predict the outcome of the maze procedure. J Am Coll Cardiol 2002;39/2:288–294.

5 Zhu F, Schneditz D, Levin NW: Sum of segmental bioimpedance analysis during ultrafiltration and hemodialysis reduces sensitivity to changes in body position. Kidney Int 1999;56:692–699.

6 Levin NW, Zhu F, Keen M: Interdialytic weight gain and dry weight. Blood Purif 2001;19/2: 217–221.

7 Shulman T, et al: Changes in blood volume compartments during hemodialysis. ASAIO J 2001; 47:615–618.

8 Sherman RA, Cody RP, Rogers ME, Solanchick JC: Interdialytic weight gain and nutritional parameters in chronic hemodialysis patients. Am J Kidney Dis 1995;25:579–583.

Nathan W. Levin, MD, Medical and Research Director, Renal Research Institute,
207 East 94th Street, Suite 303, New York, NY 10128 (USA)
Tel. +1 212 360 4954, Fax +1 212 996 5905, E-Mail nlevin@rriny.com

Ronco C, La Greca G (eds): Hemodialysis Technology.
Contrib Nephrol. Basel, Karger, 2002, vol 137, pp 279–286

Information Technology Applied to Hemodialysis

Claudio Ronco[a], *Nathan W. Levin*[b], *Massimo Milan*[a]

[a] Department of Nephrology, St. Bortolo Hospital, Vicenza, Italy;
[b] Renal Research Institute, New York, N.Y., USA

In recent years an exponential increase in the use of computers in the field of hemodialysis has occurred [1, 2]. This trend has been supported by the rush to keep pace with advances in technology and the need of substantiating the quality of centers' care often by implementation of clinical guidelines. To these aspects one must add the fact that dialysis is one of the most 'quantitative' fields in medicine with a progressive increase in patient number and files. Finally, there has been a general desire to become 'paperless' and computers seem to offer the adequate solution to all these needs. However, not always the satisfaction of the medical and nursing staff has followed the use of electronic records and computer files; on the contrary, often a sense of frustration has been experienced and computers have become useless if not a real problem.

There are several reasons why computers can be underutilized or simply inadequate to perform the originally planned task. Often hardware was purchased before the problems had been clearly defined. As a consequence the system in use does not fit the actual requirements. The collection and the entering of data may be cumbersome due to an inadequate software or interface. Moving to the following step, the management of collected data may be complex with an unfriendly and time consuming interface. The medical community may finally feel that the output is not suited for improving patient care and thus the final outputs are not offering the expected results.

In conclusion, as John Sargent has recently stated at the International Conference on Dialysis in Phoenix, Ariz., 'in spite of an increasing availability of electronic media in the dialysis centers, the use of computers to improve

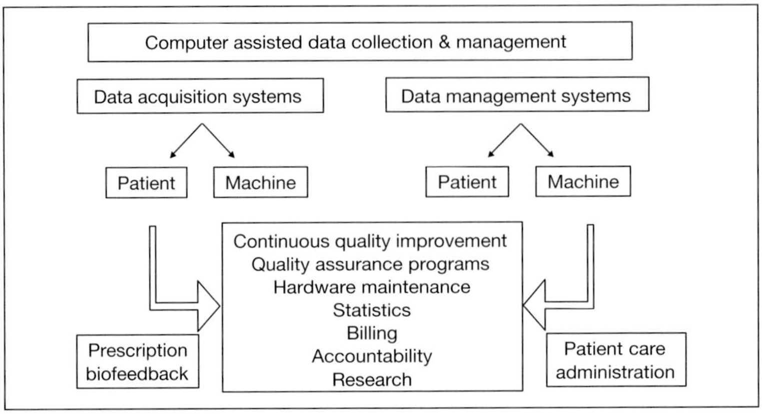

Fig. 1. Characterization of data acquisition and data management systems.

treatment care in hemodialysis has been till now limited. Many centers have invested in computerization but very few have reported the achievement of useful information to expand knowledge and improve care. Computers convert data into information: they do not create knowledge'.

Data Acquisition

There are two possible approaches for computerized data collection: one is to produce a huge database with everything inside and then analyze whatever you may be interested in: in this way, groups that tried to retrospectively analyze the database of the NCDS could not perform the analyses because pre-post urea levels had not been measured and were not included in their databases. Another approach consists of a process that decides what knowledge is desired and defines data required to produce the desired information. As the knowledge created indicates different information is needed to better understand the problem, the data requirement and collection may be altered and modified accordingly.

Considering the second approach the most wise and logical, there are some steps to undertake in order to build an adequate computerized system in dialysis. The present knowledge should be used to perform an accurate analysis of the problem. The knowledge that is contained in existing data should be used to provide the rationale for the new data collection system. The data should be utilized to build new information and knowledge possibly making periodical evaluation for quality assurance. Once the program of quality assurance is

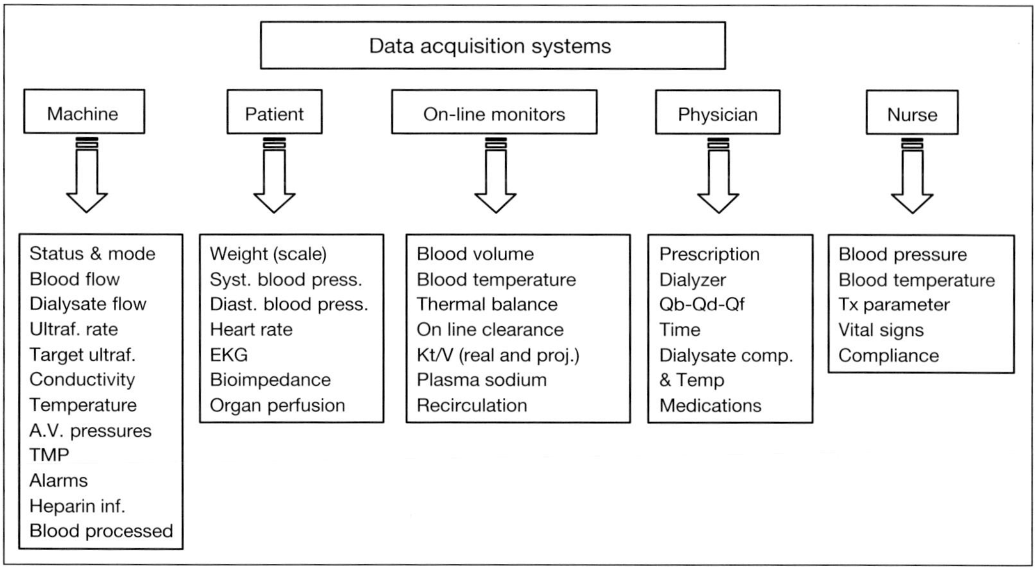

Fig. 2. Possible input sources for a data acquisition system.

implemented, the obtained knowledge should be oriented towards the generation of quality improvement programs. In all cases data collection and management must be easy.

There are on the contrary several reasons why the use of computers is limited in data collection: sometimes automation of data entry is difficult because of machine-specific codes. The integration between different inputs can be difficult or simply there is a poor and unfriendly operator interface. In conclusion, the desirable features for a data acquisition system are an easy data entry, an exchangeable format of entered data, an easy interface and a wide scalability of the system. Possibly, data entry should be automatic, minimal input from the operator should be required and finally data entry should be possible from different sources.

Data Management

The principle of monitoring in dialysis is based on the concept that the measure of one parameter can be analyzed and a feedback can be actuated according to the outcome of the analysis. Thus the original parameter can be modified if considered inadequate (fig. 3).

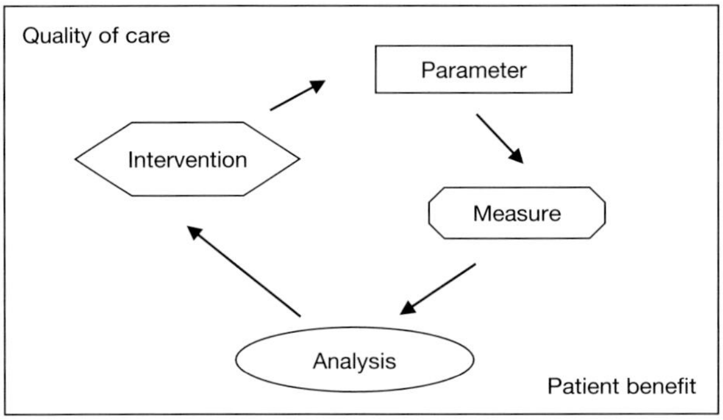

Fig. 3. Principle of monitoring in dialysis.

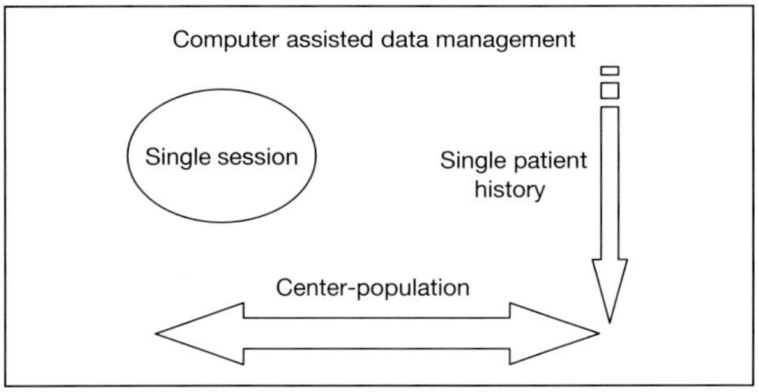

Fig. 4. Possible domains for a data management system.

Therefore, once data acquisition has been accomplished, the subsequent question is what to do with the collected data. At this point the methods of management of data are subject to the final objectives of the data collector (fig. 4). Data can refer to a single dialysis session, to a longitudinal history of sessions in a single patient, or to a cross-sectional analysis of multiple patients or even dialysis facilities. In figures 5 and 6, we report a pictorial view of the trends relative to several parameters recorded during one single session of hemodialysis (3 h) and continuous renal replacement therapy (8 h). In detail, measured parameters can be quantified at each single moment of the session, but overall and cumulative trends can also be identified. In figure 7, a 2-year longitudinal analysis of blood pressure values and pre-post dialysis body weight measurements is reported. A trend analysis can definitely be performed and correlations

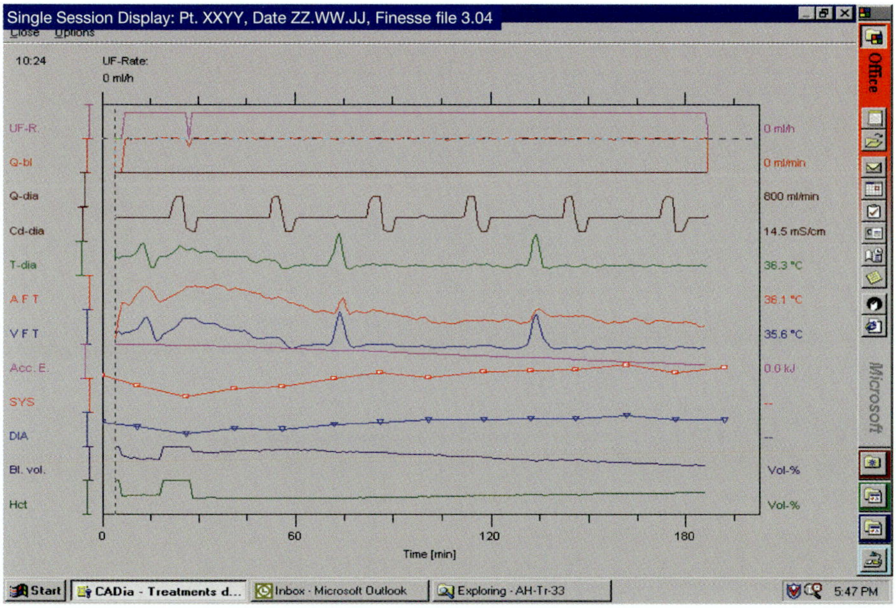

Fig. 5. File acquisition of an entire dialysis session: different parameters are displayed and the values in correspondence with the dotted line are reported on the right side of the graph.

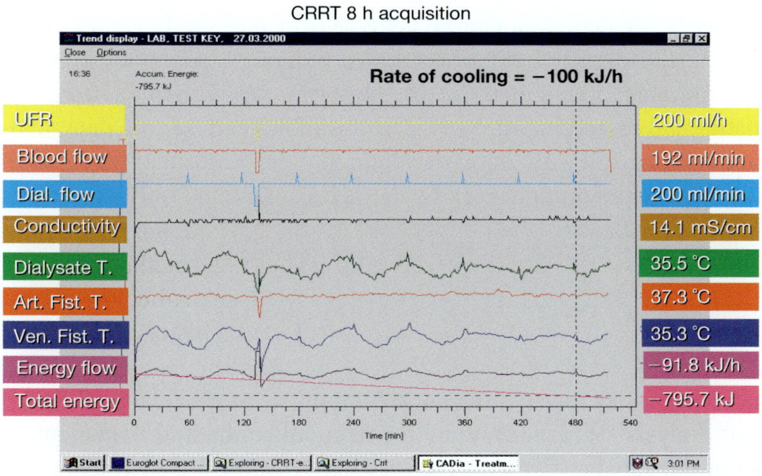

Fig. 6. File acquisition of an 8-h continuous renal replacement therapy (CRRT) session: different parameters are displayed and the values in correspondence with the dotted line are reported on the right side of the graph. Cumulative values of total energy balance are reported on the last line.

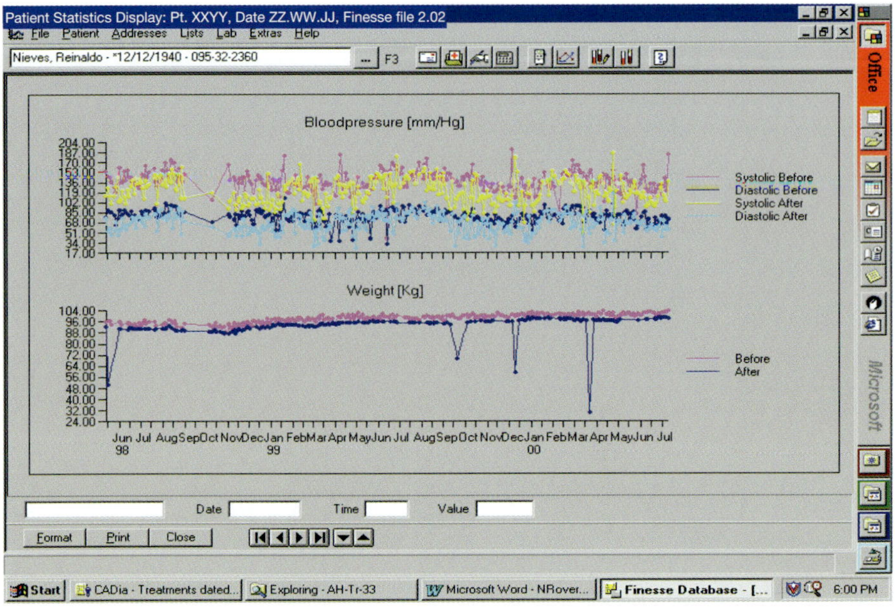

Fig. 7. 2 years' data collection for one single patient. Blood pressure and body weight are reported before and after dialysis in a 2-year period.

are made possible. Collected data can be analyzed for one single center or for a group of facilities leading to quality assurance programs, continuous quality improvement programs, trend analysis on hardware performance, financial budgets, statistics and research (fig. 8, 9). The desirable features of a data management system are the full utilization of acquired data, wide analytic capabilities, scalability with rapid outputs even for large organizations, and last but not least a friendly user interface.

Conclusions

The trend is definitely towards the use of computer-assisted data collection and analysis in dialysis. Several systems for data collection and management are available but the satisfaction with the existing systems is not always complete. Desired knowledge must be defined before starting computerization in order to purchase the most adequate system. Data acquisition systems are increasingly needed in hemodialysis because of the lack of nurses and technicians and the increased requirement for accountability and documentation.

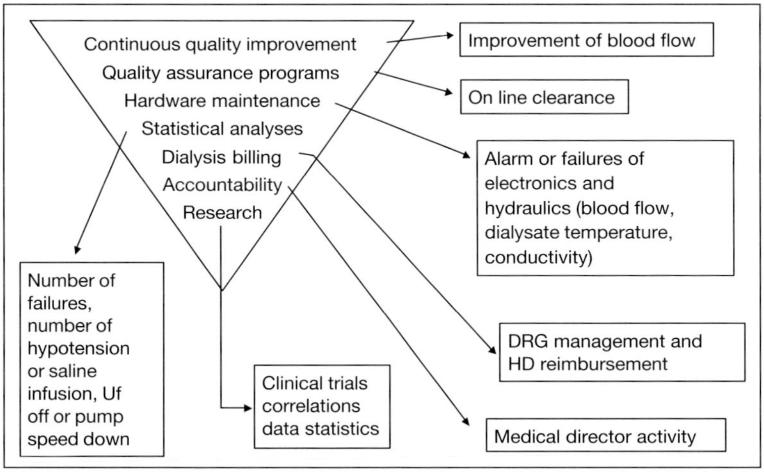

Fig. 8. Example of tasks accomplished by a good data management system.

HD station	Patient
Hours of use Mean time between failures Maintenance Quality assurance Quality improvement Equipment amortization	Demographic data Medical history, dialytic history Hemodialysis prescription & delivery Medications, hospitalizations Social condition, diet, compliance
Facility	**Network**
Demographic data Hospitalization morbidity and mortality Treatment delivery versus prescription Medications, anemia management Quality assurance programs Continuous quality improvement	Demographic and geographic distribution Standardized mortality rates Hemodialysis protocols and compliance Quality assurance programs Quality improvement programs Single center performance versus average

Fig. 9. Different domains of data management application.

Data management systems are useful for different purposes including quality assurance programs and continuous quality improvement. DRG management, billing, accountability for the personnel, and center management for dialysis providers are other options. To have a reliable system, however, data entry must be consistent and complete. Once again, compliance with the system is the key issue for a perfect functioning of the project.

References

1 Sargent JA: Identifying the value of computers in dialysis. Blood Purif 2002;20:11–19.
2 Sargent JA: Gathering data in the dialysis unit. What do you need? What do you need it for? Nephrol News Issues 1999;11:19–22.

Claudio Ronco, MD, Department of Nephrology,
St. Bortolo Hospital, Viale Rodolfi, I–36100 Vicenza (Italy)
Tel. +39 0444 993869, Fax +39 0444 993949, E-Mail cronco@goldnet.it

Ronco C, La Greca G (eds): Hemodialysis Technology.
Contrib Nephrol. Basel, Karger, 2002, vol 137, pp 287–292

Practical Approach to Data Collection in a European Dialysis Network

Jörgen Hegbrant[a,c], *Alan Alper*[c], *Juan P. Bosch*[b,c]

[a] Gambro Corporate Research, Lund, and
[b] Gambro Corporate Medical Office, Stockholm, Sweden;
[c] Gambro Healthcare International, Denver, Colo., USA

Collection of Dialysis Treatment Data and Patient-Related Information in a Single Dialysis Unit

State-of-the-art dialysis machines are capable of automatically collecting huge volumes of dialysis treatment data (blood and dialysate flow rates, venous and arterial pressures, ultrafiltration rate, ultrafiltration volume, transmembrane pressure, conductivity, etc.) and displaying the information on the monitor screen. Commercially available software allows this information to be exported to a clinical database on a server through a local network in the clinic, enabling healthcare professionals to further process, display, and evaluate the data. Moreover, on-line sensors can be used to monitor patient-related information, e.g. effective ionic dialysance as a marker of urea clearance [1–3], urea removal and additional parameters (e.g. whole-body Kt/V) based on dialysate urea measurements [4, 5], and blood volume changes [6]. Although many of these sensors are available in dialysis machines, their clinical value in routine dialysis is still subject to debate [7].

Importance of Quality Assurance in Dialysis Care

Quality assurance (QA) in dialysis care is a matter of growing concern. The release of the National Kidney Foundation Dialysis Outcomes Quality Initiative (DOQI) guidelines in 1997 drew considerable attention, and European and

Australian guidelines have followed. However, the implementation of treatment guidelines does not necessarily improve the quality of care. Implementation must be followed by the introduction of a system that can effectively monitor how the dialysis prescription is actually delivered. Thereafter, the next step in the quality cycle is to provide feedback reports and implement appropriate educational tools to improve the quality of dialysis delivery.

As discussed above, in a single dialysis facility a large volume of technical and medical information can be gathered from the individual patients. A more delicate matter is the issue of how to collect information from numerous patients treated in a dialysis network consisting of facilities located in different countries around the globe, how to process this information, and how to feed information back to the separate units in an appropriate way.

Data gathering is important in a dialysis clinic network for several reasons, e.g. to ensure that local/national/international recommendations for dialysis quality are fulfilled, and because monitoring of medical data improves quality per se, and improving the quality of dialysis care improves patient outcomes (quality of life, morbidity, mortality), and further to be able to document and demonstrate excellent quality care to patients, family members and relatives, referring nephrologists, healthcare payers, health authorities, and others.

Practical Approach to Medical Outcome Reporting in a Dialysis Clinic Network

When Gambro Healthcare International started to implement a medical QA system for its clinics, a decision was made to initially introduce a simple system that would provide information immediately rather than await the development of a sophisticated software tool. Hence, a predesigned Excel spreadsheet was used where each separate clinic manually enters the data on a monthly basis. Each patient has a specific identification code. Demographic data, e.g. date of birth, sex, height, primary renal diagnosis, date of first dialysis, etc. need to be collected only once. Certain information is collected on each occasion, such as treatment prescription data (blood flow rate, dialysate flow rate, treatment time, etc.) and pertinent physiological and laboratory parameters, including blood pressure, pre/post body weight, pre/post urea, hemoglobin, albumin, calcium, phosphorus, PTH, etc. Using the data that are manually entered into the spreadsheet, the program calculates additional information, e.g. age, time on dialysis, body mass index, urea reduction ratio, Kt/V, nPCR, mean arterial blood pressure, dialysis process variability, etc.

The anonymous information in the Excel files is forwarded to the European central office, where all the data are collected, aggregated and saved in Excel format on a server. In the central office the information is processed, 'cleaned' from 'impossible values', and finally evaluated by the medical management team. Feedback reports are submitted to every country on a regular basis, showing results of the clinics in the specific country, regional and national information, and company average data. This information is further disseminated and communicated in the countries, which makes it possible for the clinics to benchmark with the national and international results available within the network. Information relating to individuals is not provided.

Every country has a dedicated country medical director who serves as the contact person to the clinics within that country and who is responsible for the completeness and accuracy of the information that is collected and reported. The country medical director receives the feedback report and communicates this information to the clinics within the country. He/she is also accountable for implementing the company-specific treatment guidelines and the programs developed for improving medical outcomes.

As apparent from above, there are many benefits with collecting the parameters in an Excel spreadsheet. The most obvious advantage of this system is its simplicity. Other key benefits include the limited computer hardware/software requirements and the limited need for computer knowledge and experience by the user. This fairly simple QA system enabled us to acquire valid information almost immediately and, accordingly, gave us the ability to provide feedback leading to improved quality of care. The disadvantage of the system is the manual effort required, both on the clinic level and in the central office.

On-Line Access to Medical Outcome Data over the Internet

At Gambro Healthcare International, a further step has been taken to save this data in a central database. After the Excel data are 'cleaned', they are exported to a format that can be easily introduced to the database. All clinics in the group are represented in this database.

The database is Oracle 8i, running on an HP/Unix server. Through a graphical user interface, the user identifies the file to be loaded. The file already contains the clinic identifier needed by the system. As mentioned earlier, patient names are coded so that personal information about the patient cannot be identified. If the patient does not already exist in the database, then basic information is added about the patient, and the corresponding clinical and laboratory data are saved. If the patient already exists in the database, then basic data are updated (if different than before), and the clinical and laboratory data are saved.

These data are now available to be viewed over the Internet through a program called Patient Quality Tools (PQ Tools). A series of security measures ensure the confidentiality of this data. The first is the use of a secure connection (https:), a certificate that ensures the need for a user login and password, plus the required encryption of the data that are transferred over the network. This capability is the same as that used by banks and brokerage houses to ensure the confidentiality of financial transactions. As an alternative, a hardware/software solution known as VPN (Virtual Private Network) can also be used, which accomplishes an even higher level of security by requiring a 'handshaking' protocol on either end of the communication line.

Once given access to the system, another layer of security determines the access level of the user. One clinic cannot see the detailed data of another clinic. But within a given clinic, there is access to all known data about the patients, including names and other personal data.

In PQ Tools, data are aggregated to the area, country, world region, and division level. All users can view this data, but, of course, individual patient data cannot be accessed.

Data may be viewed by picking from the general parameters of geography, time frame or time span, and a clinical standard (e.g. dialysis adequacy, anemia, nutrition, bone disease, cardiovascular status). Within the latter, specific parameters are chosen, such as Kt/V, hemoglobin, albumin, phosphorus, blood pressure, etc. Once selected, the data can be viewed as mean values (fig. 1) or a categorical analysis. The categorical view (fig. 2) shows the percentage of patients, for the selected parameter, that fall into the specified range. The ranges are based on predefined company standards.

As described above, the Excel data are aggregated and graphed in many of the same ways, but the power of the central database approach is in the flexibility and delivery of the analysis, using the Internet as the delivery medium. Thus, clinics have on-line access to the information and can compare their own results with national and international average data in the internal network.

A Renal Information Management System for Use in the Clinics

This database of clinics and patients is a powerful tool for analyzing clinical parameters concerning the efficacy of the dialysis treatment process. At Gambro Healthcare International, the database has enabled the development of a program, International Renal Information Management System (*i*RIMS), that is

Fig. 1. Hemoglobin mean values for the first 9 months of 2001 for a given country.

Fig. 2. A categorical view of Kt/V values for the first 3 quarters of 2001 for a given clinic, showing the percentage of patients that fall into a specified range.

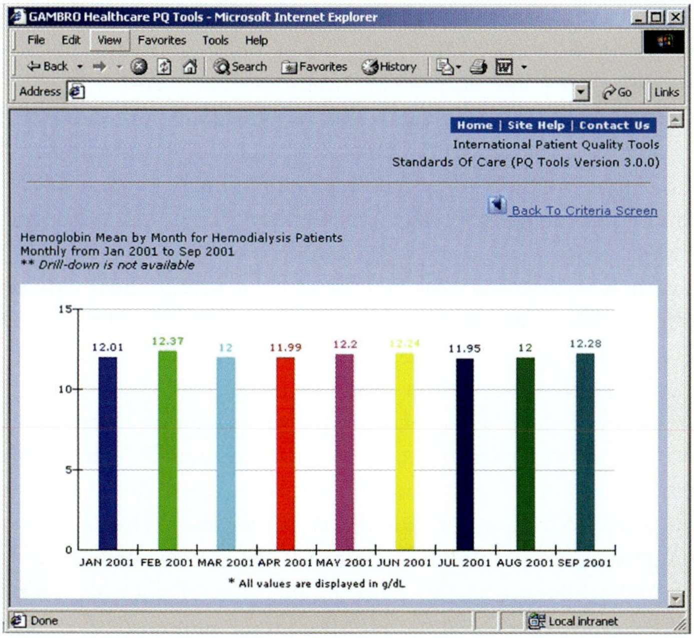
GAMBRO Healthcare PQ Tools - Microsoft Internet Explorer
Home | Site Help | Contact Us
International Patient Quality Tools
Standards Of Care (PQ Tools Version 3.0.0)
Back To Criteria Screen
Hemoglobin Mean by Month for Hemodialysis Patients
Monthly from Jan 2001 to Sep 2001
** Drill-down is not available
12.01
12.37
12
11.99
12.2
12.24
11.95
12
12.28
JAN 2001 FEB 2001 MAR 2001 APR 2001 MAY 2001 JUN 2001 JUL 2001 AUG 2001 SEP 2001
* All values are displayed in g/dL
Done
Local intranet

1

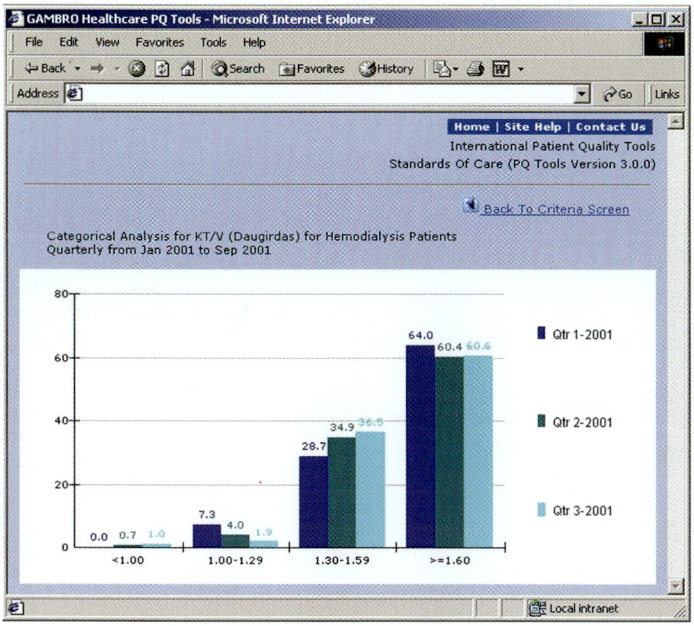
GAMBRO Healthcare PQ Tools - Microsoft Internet Explorer
Home | Site Help | Contact Us
International Patient Quality Tools
Standards Of Care (PQ Tools Version 3.0.0)
Back To Criteria Screen
Categorical Analysis for KT/V (Daugirdas) for Hemodialysis Patients
Quarterly from Jan 2001 to Sep 2001
0.0 0.7 1.0
7.3 4.0 1.9
28.7 34.9 36.5
64.0 60.4 60.6
<1.00
1.00-1.29
1.30-1.59
>=1.60
Qtr 1-2001
Qtr 2-2001
Qtr 3-2001
Local intranet

2

used in the clinics of the group to track and monitor all aspects of dialysis treatment. *i*RIMS consists of modules that track patient demographics, dialysis prescription data, medication (type and dose), progress notes (doctor, nurse), dialysis treatment parameters, physiological and laboratory parameters, etc. Reports and graphs help to monitor the patients' progress during the end-stage renal disease process. There are also many features that automate the day-to-day processes of scheduling and inventory control as well as other tools to streamline clinical operations.

The program, which is already deployed in some countries and will be deployed in all countries where Gambro Healthcare International operates, can be easily translated to the required target languages. As with PQ Tools, this program is delivered as a secure Internet connection (SSL) or using VPN. By using this program through the Internet, the only software required on the user's desktop is a web browser. Since there is no need to deploy software to local PCs, it is easy to provide enhancements and new versions of the software, rather than having a local server in each clinic. All data backups are done centrally. Hence, clinic personnel are no longer burdened with this tedious, yet critical, responsibility.

Of course, using the Internet as the delivery medium of data has some disadvantages. At times, access can be slow, and some Internet providers are not as reliable as needed. Yet, based on our experience, applying an Internet-based solution is currently the best approach when implementing a QA system in a dialysis clinic network.

References

1 Polaschegg HD: Automatic, noninvasive intradialytic clearance measurement. Int J Artif Organs 1993;16:185–191.

2 Gotch F, Peter H, Panlilio F, Folden T, Keen M: On-line measurement of delivered Kt/V during dialysis (abstract). J Am Soc Nephrol 1995;6:600.

3 Lindsay RM, Béné B, Goux N, Heidenheim P, Landgren C, Sternby J: Relationship between effective ionic dialysance and in vivo urea clearance during hemodialysis. Am J Kidney Dis 2001; 38:565–574.

4 Sternby J: Whole body Kt/V from dialysate urea measurements during hemodialysis. J Am Soc Nephrol 1998;9:2118–2123.

5 Sternby J: Urea sensors – A world of possibilities. Adv Ren Replace Ther 1999;6:265–272.

6 Santoro A, Mancini E, Paolini F, Cavicchioli G, Bosetto A, Zucchelli P: Blood volume regulation during hemodialysis. Am J Kidney Dis 1998;32:739–748.

7 Ronco C, Ghezzi PM, La Greca G: The role of technology in dialysis. J Nephrol 1999;12 (suppl 2):S68–S81.

Jörgen Hegbrant, MD, PhD, Senior Medical Director, Gambro Corporate Research,
Chief Medical Officer, Gambro Healthcare Europe, Gambro Lundia AB,
PO Box 10101, SE–220 10 Lund (Sweden)
Tel. +46 46 169 344, Fax +46 46 169 440, E-Mail jorgen.hegbrant@gambro.com

Ronco C, La Greca G (eds): Hemodialysis Technology.
Contrib Nephrol. Basel, Karger, 2002, vol 137, pp 293–299

Data Management and Quality Assurance for Dialysis Network

Daniele Marcelli[a], *Victor Moscardó*[a], *Helmut Steil*[a], *Mark Day*[b], *Judith Kirchgessner*[a], *Alexander Mitteregger*[a], *Giancarlo Orlandini*[a], *Emanuele Gatti*[c]

[a] Clinical Management Europe,
[b] Quality Regulatory Environmental Management and
[c] Management Board, Fresenius Medical Care, Bad Homburg, Germany

The relationship between medical science and computers has increased significantly over the last few decades and many management and clinical databases have been designed to address specific and defined problems, thus facilitating data management as well as developing knowledge from the collected information. The dialysis network has experienced continuous technological improvements over the past 30 years (biocompatibility of products, advances in dialysis machines), more effectively adapting the use of computers in the administrative and production field than in the clinical side of its activity. As a result of this, dialysis providers failed in both, the adoption of computers in guiding the delivery of clinical care [1] and more importantly, in the per se difficult task of converting data into knowledge [2]. More recently, the implementation of Clinical Practice Guidelines, Clinical Performance Measures, Patient Safety Initiatives and Continuous Quality Improvement (CQI) programs by dialysis providers have demanded the development of computerized monitoring systems in order to collect and supply information to increase knowledge thereby assuring a higher quality of care. Some of these systems are specifically designed for dialysis units, others are traditionally used by hospitals for acute patients, some are designed by individual nephrologists according to their own criteria or are modified systems originally used in other areas of medicine.

Fresenius Medical Care (FMC), the world's largest provider of dialysis care, has implemented in addition to its Quality Management System, a clinical database called EuCliD®[1] (European Clinical Database), as a tool to monitor the critical aspects of quality patient care [3] throughout its European clinics.

Data Collection: Just One of the First Steps on Quality Assurance

The fast development of sophisticated hardware and software over the past years eliminated the potential problem of storing a large amount of clinical information, allowing dialysis providers to collect as many parameters as they find necessary. This fact puts on the table the risk of assuming that all data is equally important and therefore, given the technological conditions, all data must be collected and monitored. If we follow this assumption, we would lose the challenge of using data to continuously provide dialysis patients with an appropriate quality of care, due to the lack of a well-defined structure for data acquisition. Thus, behind any data management system for dialysis patients, a strategy is needed which would answer important questions such as:

- What do we want to achieve?
- What sort of information do we need to meet goals?
- How are we going to integrate the data in a way that benefits both, providers and patients?

There are many different categories of data that can be collected in dialysis (all available parameters from the dialysis machine, comorbid conditions, outcome data), but there must be a reason for the data collection. This must be programmed and structured from the beginning by the provider. Without this structure, data will just be collected and no benefit either for patients (no identification of problems) or providers (no possibility to control and amortize cost) will be achieved. Another important issue to consider when identifying and selecting data is that information has, in most cases, to be collected by staff, and therefore, the introduction of a data collection and management system must comply with specific situations and requirements of the responsible personnel (structure of databases, training).

EuCliD is structured to follow a logical flow of information. In a first module, general data regarding the dialysis center itself is collected, including rather stable figures such as staff number, opening times, available technologies, modalities of treatment and water treatment devices as well as valuable information strongly influenced by the medical policy in terms of goals and desired outcomes [Kt/V, hemoglobin (Hb), treatment time]. As for patient data, EuCliD

[1]EuClid® is trademark of Fresenius Medical Care Deutschland GmbH, finally registered in Germany, provisionally registered in all (western and eastern) European countries.

collects patient description, follow-ups and outcomes. Patient description is collected at the time of admission (main demographics, anamnesis, comorbids, treatment description). Follow-ups report changes on patient health status after admission in the FMC facility (antihypertensive therapies, changes on prescribed treatment, erythropoietin, iron), lab tests (dialysis dose, electrolytes, lipid profile, nutritional parameters) and outcome (morbidity with cause of hospitalization and mortality with discharge diagnosis) is also recorded. In accordance with data protection laws, no private patient data is transferred out of the dialysis center.

Quality Assurance: The Concepts

Quality assurance (QA) could be defined as 'all those planned and systematic actions necessary to provide adequate confidence that a product or service will meet performance requirements'. In relation with data management, QA can be defined as 'the policy, procedures and actions established in an enterprise for the purpose of providing and maintaining a high degree of confidence in data integrity and accuracy throughout the lifetime of the process of data management, which includes input, update, manipulation and output'. As part of Fresenius Medical Care's Quality Management System, EuCliD handles delicate clinical data following one of the most reliable approaches on QA, CQI, a continuous way to improve outcomes, based on a continuous progress toward improved quality without establishing upper limits. Thus, EuCliD works as a tool to evaluate the implementation of such CQI programs at the same time as it provides the necessary information in order to assess and monitor the effectiveness.

Defining Targets: Guidelines and QA

Bearing in mind that creating and implementing guidelines is only a part of the whole QA system, several European medical organizations have developed their own guidelines, mainly adapting the 'Dialysis Outcome Quality Initiative Guidelines' (DOQI) [4, 5] of the National Kidney Foundation to the local conditions [6–8]. Important issues such as dialysis dose Kt/V and Hb are dealt in those guidelines, fixing minimum values to be reached as well the percentage of patients that should reach that standard (e.g. 80% of patients with $\geq$1.2 equilibrated Kt/V). Now it becomes useful to ask: how much treatment has to be delivered to achieve the goal? The European guidelines of anemia in patients with chronic renal insufficiency recommend a minimum Hb value of 11 g/dl in >85% of patients after 3 months of treatment. As in any frequency

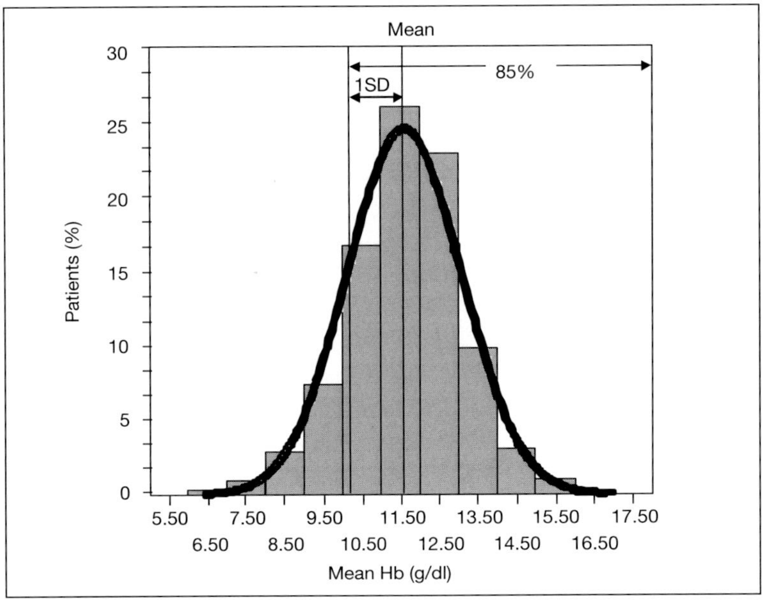

Fig. 1. Mean Hb distribution of patients monitored by EuCliD during the second half of 2001 (July to December).

distribution curve of laboratory data, with an inevitable dispersion of results, there is a tendency for values to fall away or overshoot over time on treatment (fig. 1, 2). According to the information stored in EuCliD, the mean Hb value of 85% of the population during the second part of 2001 was greater than 10.13 g/dl (mean 11.61; SD 1.61), and 68% was the percentage of patients reaching 11 g/dl (interquartile interval: 10.7–13). Therefore, and in order to achieve the minimum established by the guidelines, the target needs to be recalculated as the desired minimum (11) plus SD (1.61).

Following the CQI approach of FMC, figure 3 shows the improvements achieved in terms of Hb. In the first part of 2000, 45% of the patients evaluated had an Hb value greater than 11 g/dl. In the second part of 2001 this figure rose to 68%. Maintaining the typical distribution of the Gaussian curve, 85% of patients had an Hb value greater than 9.60 g/dl during the first half of 2000. During the second half of 2001 this value rose to 10.13 g/dl.

Another aspect that guideline culture does not reflect is the intervention model that would save patients from suffering pathological effects. Following the anemia example, the European best-practice guidelines [6] establish a minimum ferritin level of >100 ng/ml. Below this level, and according to bone marrow studies, patients fall into iron deficiency. As shown by an outpatient-based

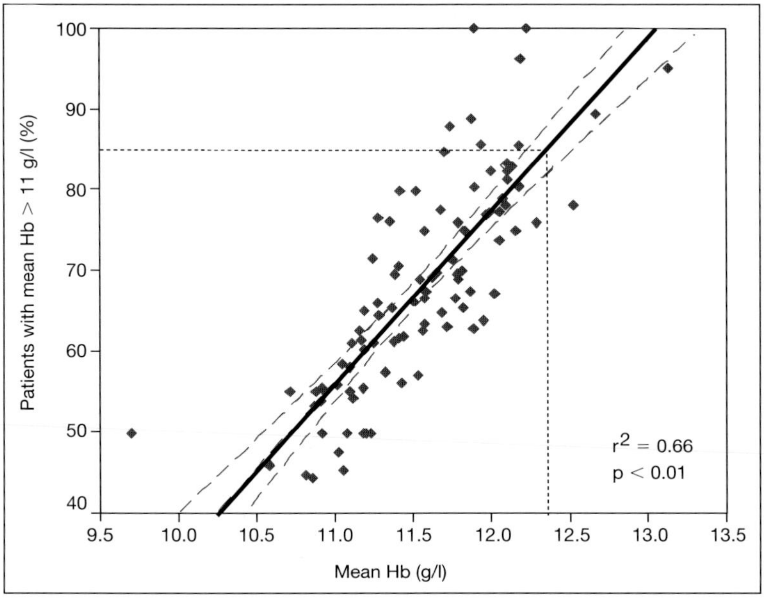

Fig. 2. Facility average of hemoglobin with corresponding proportion of patients reaching the Hb target during the second half of 2001 (July to December).

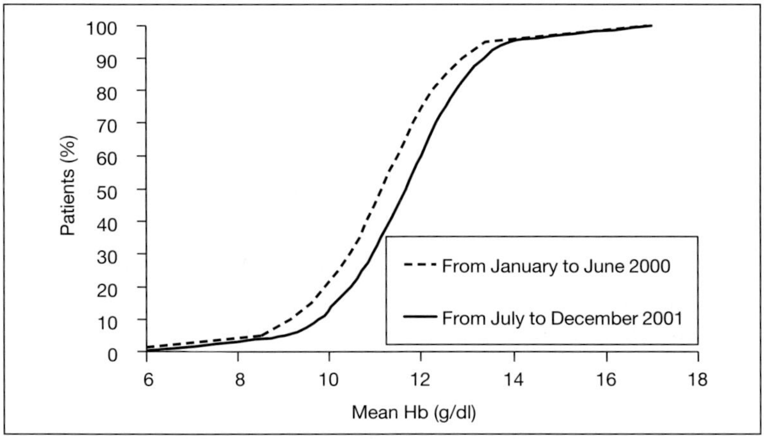

Fig. 3. Distribution of the average of Hb during the first half of 2000 and the second half of 2001.

protocol for intravenous iron in CAPD populations [9], using a proactive approach (intervention values to be set above minimum recommended) clearly shows better results than the traditional reacting model (wait until the minimum value is reached to start therapy). In this case, the early intervention improved the proportion of patients with absolute iron deficiency from 24 to 2%. Dialysis providers should integrate this concept of intervention points with the same degree of importance as the target itself in both, clinical guidelines and QA programs, containing not only desirable limits but also focusing on defining and anticipating patient distribution.

Getting Knowledge from Data Management and Human Structure

Definition of goals, development and implementation of a well-designed data management system, with the right data selection, analysis of information and preparation of final figures are only the beginning of the job. Once this huge procedure has ended, the critical stage begins with the interpretation and adoption of measures in order to get the possible benefit at the patient's level.

FMC, in its continuous search for quality improvements, has to deal with different socioeconomical situations in the different European countries included in its provider organization. The reporting activities coming from EuCliD represent a valuable tool in order to assess results, anticipate potential problems (by early detection of 'weak points') and start corrective actions to resolve current underachievement of goals. Among other annual, semiannual, and data control reports, a 'Unit-Specific Report' is produced and distributed to each center included in the system on a semiannual basis (currently over 150 dialysis units in nine European countries). This report contains the description as well as quality indicators of the patients treated in the center, comparing the result of the individual center with country averages. In addition, medical meetings are organized every year, country by country, where managers and clinicians work together, focusing on the identified problems and related issues, planning actions and finding solutions in order to assure a continuous improvement of the quality of care delivered to the patients.

Conclusion

Nowadays it is increasingly important that dialysis providers comply with QA programs and guidelines. These programs should be methodologically structured in order to answer vital questions as where to go and how to get there.

FMC works closely with the different members of the community using EuCliD, a clinical database for data management as well as CQI programs as tools for a better understanding. Far from leaving the staff to their own devices to convert data into knowledge, FMC data management and QA system support and encourage them to identify problems and find solutions, strongly involving clinicians, managers and local authorities in a global quality context.

References

1 Wriston WB: The world according to Walter. Harv Bus Rev 1986;1:64–65.

2 Sargent JA: Gathering data in the dialysis unit: What do you need? What do you need it for? Nephrol News Issues 1999;13:19, 22–28.

3 Marcelli D, Kirchgessner J, Amato C, et al: Euclid (European Clinical Database): A database comparing different realities. J Nephrol 2001;14(suppl 4):94–100.

4 European best practice guidelines for the management of anemia in patients with chronic renal failure. Nephrol Dial Transplant 1999;14(suppl 5):1–50.

5 NKF-DOQI Clinical Practice Guidelines for Haemodialysis Adequacy. New York, National Kidney Foundation, 1997.

6 NKF-DOQI Clinical Practice Guidelines for Peritoneal Dialysis Adequacy. New York, National Kidney Foundation, 1997.

7 The Renal Association. Treatment of Adult Patients with Renal Failure: Recommended Standards and Audit Measures, ed 2., 1997.

8 Gruppi di lavoro delle linee guida SIN. Linee guida della Società italiana di Nefrologia (http://www.sin-italia.org/protocol/).

9 Richardson D, Bartlett C, Jolly H, Will EJ: Intravenous iron for CAPD populations: Proactive or reactive strategies? Nephrol Dial Transplant 2001;16:115–119.

Dr. D. Marcelli, Fresenius Medical Care AG,
Else-Kröner Strasse 1, D–61362 Bad Homburg (Germany)
Tel. +49 6172 609 2153, Fax +49 6172 609 2190, E-Mail daniele.marcelli@fmc-ag.de

Ronco C, La Greca G (eds): Hemodialysis Technology.
Contrib Nephrol. Basel, Karger, 2002, vol 137, pp 300–310

Continuous Quality Improvement for a Hemodialysis Network

Juan P. Bosch, Brian A.J. Walters

Gambro Healthcare, Scientific Affairs and Clinical Research,
Fort Lauderdale, Fla., USA

It is becoming clear that as the hemodialysis (HD)population continues to increase at a rate of 5–10% each year around the world, there needs to be developed a structured approach to monitoring quality that is combined with a disciplined approach to solving problems and improving outcomes for the patients. A process is required that draws upon the leadership of the physician but at the same time empowers and encourages all healthcare personnel within the dialysis facility to participate and contribute towards improving care. At the center of such a process should be the dialysis patient whose representatives should be given the opportunity to comment and provide input to the healthcare community of the relative importance of any proposed changes to the care normally given or expected. The process that we propose recognizes that medical quality is defined as the adherence to recognized appropriate medical standards of peer-reviewed practices that have been consistently associated with the best patient outcomes. Appropriate medical standards of care address the extent to which a particular procedure, treatment, test or service is efficacious, is clearly indicated for the patient, is neither deficient nor excessive for the patient and is provided in the setting best suited for the patient's needs. This process includes three important areas of quality that must operate in harmony for continuous quality improvement in care to occur. They include the areas of cost-effectiveness, employee relations and patient care. While there exist around the world different models of health care, whether the model is based upon not-for-profit or for-profit delivery there must be accountability and balance between spending and improved outcomes for quality to have meaning.

Is this possible in a health care environment that is fiscally spiraling out of control? Is this possible where healthcare payers look at the differences

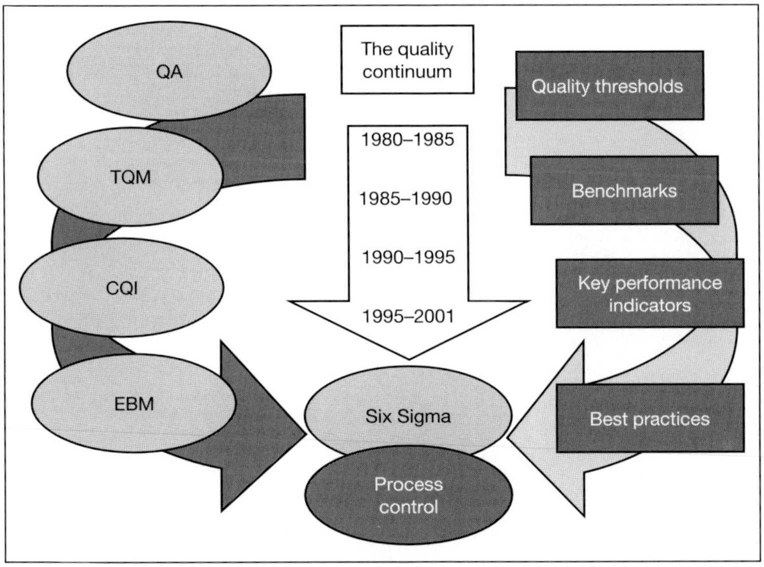

Fig. 1. Evolution of quality management.

in dialysis outcomes across the world and instead of seeing a well-ordered knowledge-based system, see variation in practice patterns and outcomes that suggest chaos? We believe it is possible by integration of the theories of total quality management (TQM) with evidence-based medicine (EBM) through the process of continuous quality improvement (CQI) refined by the application of the Six Sigma theory. The evolution of these theories in quality management is outlined in figure 1.

Quality Management Theory

The concept of TQM is borrowed from business management theory and emphasizes the commitment to the patient (customer) through continually striving for improvement through data-driven, problem-solving solutions to issues that originate and are implemented by empowered employees (fig. 2). Clinicians developed the practice of EBM as a process of arriving at medical decisions based upon not only clinical experience but also a consolidation of the best evidence from research (fig. 3). This process was used to develop the K/DOQI guidelines and in practice it means forming a healthcare team to convert problems into answerable questions, searching the medical literature for

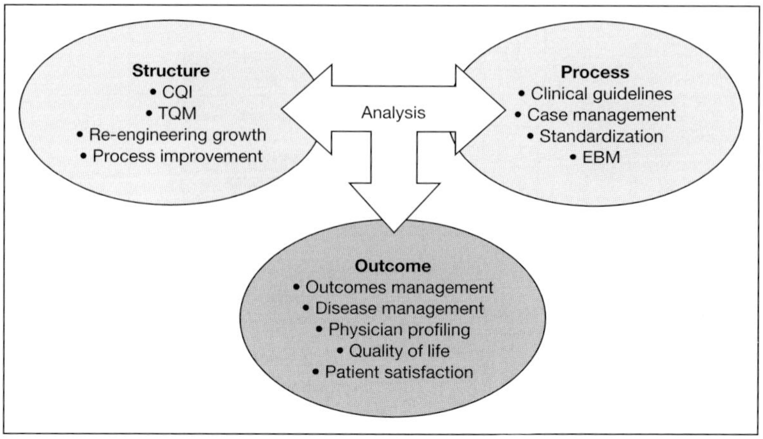

Fig. 2. Three components of quality management.

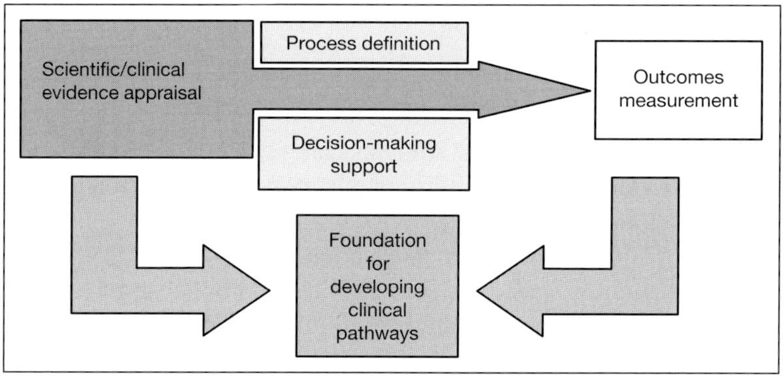

Fig. 3. Four components of EBM [adapted from 1].

the best evidence upon which to answer them, critically reviewing the evidence for accuracy, validity and integrity, applying the results to routine clinical practice and evaluating outcomes to confirm their value before communicating them back to the team and colleagues [1]. Unfortunately, EBM does not take into consideration factors outside of medical control that also impact on successful outcomes. These include a variety of dialysis facility issues that can only be addressed locally by a team of committed individuals through CQI. This process is also data-driven and involves problem-solving techniques that draw upon leadership, planning, process control and improvement.

Table 1. Differences between QA and quality improvement.

QA		CQI	
steps	characteristics	steps	characteristics
Select quality marker	Policies involve rules	Reason for improvement	Policies involve leadership
Determine threshold	Quality by inspection	Current situation	Quality by process management
Set survey frequency	Involves a quality manager	Analysis	Involves a team
Corrective actions	Simple problem solutions	Countermeasures	Complex problem solutions
Confirm effectiveness	Used for surveillance	Results	Used for improvement
		Standardization	Used as basis for clinical pathways
		Future plans	

The program utilizes a quality assurance (QA) surveillance program to identify areas of concern that are out of control or consistently do not meet an achievable benchmark to prompt intervention through the CQI team. The component steps of QA and CQI are listed in table 1 together with the essential differences between the two quality programs. The concept of the Six Sigma theory refers to a method of improving quality by reducing outcome variability within a group of patients or between two groups of patients each attending different facilities. The Six Sigma quality concept first identifies an outcome specification such as a Kt/V being between 1.2 and 1.4 or in the case of anemia management as blood hemoglobin being managed at the specification of 11.0–12.5 g/dl and then monitors the frequency of not meeting the specification (fig. 4). The program identifies and corrects those process factors that exert pressure on the variability of the outcome specification as measured by large standard deviations in the mean outcome benchmark (SD or Sigma).

Process of CQI: The Gambro Healthcare Experience

In designing a CQI program for an HD network, one first needs to choose from the medical literature a set of QA benchmarks that represents all of the comorbid conditions that influence HD outcomes and then determine the

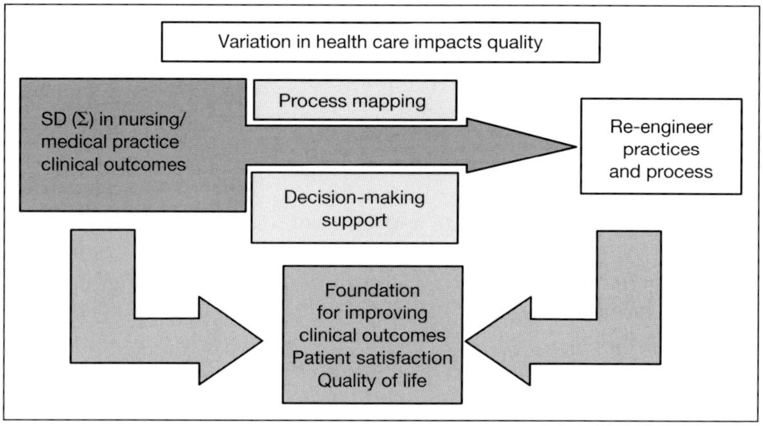

Fig. 4. Components of Six Sigma (6Σ)-based medicine.

hierarchy of importance of each so that priorities can be justified. The HD Network is also responsible for forming a peer review team of physicians and respected healthcare personnel who collect the data from each of the dialysis facilities that make up the network and provide regular feedback to the facilities as well as advice and help in designing CQI programs. In describing such a program, the authors will draw upon the lessons learned from their own experience in developing such a program within Gambro Healthcare, which began in 1992 in the United States of America but in recent years has extended into Europe and South America. The success of such a program has depended on the existence of a standardized electronic medical record for each patient, the basis of which is the Renal Information Management System (RIMS®) from which data is extracted, submitted to quality control logic and stored as the Gambro Healthcare quality dataset (Nightingale Datamart®). The data are routinely analyzed for their accuracy, validity and integrity. It includes all of the patient demographic variables as well as treatment prescriptions, medications, interventions, laboratory results and patient outcomes. The datamart interfaces with a patient quality of life (SF36) dataset, depression screening tool and a patient satisfaction dataset enabling patient input into outcome analyses.

The Department of Scientific Affairs and Clinical Research maintains responsibility for the Nightingale Datamart independent of dialysis facility operations and provides feedback reports in the form of tables to the dialysis facilities, approved by the Chief Medical Officer and the Medical Advisory Board. Each report consists of a categorical analysis of outcome benchmarks instituted to address hemodialysis CQI programs in vascular access, dialysis

Table 2. Quality markers used to monitor outcomes for patients on HD

Quality area	Primary quality marker	Secondary quality markers
Vascular access	% AVF, % graft, % catheter	Hospitalization Access survival Access interventions
Dialysis adequacy	Kt/V, urea reduction ratio	Interdyalytic weight gain Treatment time Missed treatments (%) Shortened treatments (%)
Nutrition	Serum albumin	Serum cholesterol Protein catabolic rate Serum bicarbonate
Anemia	Hemoglobin	Hematocrit Serum ferritin Transferrin saturation (%) Erythropoietin dosage Patients on iron therapy (%)
Osteodystrophy	Parathyroid hormone Serum phosphorus	Serum Calcium Alkaline phosphatase Patients on vitamin D (%) Patients on phosphate binders (%)

adequacy, anemia management, nutrition and osteodystrophy. Every Gambro Healthcare facility operating for at least one quarter is included in one of three geographic divisions but further divided into four regions for each division. The quality reports are published in rolling quarters updated each month on the Scientific Affairs and Clinical Research intranet website. The tables list for comparison, facilities with the best outcomes in descending order together with outcomes from the region, division and the entire corporation. The list of quality benchmarks representing the major complications of HD and recommended by the Gambro Healthcare Medical Advisory Board (MAB) acting as a peer review committee is shown in table 2. The choice of these benchmarks followed the implementation of a set of multidisciplinary standards of care by the Gambro Healthcare MAB in 1993 [2]. Over time other evidence-based quality markers were included following an analysis of the Gambro Healthcare dataset and after searching the medical literature. The K/DOQI guidelines were accepted as the minimum recommended quality benchmarks. In several instances, such as non-compliance with the treatment prescription that included missed treatments and shortened treatments, benchmarks were chosen based on the development of in-house statistical models [3].

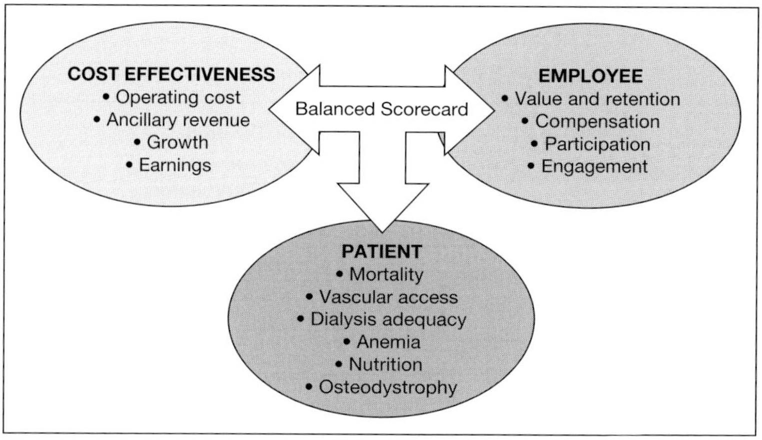

Fig. 5. Three components of quality objectives.

The multidisciplinary standards of care provide the technical recommendations by the Gambro Healthcare MAB acting as a peer review body of experts on the responsibilities of the physician, nursing staff, dietitian and the social worker in maintaining quality outcomes. While it is not the intention of this review to detail the standards used in the business and employee components of the quality continuum, it is important to state that the benchmarks used in the full continuum constitute the Gambro Healthcare Balanced Scorecard which is used to determine the hierarchy of performance by each dialysis facility within the Gambro Healthcare Corporation (fig. 5). On a quarterly basis, facilities found in the upper and lower quartile of outcome performance in all of the three components (business, employee, patient) and the individual benchmarks are studied for unique and common attributes that may be associated with their sustained presence in that quartile.

Having described the QA tool used to track and provide regular feedback to the dialysis facilities, it is important to emphasize that the data must be as recent as possible to ensure that the CQI team at the dialysis facility is exposed to clinical management behaviors and processes that are also current and can be analyzed to determine cause and effect. The objective of the QA program is to provide the CQI team with an honest accurate assessment of the current situation as it applies to the five major areas of HD patient quality. The CQI team is expected to analyze the data and determine where their facility rates when compared with facilities within their immediate region, their division and the corporation or network. Such an analysis will provide the CQI team with a priority list from which the team can begin to catalyze the improvement process.

This will be an important function of the Network. The division of Scientific Affairs and Clinical Research regularly determines the relative importance of each of the quality benchmarks by statistical analysis of the data using multiple regression analysis, Cox regression analyses or other statistical models. The results of such analyses are always being reviewed, since the relative importance of one outcome benchmark compared with another will change as quality continues to improve as a result of the program. In terms of the quality areas (benchmark) having an impact on mortality and hospitalization, the order of decreasing impact is vascular access (catheter use), dialysis adequacy (Kt/V, urea reduction ratio, missing treatments), nutrition/inflammation (serum albumin), anemia (hemoglobin), and osteodystrophy (parathyroid hormone). As the CQI program continues resulting in major improvements in the delivery of dialysis adequacy, anemia, nutrition, and vascular access, the outcome predictors change and the statistical model begins to identify other outcome markers such as hyperphosphatemia which then become important.

Quality Analysis and Planning Intervention

The description above has outlined a program in which areas of quality have been determined by a respected peer review group (HD Network Quality Committee) who have outlined a set of quality standards (based on medical evidence) and agreed on a set of quality markers and benchmarks that accurately measure performance in each quality area. While the choice of what area to focus attention upon and when to institute a CQI program will be different for different facilities it should be based upon historical data collected for at least two consecutive quarters. Such a set of markers for anemia might be hemoglobin (categories of analysis: <10, 10–11, 11–12.5, >12.5 g/dl), hematocrit (categories of analysis: <30, 30–33, 33–36.5, >36.5%), transferrin saturation (<20, 20–25, 25–30, >30%), serum ferritin (<100, 100–300, 300–800, >800 ng/ml), percentage of patients receiving erythropoietin with mean dosage per kilogram, and percentage of patients receiving iron supplements. Hemoglobin is the major quality marker for anemia while the other markers act as secondary markers allowing further analysis and insight into the quality area. Each of the categories chosen for each quality marker requires support in the medical literature or support from current medical opinion for them to be used. The facilities are arranged in descending order with the facility with the least percentage (facility >30 patients) of patients having hemoglobin <10 g/dl at the top to the facilities having the highest percentage of patients with hemoglobin <10 g/dl at the bottom. Facilities in the upper quartile are then compared with facilities in the lower quartile in respect to the other quality markers for anemia and facilities in the lower quartile submitted to the peer review committee for intervention after analysis for confounding variables that may have impacted on the analysis. Such confounders known to have an impact on quality differences between facilities include differences in acuity, abnormally high staff turnover and a sudden influx of incident patients. Assuming that this is not the case, the facilities with lower than expected outcomes are analyzed and compared with the facilities in the upper quartile of outcome performance for the root cause of the problem.

Such a process involves an open, honest dialogue with the facility identified, between the HD Network physician and the physician responsible for the facility. Experience has shown that for the CQI process to be successful there must be support from the medical leadership of the dialysis facility for the entire team that is responsible for instituting the program. Leadership includes commitment to the CQI philosophy by attending the CQI team meetings, establishing a mission statement and empowering the healthcare personnel on the CQI team. The team is responsible for identifying the patients affected, selecting the CQI methodology, training the staff and instituting the correction plan through the application of countermeasures that correct the root causes of the suboptimal outcome. The team is also responsible for monitoring the outcome performance measures following the institution of the correction plan and reporting the results back to the entire facility healthcare team and the HD Network Committee. Following the success of the CQI program, the team is responsible for standardizing the corrective plan by incorporating it into the facility medical procedures and policies. Follow-up monitoring for up to four successive quarters should be continued to ensure that the root causes do not reappear.

While what we have described assumes that the root causes are identified and corrected, it does not address unexpected problems for which solutions might not be immediately apparent. An example of such a case often encountered in anemia CQI programs is erythropoietin resistance resulting from functional iron deficiency (high serum ferritin, low % transferrin saturation) the cause of which is not immediately obvious. Other examples include low urea reduction ratio or Kt/V resulting from recirculation not immediately obvious or inaccurate collection of the post-blood urea sample. Dietary noncompliance interfering with the management of vitamin D analogue dosing in the management of hyperphosphatemia also requires innovative analysis strategies to identify and correct. In such cases, the HD Network Committee should enlist the advice and counsel from the physicians who have maintained a successful record of remaining in the upper quartile of outcome performance within the network for an extended period of time. Experience within the Gambro Healthcare network has continued to identify facilities that maintain outcomes in the upper quartile for several years. It should be recognized that the HD CQI network program described above contains an inbuilt mechanism of identifying the opinion leaders within the network for each of the quality areas monitored; these are the physicians who manage patients who consistently exceed the quality benchmarks. Analysis of practice patterns and disease management strategies utilized by these physicians should become an important process used by the HD Network Committee to foster improvement and excellence within the network.

The consistent monitoring of the selected HD quality benchmarks monthly, quarterly or as a unique time frame within any given year such as in the Core Indicators Project [4] has another important benefit. It allows conclusions to be reached regarding the consistency of the quality program. Consistent quality over time or the minimizing of variability in the quality benchmarks should become a part of the HD network culture. As each facility in the lower quartile improves resulting from the CQI program, the benchmark means improve, the differences between those facilities in the lower quartile become closer in outcomes to the facilities in the highest quartile and a culture of collaboration and mutual respect spreads within the network. It soon becomes easy for staff from one facility to operate in the environment of another within the network. Productivity improves and staff satisfaction with their responsibilities within the facility also improves.

When this level of quality performance is reached, one might consider shifting to monitoring of the standard deviation (SD) in the quality outcome mean. Studies within our own Gambro Healthcare facilities including statistical analysis using experimental models suggest that variability in outcome performance is an important predictor of not only medical outcomes but also outcome performance of cost-effectiveness. Facilities in the highest quartile of outcome performance within the HD group with the lowest SD in outcome performance usually have the lowest mortality rates, hospitalization and operate at lower cost than facilities with higher SD in outcome performance. Facilities may also be analyzed for the interpatient benchmark SD and intrapatient benchmark SD by selecting a laboratory analyte representing a quality area that is tested at regular intervals such as Kt/V, hemoglobin, albumin or phosphorus. Interpatient variation (SD) expresses the ability of the healthcare team to deliver consistent high quality care to all patients within the facility and intrapatient variation (SD) tests the ability of the healthcare team to reproduce this quality of care consistently in the same patient each month. This program is an extension of the CQI process and borrows from the Six Sigma theory that is used in manufacturing [5].

Conclusions

We have outlined the process for developing a CQI program for an HD network that begins with establishing a peer review group of committed healthcare personnel who, under the leadership of physicians, and influenced by the tenants of EBM, develop a set of standards of care that address the major complications of dialysis care and can be measured accurately, reproducibly and with precision. The data are further subjected to quality control logic that seeks to exclude measurements that are outliers or are inaccurate due to preanalytical causes (e.g. Kt/V >2.5). The process categorizes the data in a manner consistent with clinical practice and arranges the data so that underperforming facilities can be identified. A process of reporting back to the facilities over time will identify those facilities that consistently underperform their peers and who should attract the focus of the CQI program. The program from the HD network's perspective operates to enable the facility to correct its underperformance through its own CQI committee operating with help and guidance from the HD network opinion leaders, namely physicians operating facilities that consistently exceed the performance measures. This process leads to a narrowing of the gap between facilities across the spectrum of outcome performance, the raising of the quality benchmark to higher expectations and improvement in the patients' quality of life and mortality, while providing an exceptional work environment for the facility staff.

References

1 Sackett DL: Evidence-Based Medicine: How to Practice and Teach EMB. New York, Churchill Livingstone, 1997.
2 Multidisciplinary Standards of Care, Report from the Medical Advisory Board, Gambro Healthcare Internal Bulletin, 1993.
3 Walters BAJ, Ginn HE, Lin S, REN Medical Advisory Board, REN Corp: Missed treatments – Another risk determinant for hemodialysis patients (HP) (abstract). J Am Soc Nephrol 1994; 5:484.
4 HealthCare Financing Administration: 2000 Annual Report: ESRD Clinical Performance Measures Project. Am J Kidney Dis 2001;37(suppl 3):S1–S74.
5 Eckes G: The Six Sigma Revolution. New York, Wiley, 2001.

Dr. Juan P. Bosch, Director Renal Division, George Washington University,
The H.B. Burns Memorial Building, 2150 Pennsylvania Avenue,
N.W. No. 505, Washington, WA 20037 (USA)

Ronco C, La Greca G (eds): Hemodialysis Technology.
Contrib Nephrol. Basel, Karger, 2002, vol 137, pp 311–316

Pre-End-Stage Renal Disease and Dialysis Programs: The View of the Manager

Linda L. Donald

Renal Research Institute and Optimal Renal Care, New York, N.Y., USA

The end-stage renal disease (ESRD) program in the United States continues to grow at a 5–7% annual rate and this is projected to continue through 2010 (fig. 1). Costs from all insurance sources were USD 15.64 billion in 1997, USD 16.7 billion in 1998 and USD 17.9 billion in 1999.

Chronic kidney disease (CKD) is the term now used to indicate disease of the kidneys, which also may be called chronic renal insufficiency or pre-ESRD. The term reflects disease of the kidney ranging from near normal function to severe loss of function requiring hemodialysis or transplantation. The stages of CKD are delineated in table 1.

This discussion will be limited to stages 2 through 4 and referred to as CKD leading to pre-ESRD. The focus, from a manager's perspective, evolved as clinical evidence has slowly (since 1996) been presented that illustrates the myriad of medical problems dialysis patients face in the months and even years prior to having their first dialysis treatment or in a rare case a preemptive transplant. Examples of such clinical issues are now apparent: lengthy hospitalization associated with the first dialysis treatment, lack of proper access resulting in catheter placement with all of its related problems, readmissions required for proper access placement, severe anemia, malnutrition and uncorrected hyperlipidemia, hypotension, poor diabetes control and lack of investigation of coronary artery disease. Managers could instinctively realize along with the medical professionals that this was not good quality of care and an attempt to solve any of these problems 'up front' would not only improve the quality of care but also decrease the costs. Therefore, as is often the case, giving the highest quality of care, assuming the delivery system is efficient, results in

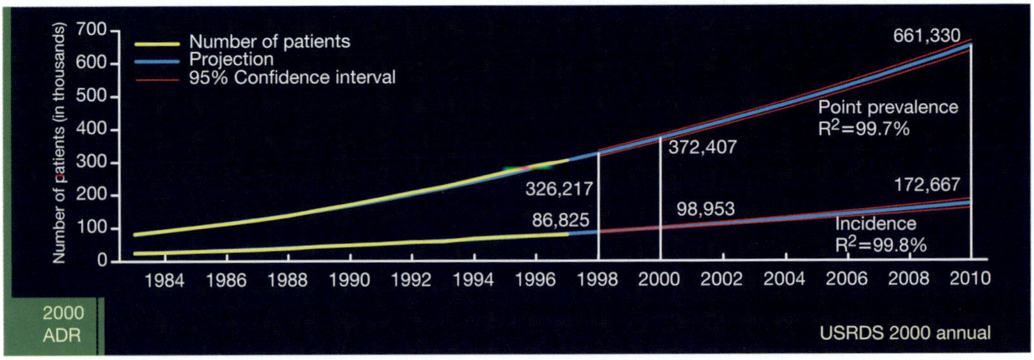

Fig. 1. Number of incidents and point prevalent patients projected to 2010.

Table 1. Stages of CKD: a clinical action plan [2]

Stage	Description	GFR (ml/min/1.73 m^2)	Action[1]
	At increased risk	>90 (CKD risk factors)	Screening, CKD risk reduction
1	Kidney damage with normal or ↑ GFR.	>90	Diagnosis and treatment, treatment of comorbid conditions, slowing progression, CVD risk reduction
2	Kidney damage with mild ↓ GFR	60–89	Estimating progression
3	Moderate ↓ GFR	30–59	Evaluating and treating complications
4	Severe ↓ GFR	15–29	Preparation for kidney replacement therapy
5	Kidney failure	<15 or dialysis	Replacement, if uremia present

[1]Includes actions from preceding stages.

decreased costs (fig. 2). Special attention has to be given to diabetes in the US. At present 40–50% of new patients coming to dialysis are diabetic. Programs aimed at rigorous control of blood sugar and early detection of complications especially cardiovascular are essential to change the very poor outcomes of diabetic dialysis patients.

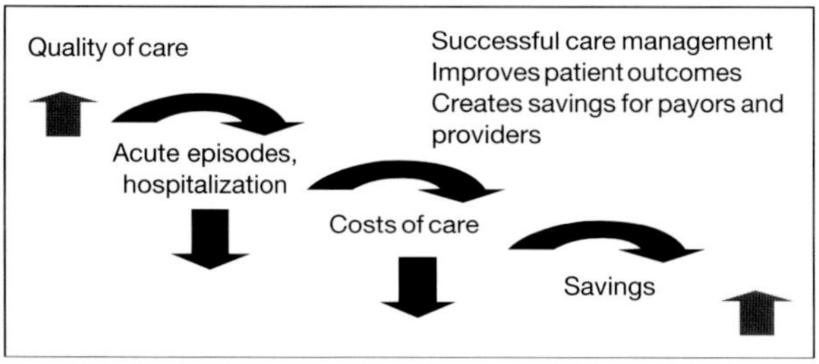

Fig. 2. Benefits of provider-based disease management.

The goals of a successful CKD program would be identified as follows: (1) Exclude reversible causes and slow the progress of kidney disease through patient education, dietary and drug management and active management of comorbid conditions. The role of the ACE inhibitor drugs appears to be particularly important. (2) Discuss dialysis modality with family and patient. (3) Arrange for preemptive transplant if appropriate. (4) Arrange timely vascular or peritoneal access according to modality. (5) Provide information and psychosocial support to patient and family.

Over the past 5 years a fairly sophisticated system has developed to encompass the care of the CKD patient in a systematic manner. Currently in the United States these systems exist as follows: (1) Disease management organizations (DMO) offering this service to insurance companies (most common). (2) Physicians – generally nephrology practices with primary care physicians (PCP) offering the service within their practice. (3) Insurance companies 'building' a disease management module specific to kidney disease as they may have done for diabetes or congestive heart failure.

Any of these approaches can be successful. The method chosen is a matter of expertise and monetary resources available to build the support structures that will deliver a well-organized plan of care to the individual patient. This can be easily monitored and applied from that specific patient to an aggregate population in a defined group, i.e. health plan or physician practice.

The manager must not only accept the philosophy that increased quality will deliver decreased morbidity but that this must be done in a systematic manner. What is needed is as follows: an allied professional multidisciplinary team consisting of a nurse, dietitian, social worker, and pharmacist; a flexible, disease management-specific clinical data system; disease management-specific claims/financial system; staff and patient education programs; and physician education program and implementation plan (PCPs, nephrologists, surgeons, specialists, internists). Having such a complex program involves an enormous amount of administrative effort.

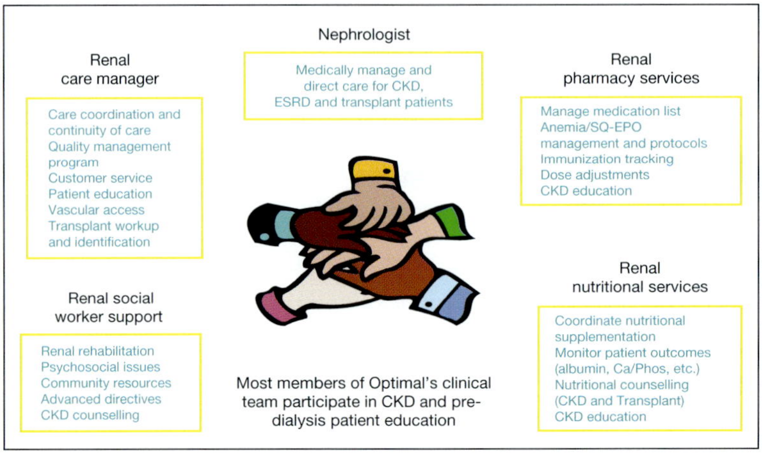

Fig. 3. Supporting the physician-patient relationship: Optimal's health management team.

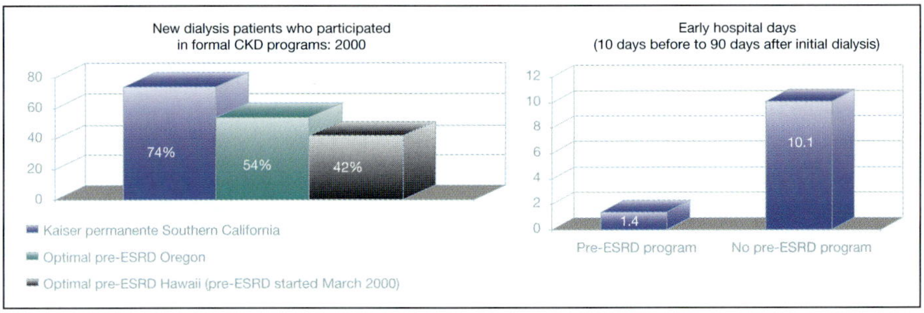

Fig. 4. Optimal renal care, LLC. Educate and empower patients.

The heart of the program lies within the multidisciplinary team. Figure 3 summarizes the various roles for each title.

The clinical database must be flexible. A web-enabled system gives availability of the data at all levels: the multidisciplinary team, physicians, health plan and individual patients: Data from the system is then used for the daily care of the patient by the team, production of standard reports for the quality assurance process at specific levels, overall population management and ad hoc reports on individual projects. The following illustrate two different examples of utilizing the database. The first illustrates in an abstract presented by Yeoh [1] at ASN 2000, the impact of pre-ESRD education of patients and hospitalizations surrounding the initiation of dialysis as seen in figure 4.

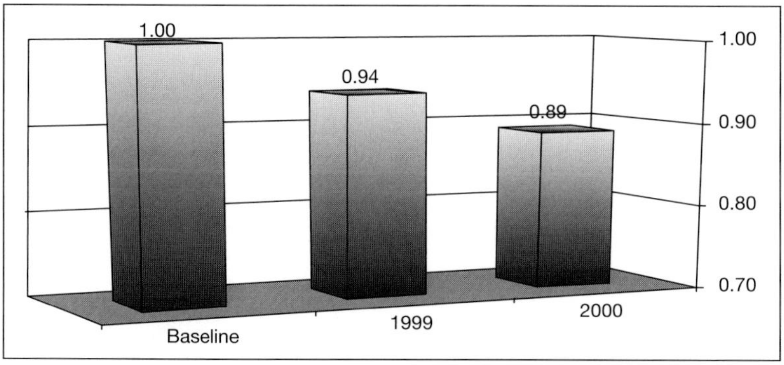

Fig. 5. Cost experience (per patient per month).

The second database that is critical to the success of a global approach to patient care in pre-ESRD is a claims/financial database. While the clinical team has specific targeted activity to effect care, the financial system must run concurrently to enable the manager to analyze the financial impact of such efforts. The system serves to store all medical claims on individual patients. This includes the cost of every single intervention a patient has, i.e. lab tests, office visits, hospitalizations, emergency room visits. Like the clinical database, the financial information must be able to be examined at the most fundamental level, i.e. what are the lab expenses for a year in a specific patient to a population level or what are the per patient per month overall medical costs for all patients in the program. For programs such as this to be successful they must decrease utilization of resources. Examples of this would be out patient access work, not admitting for first dialysis or decreased emergency room visits. Figure 5 illustrates the results of such efforts.

The combination of these systems allows the manager to assess the cost/benefit ratio of specific efforts of the team as well as overall population effects.

Finally the education program involves the following: (1) Training the multidisciplinary team in all aspects of care management for the specific area of expertise as well as the total concept. (2) Patient education as specific to the stages of CKD, modality choice and all aspects of comorbid condition management with special focus on conditions such as diabetes and high blood pressure. (3) The PCP need to be given particular and specialized attention. The development of special tools to assist in their practice (laminated information cards) are helpful. (4) Nephrologists require special attention. They are in essence the 'leader' of the multidisciplinary team and must be completely involved in the program. This requires specific presentations and continual discussions with them.

To conclude, a systematized approach to the care of the chronic kidney patient at the earliest stages is a requirement for cost-effective care at the highest quality. The manager should have this as a top priority from a business as well as marketing perspective. More research is required on the specific gains in mortality and comorbidity as the result of intervention, especially in stages 2 and 3 of the CKD progression.

References

1 Yeoh HH, Daneshvari S, Rasgon S, et al.: Impact of pre-dialysis education on clinical outcomes and hospitalization (abstract). J Am Soc Nephrol 2000;11:AO771.

2 Clinical Practice Guidelines for Chronic Kidney Disease: Evaluation, classification and stratification. Am J Kidney Dis 2002;39(suppl 1):266.

Linda L. Donald, Renal Research Institute,
207, East 94th Street, Suite 303, New York, NY 10128 (USA)
Tel. +1 212 360 4900, Fax +1 212 360 4913, E-Mail ldonald@rriny.com

Ronco C, La Greca G (eds): Hemodialysis Technology.
Contrib Nephrol. Basel, Karger, 2002, vol 137, pp 317–324

Water Treatment for Hemodialysis

Gianni Cappelli, Paola Inguaggiato, Emiliana Ferramosca, Alberto Albertazzi

Division of Nephrology, University Hospital of Modena, Italy

Water treatment represents a fundamental aspect of modern hemodialysis technology [1]. While at the beginning of chronic hemodialysis therapy, chemicals were major contaminants, over the last decade microbial contamination has become a major concern. Water supplied to hospitals is normally of a quality similar to that supplied to homes but its use in hemodialysis deserves further treatment as impurities can be responsible for many unwelcome acute side effects, including cramps, nausea, hypotension and fever. Water impurities have also resulted in epidemics of severe, occasionally fatal, disease in dialysis patients and can cause a range of clinical problems including anemia, bone disease, hyper- and hypotension, acidosis, muscle weakness, nausea, vomiting and neurological disturbance. Recently, chronic exposure to low levels of dialysate impurities has also been linked with malnutrition, heart disease and amyloidosis, which, in turn, are associated with reduced survival [2, 3].

Fatal or life-threatening mishaps still occasionally occur in the process of performing hemodialysis treatment. These events are rare, but several have been due to tragic failures in dialysis water delivery systems. Examples of actual events that serve to point out some of the avoidable causes of such disasters are reported in table 1 [4].

Standard Setting

In order to ensure that tap water is safe to drink, national agencies prescribe regulations which limit the amount of certain contaminants in water supplied to public water systems. Contaminants in drinking water sources may include microbial and inorganic contaminants, pesticides and herbicides,

Table 1. Recent failures of dialysis water delivery systems

Contaminant	Aluminum	Water	Chloramines	Fluoride	Cyanotoxin of blue algae
Date	March 1993	October 1994	September 1987	July 1993	February 1996
Place	Alentejo, Portugal	Southwestern USA	Philadelphia, Pa., USA	Chicago, Ill., USA	Caruaru, Brazil
Clinical effect	Neurological, encephalopathy	Chest pain, nausea, vomiting, cramps	Anemia, low blood pressure, acute dyspnea	Nausea, malaise, itching, severe arrhythmias	Vomiting, jaundice, ascites, high blood pressure
Prologue	Need to remove particulates from public water in a dry summer	Dialysate supplying system by two CDM working alternatively	Recent changes in water system with increased water flow rate, a single GAC filter	Unit renovations with temporary use of a water treatment system with GAC and DI tanks	Changing of water supply
Circumstances	Use of aluminum sulfate as flocculating agent, clogged RO membranes	Wrong CDM switched to rinse mode	Defect in chloramine clearance due to a too fast water flow	Leaking of fluoride from exhausted DI tank and failure to recognize the alarm light	Use of surface water supplied directly from a lake
Patients affected	71	6	44	11	108
Patients dead	25	1	0	3	60

CDM = Central dialysate machine; GAC = granular activated carbon.

organic chemical contaminants, including synthetic and volatile organic chemicals, and radioactive contaminants which can occur naturally. In contrast to a normal person who drinks around 15 liters of water per week and can inactivate toxins in the gastro-intestinal tract, a dialysis patient is exposed to 250–500 liters of water per week and contaminants are transferred directly into the blood across the dialyzer membrane. Moreover, any toxic material absorbed by normal individuals can be inactivated by first-pass metabolism in the liver or excreted by the kidney. It is, therefore, not surprising that impurities in the dialysis water as well as contamination from a failing dialysis water treatment system can cause significant problems for the dialysis patient. To assure quality, in 1970 the Association for the Advancement of Medical Instrumentation (AAMI) did the first proposal of national standards for hemodialysis systems, subsequently issued in 1981 and approved by ANSI in 1982 [5]. For several years these standards represented the only references for the whole nephrological community and finally in the 1990s some European nations started to regulate some contaminants. Nowadays water for dialysis is subject to regulatory standards but for most of them the regulations are applied, at least in Europe, on a voluntary basis. The European Pharmacopoeia (EP) monograph on water for diluting concentrated hemodialysis solutions states, in fact, that it is given for reasons of information and guidance and it does not form a mandatory part of the Pharmacopoeia [6]. To note, a further difference in the EP compared to the AAMI standards is the lack of a definition of the people carrying the responsibility for the water system. Recently, as several reports have outlined that the dialysate purity is a main factor to prevent dialysate-related microinflammation, national legislator and professional associations have focused with more attention on dialysis fluid purity. The last European contributions are represented by the EDTNA/ERCA guidelines on quality assurance for dialysis quality water and dialysis fluid [7] and the French ministry 'circulaire' on technical specifications and medical security for the 'on-line' procedures [8]. Table 2 lists allowed limits for impurities comparing EP with the recent draft from AAMI [5, 6]. It is worth noting that European standards pay more attention to microbiological contamination, even if AAMI has modified previous values (200 CFU/ml in water for diluting concentrate solutions and 2,000 CFU/ml in dialysate) and set an action level that approximates EP standards.

Water Treatment Plant

Whichever standard should be met, the same equipment required to purify the water could be used. The size, specification and maintenance schedules for the devices will depend on the quality of tap water, the rate of use and the purity required. Water treatment technology has evolved throughout the history of hemodialysis. Clinical problems associated with chemical contamination of water used for dialysis began to emerge in the pioneering days when patients were dialyzed using a bath of dialysis fluid made with untreated tap water. From this time, particle filters (beds of sand and gravel or membranes) were required to remove suspended matter as well as softener to remove calcium and other multivalent cations in exchange for sodium. Nowadays a standard water treatment plant is made of a pretreatment section including softeners, granular activated carbon and microfilters, followed by a final treatment section. To polish the pretreated water a deionizer (DI) or a reverse osmosis (RO) may be used. Recently the new DI with electrochemical regeneration

Table 2. Allowed limits for impurities (ppm)

Contaminant	EP	New AAMI (Draft RD-62[a])
Aluminum	0.01	0.01
Ammonium	0.2	
Antimony		0.005
Arsenic		0.005
Barium		0.1
Beryllium		0.0004
Cadmium		0.001
Calcium	2 (0.05 mmol/l)	2
Chloramines	0.1[b]	0.1
Total chlorine	0.1	
Free chlorine		0.5
Chlorides	50	
Chromium		0.014
Copper		0.1
Cyanide		0.002
Fluorides	0.2	0.2
Heavy metals	0.1	
Lead		0.005
Magnesium	2 (0.07 mmol/l)	4
Mercury	0.001	0.0002
Nitrates	2	2
Potassium	2 (0.1 mmol/l)	8
Sodium	50 (2.2 mmol/l)	70
Selenium		0.09
Silver		0.005
Sulfates	50	100
Thallium		0.002
Zinc	0.1	0.1
Bacteria	100 CFU/ml	200 CFU/ml (action at 100)
Endotoxin	0.25 EU/ml	2.0 EU/ml (action at 1.0)

[a]RD-62 water treatment equipment for hemodialysis applications.
[b]Not included in EP but introduced as suggestion by national authorities in some countries [13].

(electrodialysis) has made it possible to avoid the trouble of using chemicals for regeneration but its use, in spite of a greater chemical quality, needs a further ultrafiltration to remove potential microbial contamination. As a result usually two RO modules in series are preferred and this combination represents the optimal configuration to preserve microbiological quality of the treated water. Finding the best assembly of the different components in terms of size (volume, fluxes, treatment capacity) and position in the chain is a major task for water engineering. To assure a consistent production of high-grade quality water, it is necessary to optimize the design of the water plant and a direct delivery to the loop is mandatory to preserve the microbiological quality of the treated water. A fundamental issue has been the discovery that microbial growth is enhanced by low flux and stagnation [9, 10]. This has changed the water distribution system from a dead-end pipeline to a distribution loop with a continuous water flow even during a period of no use; unused water enters a partial reuptake inside of the system. Material and modalities of installing a distribution loop form a critical point. For preserving water purity results depend on pipeline plumbing where high flow rate (high shear rate), avoidance of dead space and lateral arms, prevention of stagnation and possible contamination are the issues to be dealt with [1, 11]. Unprotected sampling or drain ports should be abandoned, and the pipe should be provided with adequate drainage. Medical grade polyvinyl chloride (PVC) has been the most frequently used material for piping but nowadays, based on results in pharmaceutical plants, new materials are in use. AISI 316 stainless steel, polyvinylidene fluoride (PVDF), and cross-linked polyethylene (PEX) are substituting PVC as they offer a better resistance to disinfection, the avoidance of particles or chemicals leaching, and a smooth surface able to avoid bacterial adhesion [12]. Modern technology has only a modest impact on the final cost of the hemodialytic treatment [13]. Water cost for a single dialysis treatment may vary from 1.8 to 3.1 Euro depending on the type of water treatment plant, material in use and system of disinfection. Considering a dialysis unit working on two shifts a day, table 3 reports results on costs of a single treatment comparing a standard hemodialysis (Cuprophan membrane, water treatment plant with a PVC distribution loop and chemical disinfection) with a biocompatible hemodialysis ('high-flux' membrane, ultrapure dialysate, water treatment plant with an AISI 316L stainless steel distribution loop and steam disinfection). The percentage of total costs of a water plant is minimal if considering the amount spent on a biocompatible treatment where water represents a fundamental factor.

Quality Control

Whatever the water treatment system or the disinfection protocol in use, the only way to assure a proper water quality is to have a maintenance and quality control program [7, 8, 11]. Some parameters may be checked continuously with an automatic device while for most of them there should be a periodical

Table 3. Cost analysis of a single hemodialysis treatment from different water treatment plants (see text for details)

	Standard hemodialysis	Biocompatible hemodialysis
Treatment		
Materials		
Staff	182 Euro	245 Euro
Maintenance and technical costs		
General costs		
Water treatment plant (A)		
Double RO	1.8 Euro	
PVC distribution loop		
Chemical disinfection		
Water treatment plant (B)		
Double RO		
AISI 316L stainless steel distribution loop		3.1 Euro
Steam disinfection		
Water cost as % of total treatment	0.98%	1.26%

monitoring. Frequency is regulated on manufacturer's and water engineering recommendations and on suggestions from reference standard authorities. The control program in a particular dialysis unit should be based not only on these suggestions but also on knowledge of local contaminants, specific to the area, on historical results, on clinical indications and on balance with cost [14]. Some indications may be derived from the literature and in table 4 we summarize the most recent suggestions [7, 8, 15]. For successful results water quality has to be guaranteed at the point of use and, microbiological contamination being the most important issue, the lack of real-time monitoring possibilities makes the problem worse. In some industrial fields, systems are used to rapidly detect the degree of microbial contamination: these systems are actually not sensitive enough to test real-time sterility and apirogenicity. Therefore a quality control program with periodical audit will assure the effectiveness of maintenance, cleaning and disinfection procedures. In contrast to the natural human tendency to have faith in sophisticated equipment and new technology, a quality control program should include a documented procedure for characterization of the process and involved parameters, definition of methods and tests to check the process, definition of the accepted limit values for each part of the process and for final water product results. Last but not least the quality procedure should

Table 4. Frequency of sampling for routine quality monitoring of water

	EDTNA/ERCA guidelines	Renal association	French regulations for 'on-line' treatments
Acidity or alkalinity	3-monthly	3-monthly	3-monthly
Aluminum	3-monthly	3-monthly	3-monthly
Ammonium	3-monthly	3-monthly	3-monthly
Calcium	3-monthly	3-monthly	3-monthly
Chloramines	3-monthly	3-monthly	3-monthly
Total chlorine	3-monthly	monthly	3-monthly
Chlorides	3-monthly	3-monthly	3-monthly
Conductivity	n.i.	n.i.	daily
Copper	3-monthly	3-monthly	3-monthly
Fluorides	3-monthly	3-monthly	3-monthly
Heavy metals	3-monthly	3-monthly	3-monthly
Lead	3-monthly	3-monthly	3-monthly
Magnesium	3-monthly	3-monthly	3-monthly
Mercury	3-monthly	3-monthly	3-monthly
Nitrates	3-monthly	3-monthly	3-monthly
Oxidizable substances	3-monthly	3-monthly	3-monthly
Potassium	3-monthly	3-monthly	3-monthly
Sodium	3-monthly	3-monthly	3-monthly
Silver	3-monthly	3-monthly	3-monthly
Sulfates	3-monthly	3-monthly	3-monthly
Zinc	3-monthly	3-monthly	3-monthly
Bacteria	monthly	weekly	monthly
Endotoxin	monthly	weekly	monthly

n.i. = Not indicated.

include an operational problem analysis, taking into account abnormal test results as well as clinical side effects eventually reported.

Conclusion

Modern technology allows to improve water quality and to assure a water product within the current standards. Success will depend not only on excellent technology but also on procedures and policies tailored to the individual units. This requires an absolute compliance with quality control procedures and testing and a trained and educated staff vigilant at all times.

References

1 Canaud BJ, Mion CM: Water treatment for contemporary hemodialysis; in Jacobs C, Kjellstrand CM, Kock KM, Winchester JF (eds): Replacement of Renal Function by Dialysis. Dordrecht, Kluwer Academic Publishers, 1996, pp 231–255.

2 Brunet P, Berland Y: Water quality and complications of haemodialysis. Nephrol Dial Transplant 2000;15:578–580.

3 Kaysen GA: Inflammation nutritional state and outcome in end stage renal disease. Miner Electrolyte Metab 1999;25:242–250.

4 Ward DM: Water disasters: Pitfalls and precautions. Contemp Dial Nephrol 1999;12:24–28.

5 AAMI: Standard/American National Standard: Water Treatment Equipment for Hemodialysis Applications. AAMI/DS RD62, 2000.

6 European Pharmacopoeia: Haemodialysis Solutions, Concentrated, Water for Diluting. Monograph 1997: 1167, ed 3. Council of Europe, Strasbourg 1996.

7 EDTNA/ERCA: European best practice guidelines for haemodialysis. 8. Dialysis fluid purity. Nephrol Dial Transplant, in press.

8 Ministère de l'Emploi et de la Solidarité: Circulaire relative aux spécifications techniques et à la sécurité de la pratique de l'hémofiltration et de l'hémodiafiltration en ligne dans établissements de santé. République Française, Circulaire DGS/DH/AFSSAPS No 311, June 7, 2000.

9 Man NK, Degremont A, Darbord JC, Collet M, Vaillant P: Evidence of bacterial biofilm in tubing from hydraulic pathway of hemodialysis system. Artif Organs 1998;22:596–600.

10 Cappelli G, Ballestri M, Perrone S, Ciuffreda A, Inguaggiato P, Albertazzi A: Biofilms invade nephrology: Effects in hemodialysis. Blood Purif 2000;18:224–230.

11 Cappelli G, Perrone S, Ciuffreda A: Water quality for on-line hemodiafiltration. Nephrol Dial Transplant 1998;13(suppl 5):12–16.

12 Cappelli G, Ballestri M, Facchini F, Carletti P, Lusvarghi E: Leaching and corrosion of polyvinyl chloride (PVC) tubes in a dialysis water distribution system. Int J Artif Organs 1995;18:261–263.

13 Commissione dialisi SIN: Rapporto della commissione dialisi sui costi della terapia dialitica. G Ital Nefrol 1997;14:321–338.

14 Cappelli G, Lusvarghi E: La qualità delle acque per dialisi: normativa italiana e proposta operativa di controllo periodico. G Ital Nefrol 1990;7:165–170.

15 The Renal Association: Treatment of Adult Patients with Renal Failure: Recommended Standards and Audit Measure, ed 2. London, Royal College of Physicians, 1997.

Prof. Gianni Cappelli, Division of Nephrology, Dialysis and Transplantation,
University Hospital of Modena, Via Del Pozzo, 71, I–41100 Modena (Italy)
Tel. +39 059 4222481, Fax +39 059 4222167, E-Mail cappelli@unimo.it

Ronco C, La Greca G (eds): Hemodialysis Technology.
Contrib Nephrol. Basel, Karger, 2002, vol 137, pp 325–331

Dialysate Purity: A Must

Rafael Ramírez, Julia Carracedo, Alejandro Martín-Malo, Mariano Rodríguez, Pedro Aljama

Servicio de Nefrología, Unidad de Investigación,
Hospital Universitario Reina Sofía, Córdoba, Spain

The inflammatory process is inherent to the immune response against injury. However, when the inflammatory response is inappropriate or excessively activated, it may result in a state of uncontrolled systemic inflammation which may lead to a chronic inflammatory state with obvious deleterious consequences. Despite the advance in end-stage renal disease (ESRD) therapy, a subclinical inflammatory state and a disproportionately high risk for developing cardiovascular disease (CVD) are still two important problems in hemodialysis populations. Furthermore, a large amount of clinical and experimental evidence supports an association between inflammation and risk of CVD [1, 2], and particularly in ESRD patients inflammation has been associated to cardiovascular mortality [3–5]. The interactions of blood with hemodialysis membrane may induce activation in mononuclear cells to produce proinflammatory cytokines. In addition, other factors that may be generated during the hemodialysis session such as fractions of the complement also may induce inflammation. Finally exogenous factors such as contamination by endotoxins may amplify the inflammatory response induced by the hemodialysis therapy.

An effective inflammatory response requires cooperation among numerous components including immune cells (namely neutrophils and macrophages), endothelial cells and multiple mediator networks that act coordinately in the inflammatory cascade. In this regard, macrophages may be considered as one of the principal component in the inflammatory response because in addition to their ability to kill and digest micro-organisms, they present their foreign antigen to lymphocytes and engender highly specific adaptive immune responses. Inflammatory cells also release a wide range of mediators which act to regulate the whole inflammatory process [6].

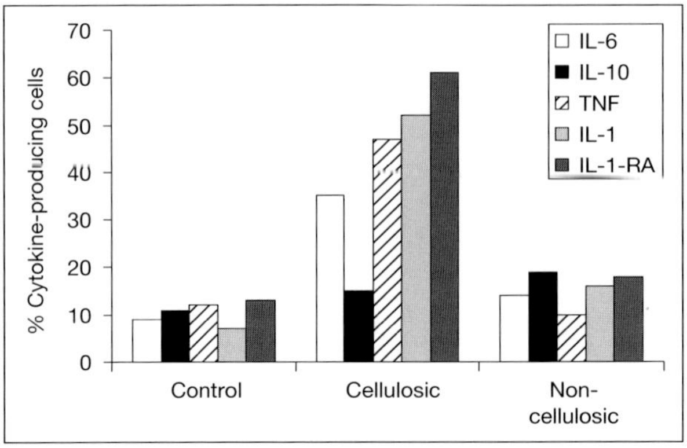

Fig. 1. Intracytoplasmic cytokines expression in mononuclear cells from controls and hemodialysis patients. Cells were washed, fixed and permeabilized, and intracellular cytokine production was determined using specific monoclonal antibodies. The data represent the mean ± SE from 10 controls and 26 hemodialysis patients (13 treated with cellulosic membrane and 13 with noncellulosic hemodialysis membrane).

Normally in the bloodstream macrophages exist in a nonactivated state (monocytes) and in the absence of stimulation they have a relatively short lifespan limited by apoptosis to 3–5 days [7]. However, numerous stimuli including specific bacterial products (mainly the lypopolysaccharide; LPS), or proinflammatory cytokines may activate macrophages prolonging their lifespan to maintain an effective response until the resolution of inflammation [8].

Hemodialysis Membranes Induce Proinflammatory Activity in Mononuclear Cells

Interaction of monocytes with hemodialysis membranes, mainly with non biocompatible membranes, induce activation of mononuclear cells which results in phosphorylation of cellular proteins [9], increased expression of adhesion molecules, increased expression of some activation markers such as the LPS (CD14) receptor, and formation of cellular aggregates [10–12]. In addition, increased levels of proinflammatory cytokines, oxidative products or lysosomal enzymes have been reported to be associated to hemodialysis with cellulosic membranes [13]. Furthermore, using single-cell cytokine determination, we have observed that cellulosic membranes induce the production of proinflammatory cytokines by mononuclear cells from healthy subjects (fig. 1).

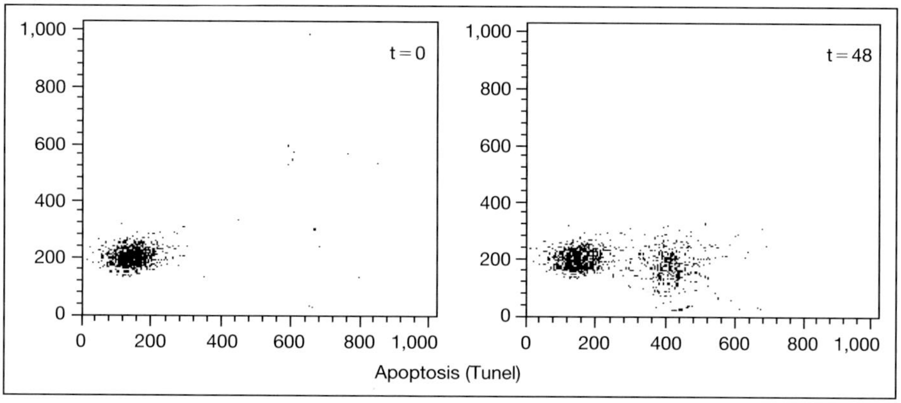

Fig. 2. Representative flow cytometric study of apoptosis in mononuclear cells from a patient on hemodialysis with cellulosic membranes. Cells were cultured during 48 h in complete medium, and apoptosis studied by Tunel assay.

Previous reports demonstrated that pro-inflammatory cytokines as well as LPS prolong the normal monocyte life-span [7]. Macrophages from cellulosic hemodialysis patients exhibit characteristics of cells with prolonged life-span such as: decreased telomere length, increased percentage of cells CD14dim/CD16bright and increased production of IL-1β and IL6 cytokines, supporting that inflammatory stimuli associated to hemodialysis, may act on macrophages prolonging their life-span [14].

Monocytes that Have Been in Contact with Cellulose Membranes Are More Likely to Undergo Spontaneous Apoptosis after Culture 'ex vivo'

It is reasonable to think that the excessive permanence of activated macrophages in the inflammatory site may became detrimental. In order to prevent the perpetuation of activated cells after inflammatory stimuli has been finished, macrophages rapidly undergo apoptosis due to the presence of anti-inflammatory cytokines. Alternatively, these cells undergo spontaneous apoptosis when deprived of pro-inflammatory factors. Macrophages from patients dialyzed with cellulosic membranes undergo spontaneous apoptosis when cultured in vitro (fig. 2) [15]. Furthermore, apoptosis is mainly observed in cells producing proinflammatory cytokines (fig. 3), indicating that apoptosis may be involved in the regulation of inflammation [14].

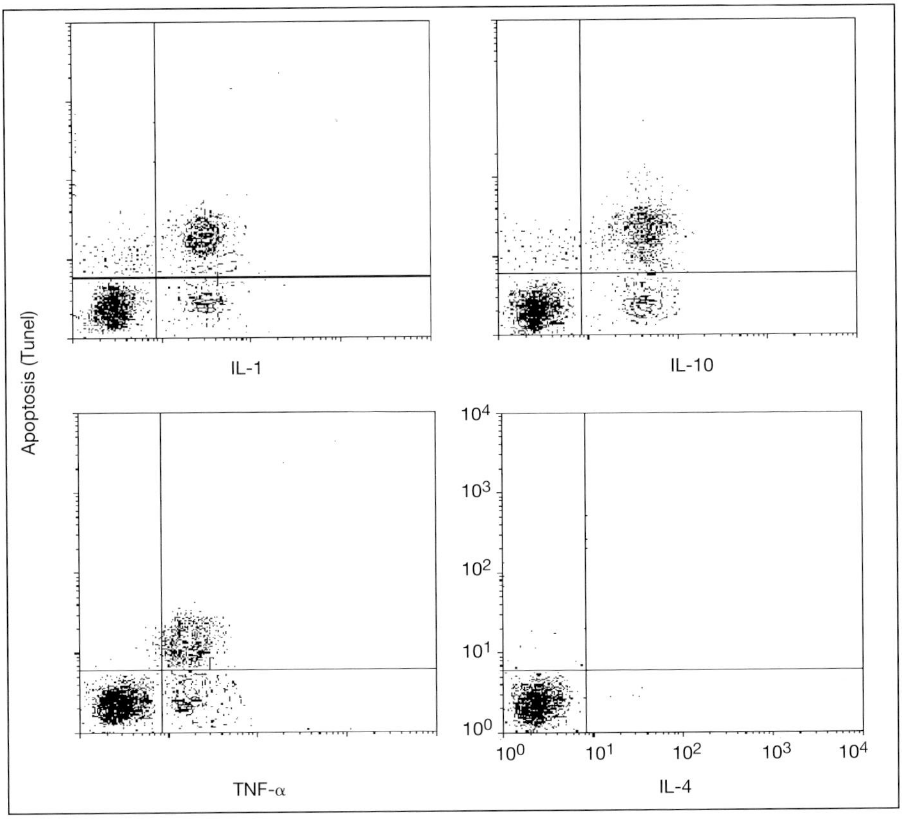

Fig. 3. Representative dot plots study of intracytoplasmic cytokine production and apoptosis in cells from a patient hemodialyzed with a cellulosic membrane. After culture, cells were permeabilized and labeled simultaneously with Phycoerithrin (PE)-conjugated anti-cytokine antibodies and TUNEL, using the respective PE and TUNEL labeled controls.

Effect of Bacterial Contamination in the Inflammatory Activity Induced by Hemodialysis Membranes in Mononuclear Cells

The results described above suggest that apoptosis of pro-inflammatory cells may have a beneficial effect by preventing the supervivence of dangerous/harmful cells in hemodialysis patients. However, bacterial products such as LPS may prevent macrophage apoptosis. To investigate the effect of bacterial contamination on mononuclear cell apoptosis associated to hemodialysis, mononuclear cells from patients dialyzed with cellulosic membranes were cultured with LPS. As shown in figure 4, the presence of LPS in culture medium prevented

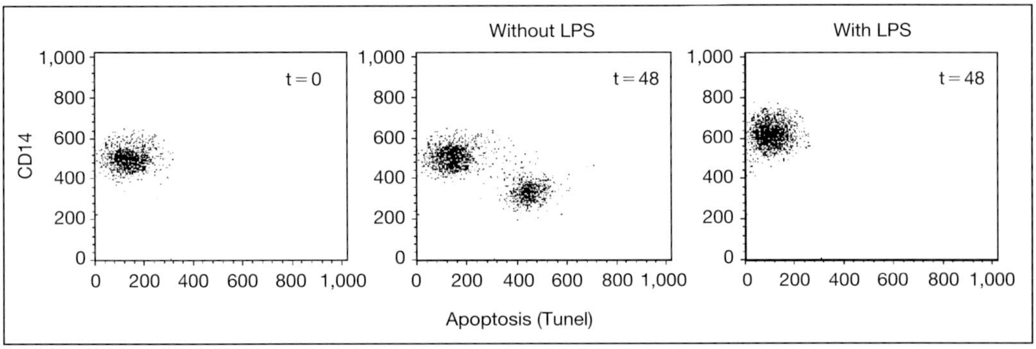

Fig. 4. Representative scatter plots obtained by flow cytometry. This figure shows the relation between CD14 expression and apoptosis in cells from a patient on hemodialysis with a cellulosic membrane cultured during 48 h in complete medium alone or with the addition of LPS (10 ng/ml).

spontaneous apoptosis in mononuclear cells. Furthermore, when cytokine production was studied in these cells by intracellular staining, production of proinflammatory activity was maintained. This suggests that bacterial contamination may perpetuate the presence of macrophages with inflammatory activity by preventing apoptosis.

Most of the results presented above are only observed in the presence of nonbiocompatible hemodialysis membranes. Biocompatible hemodialysis membranes induce a moderate monocyte activation (increase phosphorylation of proteins, expression of some activation molecules) without significant repercussion in the production of inflammatory cytokines or apoptosis [9, 14]. One of the characteristics of bacterial products is that when used at sub-stimulating concentrations, it may 'prime' immune cells, making these cells more susceptible to be stimulated by other signals. The term 'to prime' is being used to define a process whereby the response of an inflammatory cell to an activating stimulus is significantly potentiated by costimulation with a determined agent. This is an important consideration because various research groups have demonstrated that some substances like complement factors [16, 17] or bacterial endotoxins (namely LPS) [18, 19] may amplify the activation of mononuclear cells induced by hemodialysis membranes. In order to explore whether LPS is priming monocytes to increase the activation signals generated by the biocompatible hemodialisis membrane, we have performed some experiments in which monocytes were cultured with a biocompatible noncellulosic hemodialysis membrane and LPS at nonstimulating doses. The results obtained demonstrated that monocytes primed by LPS display a proinflammatory activity which is similar to that observed using nonbiocompatible cellulosic membranes (fig. 5); including monocyte life-span.

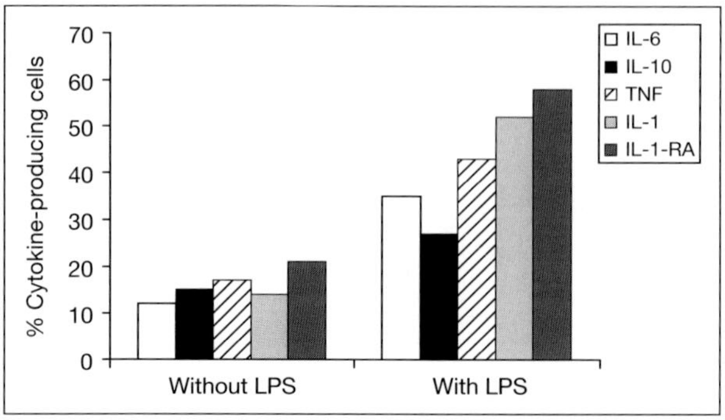

Fig. 5. Effect of LPS in the intracytoplasmic cytokines expression in mononuclear cells from 15 patients in hemodialysis with noncellulosic membranes. Cells were cultured in the presence of 10 ng/ml of LPS. After 48 h of culture cells were washed, fixed and permeabilized, and intracellular cytokine production was determined using specific monoclonal antibodies.

Conclusions

Nonbiocompatible hemodialysis membranes may activate monocytes to produce proinflammatory cytokines, and prolong their life-span. This process is limited by the increased susceptibility of senescent macrophages to undergo apoptosis when deprived of proinflammatory factors, which likely occurs when the hemodialysis session is finished. However, bacterial contamination may alter this equilibrium, since bacterial products (not only LPS, easily detected by microbiological test, but also bacterial DNA) may prime macrophages. Thus, stimulated cells did not undergo apoptosis and the inflammatory process remained after the hemodialysis session. Furthermore, priming of monocytes by contaminating factors may have important clinical consequences because 'priming monocytes' respond to biocompatible membranes with a proinflammatory activity similar to that observed with nonbiocompatible membranes. These findings may explain at least in part some of the clinical alterations induced by biocompatible membranes.

Acknowledgements

This study was supported by the Fondo de Investigación Sanitaria (FIS 98/0423, 00/0788, 00/0701), the Junta de Andalucía (213/00 and 72/00). R.R. is supported by FIS contract 00/3030, and J.C. is supported by FIS contract 98/3123.

References

1 Plutzky J: Inflammatory pathways in atherosclerosis and acute coronary syndromes. Am J Cardiol 2001;88:10–15.
2 Selzman CH, Miller SA, Harken AH: Therapeutic implications of inflammation in atherosclerotic cardiovascular disease. Ann Thorac Surg 2001;71:2066–2074.
3 Kaysen GA: The Microinflammatory state in uremia: Causes and potential consequences. J Am Soc Nephrol 2001;12:1549–1557.
4 Levin A, Djurdjev O, Barrett B, Burgess E, Carlisle E, Ethier J, Jindal K, Mendelssohn D, Tobe S, Singer J, Thompson C: Cardiovascular disease in patients with chronic kidney disease: Getting to the heart of the matter. Am J Kidney Dis 2001;38:1398–1407.
5 Mezzano D, Pais EO, Aranda E, Panes O, Downey P, Ortiz M, Tagle R, Gonzalez F, Quiroga T, Caceres MS, Leighton F, Pereira J: Inflammation, not hyperhomocysteinemia, is related to oxidative stress and hemostatic and endothelial dysfunction in uremia. Kidney Int 2001;60:1844–1850.
6 Hansson GK: Inflammation and immune response in atherosclerosis. Curr Atheroscler Rep 1999; 1:150–155.
7 Heidenreich S, Schmidt M, August C, Cullen P, Rademaekers A, Pauels HG: Regulation of human monocyte apoptosis by the CD14 molecule. J Immunol 1997;159:3178–3188.
8 Mangan DF, Wahl SM: Differential regulation of human monocyte programmed cell death (apoptosis) by chemotactic factors and pro-inflammatory cytokines. J Immunol 1991;147:3408–3412.
9 Carracedo J, Ramírez R, Martin-Malo A, Rodríguez M, Aljama P: Nonbiocompatible hemodialysis membranes induce apoptosis in mononuclear cells: The role of G-proteins. J Am Soc Nephrol 1998;9:46–53.
10 Carracedo J, Ramirez R, Pintado O, Gomez-Villamandos J, Martín-Malo A, Rodríguez M, Aljama P: Cell aggregation and apoptosis induced by hemodialysis membranes. J Am Soc Nephrol 1995;6:1586–1591.
11 Carracedo J, Ramirez R, Martin-Malo A, Rodriguez M, Madueño JA, Aljama P: Role of adhesion molecules in mononuclear cell apoptosis induced bycuprophan hemodialysis membranes. Nephron 2001;89:186–193.
12 Carracedo J, Ramirez R, Martin-Malo A, Rodriguez M, Aljama P: The effect of LPS, uremia and haemodialysis membrane exposure on CD14 expression in mononuclear cells and its relation to apoptosis. Nephrol Dial Transplant 2002;17:428–434.
13 Schwedler S, Schinzel R, Vaith P, Wanner C: Inflammation and advanced glycation end products in uremia: Simple coexistence, potentiation or causal relationship? Kidney Int 2001;78(suppl):S32–S36.
14 Carracedo J, Ramirez R, Madueño JA, Soriano S, Rodríguez-Benot A, Rodriguez M, Martin-Malo A, Aljama P: Cell apoptosis and hemodialysis-induced inflammation. Kidney Int, in press.
15 Martín-Malo A, Carracedo J, Ramirez R, Rodríguez-Benot A, Soriano S, Rodriguez M, Aljama P: Effect of uremia and dialysis modality on mononuclear cell apoptosis. J Am Soc Nephrol 2000;11: 936–942.
16 Craddock PR, Fehr J, Dalmaso AP, Brigham KL, Jacob HS: Hemodialysis leukopenia: Pulmonary vascular leukostasis resulting from complement activation by dialyzer cellophane membranes. J Clin Invest 1977;59:879–888.
17 Cheung AK, Parker CJ, Wilcox LA, Janatoba J: Activation of complement by hemodialysis membranes: Polyacrylonitrile binds more C3a than cuprophan. Kidney Int 1990;37:1055–1059.
18 Lonnemann G, Bingel M, Floege J, Koch KM, Shaldon S, Dinarello CA: Detection of endotoxin like interleukin-1-inducing activity during in vitro dialysis. Kidney Int 1988;33:29–35.
19 Laude-Sharp M, Caroff M, Simard L, Pusineri C, Kazatchkine MD, Haeffner-Cavaillon N: Induction of IL-1 during hemodialysis: transmembrane passage of intact endotoxins (LPS). Kidney Int 1990;38:1089–1094.

Dr. Pedro Aljama, Servicio de Nefrología, Hospital Universitario Reina Sofía,
Avda Menendez Pidal s/n, E–14004 Córdoba (Spain)
Tel. +34 957 010143, E-Mail paljama@hrs.sas.junta-andalusia.es

Ronco C, La Greca G (eds): Hemodialysis Technology.
Contrib Nephrol. Basel, Karger, 2002, vol 137, pp 332–337

On-Line Fluid Preparation

Gerhard Lonnemann

Gemeinschaftspraxis Nephrologie, Langenhagen, Germany

The preparation of substitution fluid for hemofiltration (HF) and hemodiafiltration (HDF) by the hemodialysis monitor (on-line preparation) became popular during the last decade for several reasons. First of all, high-flux treatment modalities with a high degree of convective transmembrane transport in order to improve middle molecule clearances require large volumes of substitution fluid. In conventional treatment modalities of HF and HDF the ultrafiltrate is replaced by intravenous infusion of sterile replacement fluid which is provided in sterile bags of 2–5 liters each by the pharmaceutical industry. In particular when high volume HF or HDF with ultrafiltration volumes as high as 50 liters per treatment are performed and bicarbonate instead of lactate buffer is used, expenses for replacement fluid increase tremendously. Alternatively, the on-line preparation of substitution fluid, in other words the use of fluid produced by the dialysis monitor for intravenous infusion, could provide the opportunity of cost-effective convective high-flux therapies. The problem of on-line preparation of infusion fluid is to ensure sterility. To address this issue, bacterial and pyrogen contamination of dialysis water, the role of biofilm formation in dialysis tubing and measures to produce ultrapure infusion fluid from bicarbonate-buffered dialysis fluid are discussed below.

Microbiological Quality of Dialysis Water

State-of-the-art preparation of water for dialysis involves several steps of filtration to remove organic particles, a softener to remove bivalent ions such as calcium and magnesium, and a reverse osmosis unit to produce pure H_2O containing no heavy metals or trace elements, no microorganisms and no bacterial products such as endotoxin. The reverse osmosis unit is connected to a loop pipe to supply the dialysis monitors with water to produce dialysis fluid from

Table 1. Standards for the bacteriological quality and pyrogen contamination of dialysis fluid

	Bacterial growth CFU/ml	Endotoxin EU/ml	Cytokine induction
Tap water (pharmacop)	100	0.25	±
Water (DAKN)	100	0.25	±
Dialysis fluid (DAKN)	1,000	0.50	+
Ultrapure fluid	<0.1	<0.03	–
Sterile fluid	<0.000001	<0.03	–

pharmacop = European Pharmacopoeia; DAKN = Deutsche Arbeitsgemeinschaft für klinische Nephrologie; + = yes; – = no.

processed water and salt concentrates. In the described system, freshly produced reverse osmosis water should be ultrapure with a bacterial growth of less than 0.1 colony-forming units (CFU)/ml, and an endotoxin concentration of less than 0.03 endotoxin units (EU)/ml when it enters the loop pipe (table 1). Bacterial contamination of reverse osmosis water occurs predominantly in the connecting tubes between the loop pipe and the dialysis monitor and inside the monitor. Connection sites and dead-end tubes are locations of entry and growth of microorganisms. Retrograde contamination of the loop pipe with bacteria and bacterial products derived from the connecting tubes may occur.

Monitoring microbiological quality of dialysis water has several pitfalls. Adequate determination of bacterial growth in water requires special agars (R2A, tryptone glucose extract), room temperature and prolonged incubation time (7 days) [1]. Using these methods, bacterial growth in dialysis water is detectable and may exceed recommended standards for dialysis water which is equal to the European Pharmacopoeia for tap water (bacterial growth <100 CFU/ml; endotoxin <0.25 EU/ml) (table 1). However, the measured contamination in water samples may only represent the peak of the iceberg of dialysis water contamination because of the phenomenon of biofilm formation. A biofilm consists of microorganisms immobilized at the inner surface of water and dialysate tubing in an organic polymer matrix of bacterial origin. Discharge of bacterial products from biofilm may act as a reservoir for continuous contamination of dialysis water [2]. Attempts to remove the biofilm using daily heat or chemical disinfection of the loop pipe may reduce the thickness of the biofilm but cannot prevent its formation completely.

Taken together, even with state-of-the-art technology significant contamination of dialysis water cannot be excluded. Therefore, if on-line produced dialysis fluid is intended to be used for intravenous infusion, special measures to ensure sterility or ultrapure quality (see table 1) have to be applied.

On-Line Preparation of Ultrapure Dialysis Fluid

By definition, sterile fluid should contain less than 1 CFU in 1,000 liters and no detectable endotoxin activity with the limulus amebocyte lysate (LAL) assay (table 1). Since 1,000 liters of dialysis fluid are never produced by a dialysis monitor in a single treatment session, the term 'sterile' cannot be applied to describe the microbiological quality of dialysis water. In order to overcome the problem of adequately describing the superior quality of the dialysis fluid the term 'ultrapure' was created [3]. Ultrapure fluid should contain less than 0.1 CFU/ml and no detectable endotoxin using the LAL test (lower detection limit at least 0.03 EU/ml).

Ultrafiltration through Pyrogen-Adsorbing High-Flux Membranes

In vitro ultrafiltration experiments were performed using culture filtrates of *Escherichia coli* and *Pseudomonas* species to challenge high-flux filter membranes and the incubation of human peripheral blood mononuclear cells to measure the cytokine-inducing activity of bacterial culture filtrates in addition to their LAL activity. These experiments demonstrated that the synthetic high-flux membranes polysulfone and polyamide retain cytokine-inducing substances (CIS) derived from bacterial cultures by size exclusion and, more importantly, by adsorption [4, 5]. In particular the common waterborne *Pseudomonas* species release CIS of a small molecular weight (<5,000 kD) which can only be rejected by adsorption. Adsorption involves binding of the lipid-like small CIS to hydrophobic domains of the synthetic polymers, a mechanism called hydrophobic interaction. In comparison to other synthetic high-flux membranes, the sponge-like support structure of polysulfone and polyamide bears relatively large hydrophobic domains which are responsible for their superior adsorptive capacity. An endotoxin concentration of 500 EU/ml in dialysis fluid, which is 1,000-fold in excess of the upper limit of recommended standards (table 1), does not lead to detectable CIS or LAL activity in the ultrafiltrate of polysulfone or polyamide ultrafilters [4, 5].

These in vitro data indicate that ultrafiltration through CIS-adsorbing synthetic high-flux membranes provides an effective measure to produce ultrapure dialysis fluid with a sufficiently high margin of safety.

Clinical studies using polysulfone and polyamide ultrafilters in the dialysis fluid circuit showed that moderately contaminated dialysis fluid (bacterial contamination <1000 CFU/ml; LAL <0.5 EU/ml) is improved to ultrapure

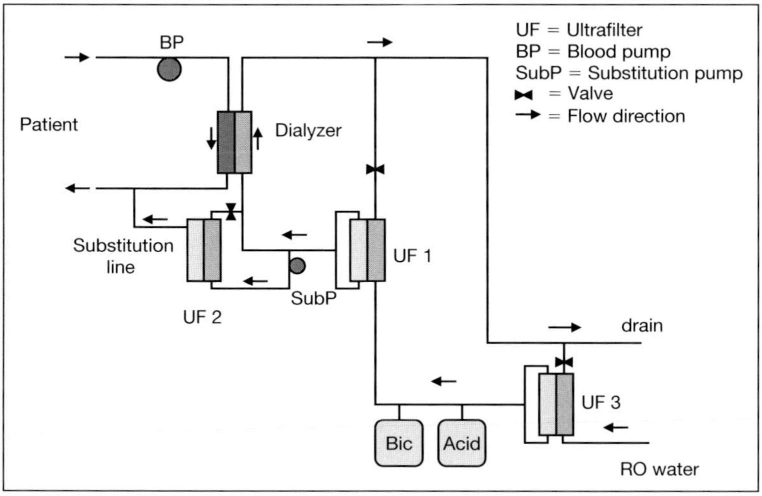

Fig. 1. On-line preparation of ultrapure pyrogen-free substitution fluid.

quality. There was no evidence of a breakthrough of LAL activity or CIS when the ultrafilters had been installed for up to 3 months filtering as much as 18,000 liters of moderately contaminated dialysis fluid [6, 7]. Several subsequent studies demonstrated that the use of ultrafilters does not only produce ultrapure dialysis fluid but also reduces the release of cytokines (such as tumor necrosis factor-α and interleukin-1 receptor antagonist) and C-reactive protein in hemodialysis patients [6–8].

Double Cascade Filtration for On-Line Production of Infusion Fluid

For on-line production of infusion fluid low grade contamination of reverse osmosis water provided by the loop pipe is a precondition. The water quality should be controlled on a regular basis and has to fulfil recommended standards (table 1). Single-step ultrafiltration is able to ensure ultrapure quality of dialysis fluid for hemodialysis. In order to further improve ultrapure fluid, double filtration of dialysis fluid through two synthetic high-flux filters in a cascade mode has been introduced [9]. Today, there are several modifications of on-line HDF machines available. All systems use two ultrafilters in a row to filter the dialysis fluid freshly mixed from ultrapure water, acid and bicarbonate concentrates (fig. 1). In all systems, one ultrafilter (UF 1) is installed in the dialysis fluid circuit and is included in the rinsing and disinfection program of the dialysis monitor. The second ultrafilter (UF 2) is either also integrated in the dialysis fluid circuit and replaced together with UF 1 every 100 treatments, or is a disposable filter for single use. In all systems, single-filtered fluid is used as dialysate and double-filtered fluid is used for intravenous substitution in on-line HF or HDF. To ensure ultrapure quality of reverse osmosis water before mixing dialysis fluid, one on-line system employs an additional ultrafilter (UF 3) at the water entry of the dialysis monitor (fig. 1).

All modifications of on-line systems have been used for high volume HDF and the bacteriological quality as well as the endotoxin concentration (using a very sensitive LAL assay, detection limit 0.005 EU/ml) and the cytokine-inducing activity of ultrafiltered dialysis fluid were repeatedly tested in samples from the substitution line [10–12]. Over study periods of up to 12 months and routine replacement of ultrafilters every 100 sessions, neither bacterial growth nor endotoxin nor cytokine induction was detected in samples of single-step-filtered dialysis fluid and two-step-filtered infusion fluid [10–12]. Comparing these parameters to those in commercially available sterile infusion solutions, on-line prepared substitution fluid can be referred to as sterile and pyrogen-free [3, 7].

Conclusion

On-line preparation of substitution fluid for intravenous infusion requires a good quality of reverse osmosis water as a precondition and two-step filtration of dialysis fluid mixed from RO water, dry bicarbonate powder and liquid acid concentrates. Today, double filtration through pyrogen-adsorbing synthetic membranes is a practical, safe and cost-effective approach to produce pyrogen-free substitution fluid on-line.

References

1 Lonnemann G: Assessment of quality of dialysate. Nephrol Dial Transplant 1998;13(suppl 5): 17–20.

2 Man NK, Degremont A, Darbord JC, Collet M, Vaillant P: Evidence of bacterial biofilm in tubing from hydraulic pathway of hemodialysis system. Artif Organs 1998;22:596–600.

3 Ledebo I, Nystrand R: Defining the microbiological quality of dialysis fluid. Artif Organs 1999; 23:37–43.

4 Dinarello CA, Lonnemann G, Maxwell R, Shaldon S: Ultrafiltration to reject human interleukin-1-inducing substances derived from bacterial cultures. J Clin Microbiol 1987;25:1233–1238.

5 Schindler R, Dinarello CA: Ultrafiltration to remove endotoxins and other cytokine-inducing materials from tissue culture media and parenteral fluids. Biotechniques 1990;8:408–413.

6 Schindler R, Lonnemann G, Schäffer J, Shaldon S, Koch KM, Krautzig S: The effect of ultrafiltered dialysate on the cellular content of interleukin-1 receptor antagonist in patients on chronic hemodialysis. Nephron 1994;68:229–233.

7 Vaslaki L, Karatson A, Vörös P, Major L, Pethö F, Ladanyi E, Weber C, Mitteregger R, Falkenhagen D: Can sterile and pyrogen-free on-line substitution fluid be routinely delivered? A multicentric study on the microbiological safety of on-line haemodiafiltration. Nephrol Dial Transplant 2000;15(suppl 1):74–78.

8 Sitter T, Bergner A, Schiffl H: Dialysis related cytokine induction and response to recombinant human erythropoietin in haemodialysis patients. Nephrol Dial Transplant 2000;15:1207–1211.
9 Canaud B, Bosc JY, Leray-Moragues H, Stec F, Argiles A, Leblanc M, Mion C: On-line haemodiafiltration. Safety and efficacy in long-term clinical practice. Nephrol Dial Transplant 2000; 15(suppl 1):60–67.
10 Canaud B, Wizemann V, Pizzarelli F, Greenwood R, Schultze G, Weber C, Falkenhagen D: Cellular interleukin-1 receptor antagonist production in patients receiving on-line haemodiafiltration therapy. Nephrol Dial Transplant 2001;16:2181–2187.
11 Ward RA, Schmidt B, Hullin J, Hillebrand GF, Samtleben W: A comparison of on-line hemodiafiltration and high-flux hemodialysis: A prospective clinical study. J Am Soc Nephrol 2000; 11:2344–2350.
12 Lin CL, Yang CW, Chiang CC, Chang CT, Huang CC: Long-term on-line hemodiafiltration reduces predialysis beta-2-microglobulin levels in chronic hemodialysis patients. Blood Purif 2001;19:301–307.

Gerhard Lonnemann, MD, Gemeinschaftspraxis für Nephrologie/Dialyse,
Eickenhof 15, D–30851 Langenhagen (Germany)
Tel. +49 511 786560, Fax +49 511 7865625, E-Mail GLonnemann@t-online.de

Ronco C, La Greca G (eds): Hemodialysis Technology.
Contrib Nephrol. Basel, Karger, 2002, vol 137, pp 338–343

Sodium Content and Profiling

Francesco Locatelli, Sara Colzani, Pietro Pozzoni, Celestina Manzoni, Salvatore Di Filippo

Department of Nephrology and Dialysis, Azienda Ospedale di Lecco, Italy

It is well known that dialytic sodium removal has very important clinical implications. Changes in the body sodium pool play a role in the pathogenesis of intradialytic cardiovascular instability, interdialytic overhydration and hypertension [1]. Despite technological advances in hemodialysis (HD) equipment and modalities, cardiovascular instability during HD treatment remains an important clinical problem. This is due to several factors: progressive aging of the dialysis population, increased frequency of cardiovascular risk factors, and tendency to shorten each HD treatment by increasing blood flow, dialyzer surface and ultrafiltration rate.

Despite improved pharmacological therapy, hypertension is epidemic among HD patients. In fact, 90% of this population is either hypertensive or on antihypertensive therapy. Together with anemia and cardiovascular calcifications, hypertension is the major determinant of cardiovascular disease, accounting for more than 50% of deaths of HD patients. The high prevalence of hypertension in the HD population may be attributed to excessive interdialytic sodium intake, inability to control volume with 'ultrashort' dialysis. Finally, therapy with erythropoietin is now considered a possible additive factor.

With the aim of improving blood pressure control while maintaining a comfortable dialysis, several methods have been proposed. It has to be noticed that not all of these are equally efficient and safe. Different parameters in the HD prescription can be modified: dialysate sodium content, ultrafiltration rate, dialysis time, dialysis technique. Each of these factors certainly affects the cardiovascular state of the patient. Hence, it is clear that the dialysis prescription must be individualized for each patient and his specific needs. Given the daily fluctuations in individual dietary sodium and water intake, HD prescription should be different not only among patients, but also intra-patient from one dialysis session to another. Finally, the development of technology and software processors have opened the doors to control systems that automatically modify dialytic parameters according to individual changes during the same dialytic session.

Dialysate Sodium Content

Sodium crosses dialysis membranes by two mechanisms: diffusion and convection. It is well known that the sodium fractions involved in these mechanisms are not the same [2]. In the past some difficulties came from the laboratory methods used to measure the blood and dialysate sodium concentrations (flame photometry or ionometry). Presently dialysis centers generally use the ionometry method, simplifying communication among nephrologists of different centers. Direct ionometry measures the ionized plasma water sodium concentration in the blood and ionized sodium concentration in the dialysate. It is acceptable to assume for clinical purposes that the plasma water sodium concentration measured by direct ionometry corresponds to the total ultrafiltrable sodium. Diffusive sodium transport depends on the difference between the sodium concentration in blood and dialysis fluid. Given the Donnan effect, the blood sodium concentration measured by direct ionometry should be corrected for a Donnan factor of 0.967 to obtain sodium available for diffusion. In contrast, as the dialysate is protein-free, the ionized sodium concentration measured by direct ionometry can be considered the concentration available for diffusion.

When the blood sodium concentration available for diffusion is known, it is possible to change the dialysate sodium concentration in order to obtain an 'isonatric', 'hyponatric' or 'hypernatric' dialysis. A low sodium dialysate can theoretically be used if we want the patient to lose sodium by diffusion (e.g. when the programmed ultrafiltration is insufficient to remove the amount of accumulated sodium). However, because of the risk of cellular overhydration, considered to be responsible for the disequilibrium syndrome, we feel that this practice should be avoided. A high dialysate sodium concentration is more frequently needed in order to avoid excessive sodium losses due to ultrafiltration and prevent cardiovascular instability. However, a 'hypernatric dialysis' can lead to insufficient sodium removal and increase the risk of hypertension, pulmonary edema and cardiac failure.

Sodium Profiling

In order to obtain good conditions during the hemodialysis treatment and optimal postdialysis volume and electrolyte concentrations, the use of sodium profiles has been proposed. The purpose of these sodium profiles is to determine, and in some cases automatically modify, the dialytic parameters for each patient, in each dialysis session and at different times during the same dialysis session. Some authors [3, 4] have proposed the so-called 'sodium ramping' profile. In the early phase of the HD treatment a dialysate with sodium concentration higher than that found in the blood is used. As the session progresses, the dialysate sodium concentration is decreased, either continuously or in a stepwise manner.

Frequently, these sodium profiles combine a variation of dialysate sodium concentration during dialysis session with a variation of ultrafiltration rate. Generally, a higher ultrafiltration rate is combined with a higher dialysate sodium concentration in the first phase of HD, which reversed in the final phase [5]. Given the role of hypovolemia in the genesis of intradialytic hypotension, the introduction of on-line blood volume continuous monitoring has offered the opportunity of changing both the ultrafiltration rate and the dialysate sodium concentration in order to maintain a constant blood volume reduction rate [6, 7].

When these sodium profiles were compared with standard dialysis, an improvement in cardiovascular stability was generally shown. However, frequently this was only an apparent improvement as higher postdialysis plasma sodium concentration, predialysis body weight and blood pressure values, resulting from a reduced sodium removal, were also demonstrated [4, 5]. A positive sodium balance can lead to side effects such as thirst, hypertension, fluid overload and pulmonary edema.

Several studies that evaluated the effect of different sodium profiles on cardiovascular instability did not take into account the sodium balance (table 1). In fact, in some cases the information necessary to calculate the sodium removal, including the technique used to measure sodium concentrations, were not reported.

The purpose of a correct hemodialysis treatment being to reproduce normal kidney function, the water and sodium removal during each dialysis session has to correspond to water and sodium accumulation during the interdialytic period.

Intradialytic water and sodium removal are equal to the interdialytic accumulation when the water/sodium balance is zero, that is, when final dry body weight is reached and the final plasma water sodium concentration is constant. For this purpose, the required water removal can be easily determined, as it corresponds to the interdialytic increase in body weight. In contrast, a mathematical kinetic model must be used at the start of treatment in order to predict the final plasma water sodium concentration and to calculate the needed dialysate sodium concentration.

Table 1. Evaluation of sodium removal in different dialytic treatments

Study	Treatment	Na measurement	Na pre-HD mmol/l	Na post-HD mmol/l	Pre-HD body weight kg	Post-HD body weight kg	Total UF liters	Na removal mEq/session
Levin et al. [3]	standard	√	136 ± 0.4	136 ± 0.5	73.7 ± 0.17	71.5 ± 0.17	2.2	√
	ramped	√	137 ± 0.4	140 ± 0.5	73.9 ± 0.17	71.4 ± 0.17	2.5	√
Lam Sui Sang et al. [4]	standard	√	137 ± 5	139 ± 2	√	√	√	√
	ramped	√	138 ± 4	145 ± 3	√	√	√	√
Oliver et al. [5]	standard	√	137.0	139.7	71.7	69.1	2.6	√
	profiled	√	137.3	141.0	72.1	69.2	2.9	√
Santoro et al. [6]	standard	direct ionometry	√	146 ± 1.5	√	68 ± 6.2	3.1 ± 0.6	√
	feed-back	direct ionometry	√	146.2 ± 1.1	√	67.2 ± 5.7	3.5 ± 0.4	√
Ronco et al. [7]	standard	√	√	√	√	√	3.6 ± 0.7	√
	feed-back	√	√	√	√	√	3.7 ± 0.7	√

Sodium Kinetic Model

By using flame photometry, Gotch developed a single pool sodium kinetic for hemodialysis. Di Filippo et al. [8] applied this model but measured sodium levels by direct potentiometry rather than flame photometry. Because of the greater precision of direct potentiometry, these authors were able to make a more accurate calculation of sodium balance. Unfortunately, neither of these models are suitable for routine clinical use because of the need for blood sampling and laboratory determinations at each dialysis session.

Given the linear correlation between the conductivity of an electrolyte solution and its sodium content, the conductivity values can be used as an estimate of sodium concentration. According to the theory developed by Polashegg [9] and Peticlerc et al. [10], ionic dialysance may be easily calculated from the dialysate conductivity measured at the dialyzer inlet and outlet ports, at two different inlet conductivity values. Then, plasma water conductivity can also be calculated. Therefore, the sodium kinetic model can be changed into the conductivity kinetic model. This allows to predict the final plasma water conductivity when the dialysate conductivity is known, and to determine the dialysate conductivity needed to obtain the desired final plasma water conductivity.

The sodium and conductivity kinetic models cannot be applied in hemodiafiltration, as sodium removal is derived not only from the sodium concentration in the dialysate, but also from that in the reinfusion fluids. Di Filippo et al. [11] developed a single-pool sodium kinetic model, and consequently a conductivity kinetic model, that can be applied in paired filtration dialysis (PFD), a hemodiafiltration technique in which convection and diffusion take place

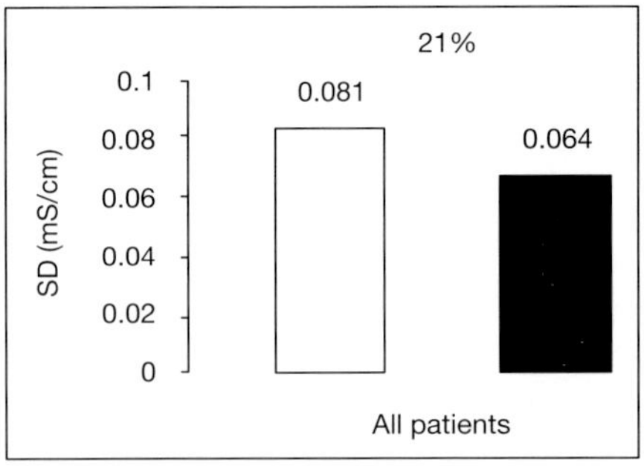

Fig. 1. Reduction of the final plasma water conductivity variability (expressed by standard deviation reduction) by applying the conductivity kinetic model in paired filtration dialysis. □ = Conventional paired filtration dialysis; ■ = paired filtration dialysis with the use of the kinetic modeling.

separately [11]. This made it possible to evaluate whether the clinical application of these models actually reduces intradialytic morbidity. A multicenter prospective controlled randomized trial [12] demonstrated that, in comparison with conventional PFD, the application of the conductivity kinetic improved cardiovascular stability in hemodialysis patients prone to dialysis hypotension combined to a reduction of the variability of the final plasma water conductivity (fig. 1).

Conclusions

The progressive development of automatic systems will allow in the future a combination of the benefits of the sodium kinetic model and those of sodium modelling. In order to obtain a sodium removal equal to the interdialytic sodium intake and the correct dry body weight, the ultrafiltration rate and the dialysate conductivity can be modulated during the dialysis session. These systems consist of software loops designed to actuate a biofeedback response based on signals derived on-line from the patient/machine complex. The integrated multi-input–multi-output controller and its software are the heart of these biofeedback systems. Today, online monitoring is possible for different parameters, such as conductivity, body weight loss, relative blood volume changes, thermal balance, urea kinetics, and access recirculation.

References

1 Locatelli F, Di Filippo S, Manzoni C: Relevance of the conductivity kinetic model in the control of sodium pool. Kidney Int 2000;58(suppl 76):S89–S95.

2 Locatelli F, Colzani S, D'Amico M, Manzoni C and Di Filippo S: Dry weight and sodium balance. Semin Nephrol 2001;21:291–297.

3 Levin A, Goldstein MB. The benefits and side effects of ramped hypertonic sodium dialysis. J Am Soc Nephrol 1996;7:242–246.

4 Lam Sui Sang G, Kovithevongs C, Ulan R, Kjellstrand CM: Sodium ramping in hemodialysis: A study of beneficial and adverse effects. Am J Kid Dis 1997;29:669–677.
5 Oliver MJ, Edwards LJ, Churchill DN: Impact of sodium and ultrafiltration profiling on hemodiaysis-related symptoms. J Am Soc Nephrol 2001;12:151–156.
6 Santoro A, Mancini E, Paolini F, Cavicchioli G, Bosetto A, Zucchelli P: Blood volume regulation during hemodialysis. Am J Kidney Dis 1998;32:739–748.
7 Ronco C, Brendolan A, Milan M, Rodeghiero MP, Zanella M, La Greca G: Impact of biofeedback-induced cardiovascular stability on hemodialysis tolerance and efficiency. Kidney Int 2000;58: 800–808.
8 Di Filippo S, Corti M, Andrulli S, Manzoni C, Locatelli F: Determining the adequacy of sodium balance in hemodialysis using a kinetic model. Blood Purif 1996;14:431–436.
9 Polashegg HD: Automatic non-invasive intradialytic clearance measurements. Int J Artif Organs 1993;16:185–191.
10 Peticlerc T, Goux N, Reynier AL, Benè B: A model for non-invasive estimation of in vivo dialyzer performances and patient's conductivity during hemodialysis. Int J Artif Organs 1993; 16:585–591.
11 Di Filippo S, Corti M, Andrulli S, Pontoriero G, Manzoni C, Locatelli F: Optimization of sodium removal in paired filtration dialysis by single pool sodium and conductivity kinetics models. Blood Purif 1997;15:34–44.
12 Locatelli F, Andrulli S, Di Filippo S, Redaelli B, Mangano S, Navino C, Ariano R, Tagliaferri M, Fidelio T, Corti M, Civardi S, Tetta C: The effect of on-line conductivity plasma ultrafiltrate kinetic modeling on cardiovascular stability of hemodialysis patients. Kidney Int 1998;53:1052–1060.

Prof. Francesco Locatelli, MD, Divisione di Nefrologia e Dialisi,
Azienda Ospedale 'A. Manzoni', Via dell'Eremo 9–11, I–23900 Lecco (Italy)
Tel. +39 0341489850, Fax +39 0341489860, E-Mail nefrologia@ospedale.lecco.it

Ronco C, La Greca G (eds): Hemodialysis Technology.
Contrib Nephrol. Basel, Karger, 2002, vol 137, pp 344–349

Dialysate/Infusate Composition and Infusion Mode in On-Line Hemodiafiltration

Luciano A. Pedrini, Vincenzo De Cristofaro, Bruno Pagliari, Pio Ruggiero

Nephrology and Dialysis Unit, Ospedale di Sondrio, Bergamo, Italy

The growth in the application of hemodiafiltration (HDF), due to its ability to increase convective removal of both small and medium-high molecular weight toxins, has been encouraged further by the availability of unlimited quantities of sterile substitution fluid produced on-line at low cost. In on-line HDF infusion of large amounts of a solution with the same electrolyte and buffer concentration as the dialysate modifies the dynamics of ionic transmembrane exchanges, thus influencing the final balance of the sessions. A crucial role may also be exerted by the infusion method. These factors may unpredictably affect the solute flux across the membrane and prevent the attainment of the planned session balance when patients are switched from hemodialysis (HD) to HDF or from one HDF infusion technique to another.

Sodium

Sodium is removed mainly by convection during extracorporeal treatment. Isolated ultrafiltration has an Na retentive effect (sieving effect), related to the electrical attraction of the negatively charged proteins. During dialysis, diffusion transfer across the membrane increases or counteracts sodium loss by convection depending on the direction of the gradient of sodium activity between blood and dialysate. Eventually, this mechanism determines the final balance of the session [1, 2]. In HDF additional factors, such as the sodium content of the replacement fluid and the rate and site of its infusion, contribute to the final

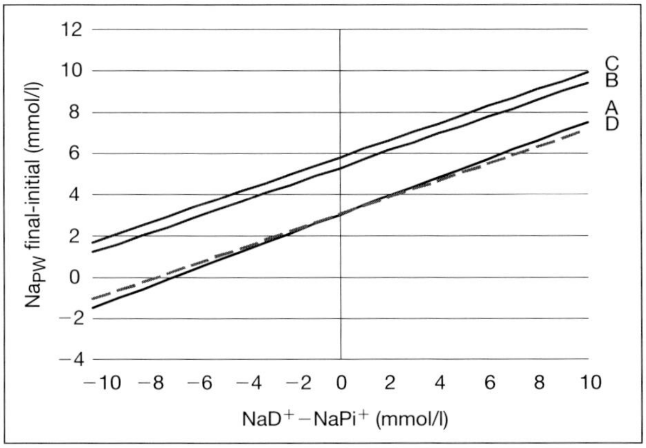

Fig. 1. Relation between plasma water Na changes during the session and dialysate-blood Na activity gradient. The regression lines C (for AFB), B (postdilution HDF) and A (HD) were derived from the statistical model developed by Pedrini et al. [3]. The general equation of the model was: $[Na_{pw}\ f - Na_{pw}\ i] = a + b\ [NaD - NaP] + c\ [NaR] + d\ QUF$, where D, P and R are dialysate, plasma and reinfusion fluid, respectively. Coefficient values and significance are reported by Pedrini et al. [3]. The dotted line (D) refers to on-line postdilution HDF, and was derived from the general equation of the model by imposing NaR = NaD, and QUF = 100 ml/min.

balance [3]. In postdilution HDF and in acetate-free biofiltration (AFB), solutions containing 140–145 and 167 mmol/l of Na (photometry measurements) infused at about 60 and 35 ml/min, respectively, resulted in a final plasma water Na concentration similar to that in HD only when the sodium gradient between dialysate and plasma was decreased by 2.7 mmol/l in HDF and by about 10 mmol/l in AFB compared to HD (fig. 1). No studies have yet been published comparing Na balance with traditional techniques and with on-line HDF, in which the infusate has the same composition as the dialysate. When simulated with a statistical model [3], the relationship between plasma-dialysate/infusate Na gradient and plasma water Na changes is similar in on-line postdilution HDF and in HD, and the two regression lines overlap (fig. 1). Comparable results have been obtained in another set of patients (fig. 2), in whom the effects of on-line predilution were examined as well. In the same patient and at similar operating conditions, significantly lower net Na removal was observed in pre-HDF versus post-HDF (fig. 2). Indeed, the two infusion modes produce different hydraulic conditions within the dialyzer. Predilution flow modifies the activity of plasma sodium ions and of other dissolved solutes which interact with sodium (bicarbonate, carbonate, sulfate). The increased water flow entering the filter dilutes proteins and exerts an increased shear stress. This reduces

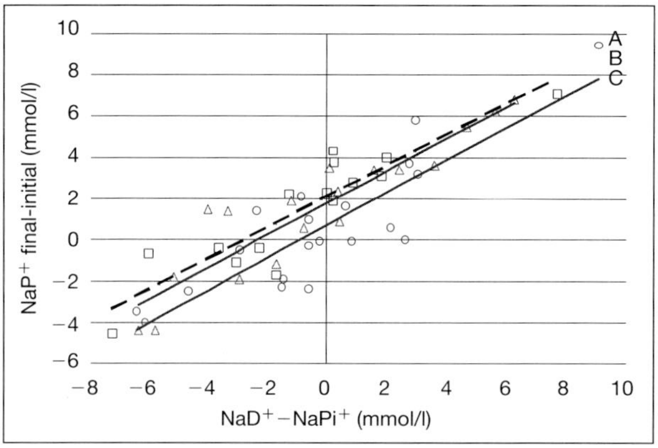

Fig. 2. The same relation as in figure 1 in 20 patients submitted to HD (□, dotted line = A), on-line post-HDF (△ = B) performed at a filtration fraction of 0.5, and on-line pre-HDF (○ = C) performed at $Q_{UF} = Q_{PW}$ (comment in the text).

the thickness of the secondary protein layer and thus the electrical barrier that opposes the Na flux. Temperature and pH influence sodium activity as well. All these effects together modify the ionic activity available for diffusion and convection. Moreover, Na activity changes continuously along the dialyzer from blood entry to exit, in relation to the effects of Q_{UF} on protein concentration. The resultant net Na flux across the membrane is not easily predictable. Available statistical models [3] suggest that, if the same plasma-dialysate Na activity gradient is maintained, the final Na balance in on-line post-HDF is not significantly different from that in HD, possibly as a result of a compensatory mechanism between Na flux by convection and diffusion. The rate of ultrafiltration has a minor influence on the final result. In the same basal conditions, Na removal in on-line predilution HDF is higher than in post-HDF. Similarly to the other strategies, the plasma-dialysate Na activity gradient is the main factor determining the amount of sodium removed, but its relation to changes in plasma sodium activity is reset to a lower level, due to the previously mentioned flux conditions produced by the predilution of blood entering the filter.

Bicarbonate

During bicarbonate dialysis a positive HCO_3^- balance is induced by a diffusive anion flux from the dialysate to plasma, along the HCO_3^- concentration gradient across the membrane. When low Q_{UF} are applied, a decrease in the net transfer occurs, due to the opposing direction of HCO_3^- convective flux. With higher Q_{UF}, as in HDF, the net HCO_3^- transfer becomes negative, due to the outstanding loss by convection. The profound influence of Q_{UF} on net HCO_3^- transport has been clearly demonstrated in HDF [4]. In this case the anion gain by diffusion, even with the highest concentration gradients, is insufficient to compensate for the loss caused by convection and a positive balance is achieved only with the amount of bases infused with the replacement fluid. During traditional HDF the fixed buffer concentration in replacement fluid bags may sometimes prevent the reaching of an adequate balance. Individual clinical requirements are more easily accomplished in on-line HDF, which allows a more precise modulation of the dialysate/infusate HCO_3^- concentration taking into account the mode and the rate of infusion. The infusion mode per se was shown to influence significantly the final balance of bicarbonate [5]. When different infusion modes in on-line HDF were compared in the same patients with similar basal acid base status and operating conditions (Q_{UF}, Q_B, Q_D and dialysate HCO_3^-), the final blood HCO_3^- concentration, and thus the final HCO_3^- balance of the sessions were found to be different. A significantly lower HCO_3^- gain was observed in pre-HDF, compared to post-HDF, while the difference between post-HDF and mixed HDF was not significant [6]. As observed in HD, changes in blood HCO_3^- concentration during the session correlated significantly with the difference between the mean dialysate/infusate HCO_3^- and the baseline blood concentration in all the three tested infusion modes. However, the parallel regression lines generated by multiple regression analysis showed that same final blood HCO_3 concentration and balance as in post-HDF may be obtained by increasing the dialysate HCO_3^- by about 2 mmol/l in pre-HDF and 1 mmol/l in mixed HDF.

The mechanisms underlying these different balances may be clarified by analyzing the instantaneous HCO_3^- transfer across the dialyzer membrane during the three infusion modes. When compared to post-HDF, during pre-HDF and mixed HDF, infusion of a solution at a higher HCO_3^- concentration than systemic blood increased HCO_3^- blood concentration entering the dialyzer, producing two opposite effects on ion transport across the membrane: ion loss by convection was enhanced, while gain by diffusion was reduced, due to a lower dialysate-blood HCO_3^- gradient, the driving force for diffusive exchanges.

Calcium

Calcium transfer by diffusion depends on the concentration gradient between dialysate calcium (ionized and bound) and ultrafiltrable blood calcium. Transfer from dialysate to blood can be expected in HD, provided that the dialysate calcium concentration is higher than 1.6 mmol/l [7]. The overall mass balance, derived from the algebraic sum of diffusive gain and convective loss may be adapted to individual needs by modulating calcium dialysate concentration. When dialysate calcium is lower than 1.5 mmol/l, a negative mass balance is usually achieved. In HDF convective calcium loss may overcome the patient's calcium gain by diffusion. Mass balance may still be weakly positive with Q_{UF} up to 60 ml/min provided that the substitution fluid contains calcium (at least 1.75 mmol/l). Otherwise, if the substitution fluid is calcium-free, a negative balance is the rule, and calcium loss is directly related to Q_{UF} [8]. Calcium kinetics becomes more complex in on-line HDF with high Q_{UF}. Mass balance is still dependent on the concentration gradient between blood and dialysate/infusate and on Q_{UF}, but it may be affected by the infusion mode, as in the case of sodium and bicarbonate. In predilution HDF calcium blood uptake by diffusion is significantly lowered as a result of both the increase in blood calcium concentration entering the dialyzer and the dilution of plasma proteins binding calcium [9]. For the same reason calcium loss by convection is enhanced. Consequently, for any given calcium gradient, calcium mass balance in on-line predilution HDF is expected to be lower than in HD. Opposite mechanisms seem to take place in postdilution HDF: no wasting of calcium gradient and a considerable increase in plasma protein concentration which limits calcium loss by convection. The negative net calcium balance across the dialyzer is counterbalanced by the direct infusion of large amounts of calcium with the replacement solution. The final balance for a given blood-dialysate gradient does not differ from HD [10]. No studies are available concerning the use of very high replacement volumes (up to 300ml/min) in on-line predilution or mixed pre- and postdilution HDF. It is likely that in spite of larger amounts of substitution fluid, the calcium dialysate/infusate concentration has to be increased in order to avoid a negative calcium mass balance.

References

1 Locatelli F, Ponti R, Pedrini L, Costanzo R, Di Filippo S, Marai P, Pozzi C: Sodium kinetics across dialysis membranes. Nephron 1984;38:174–177.

2 Gotch FA, Evans MC, Keen ML: Measurement of the effective dialyzer Na diffusion gradient in vitro and in vivo. Trans Am Soc Artif Intern Organs 1985;31:354–358.

3 Pedrini LA, Ponti R, Faranna P, Cozzi G, Locatelli F: Sodium modeling in hemodiafiltration. Kidney Int 1991;40:525–532.

4 Feriani M, Ronco C, Biasioli S, Bragantini L, La Greca G: Effect of dialysate and substitution fluid buffer on buffer flux in hemodiafiltration. Kidney Int 1990;39:711–717.

5 De Cristofaro V, Pagliari B, Pedrini L: Acid-base balance in pre- and post-dilution on-line hemodiafiltration; in De Santo NG (ed): Acid-Base Balance: From Bench to Bedside. Proceedings of the 3 G.A. Borelli Conference, Anacapri. Editoriale BIOS, 1999, pp 209–217.

6 Pedrini LA, De Cristofaro V, Masa A, Pagliari B, Samà F, Colturi C, Filippini M: Effects of the infusion mode on bicarbonate balance in on-line hemodiafiltration. Int J Artif Organs 2002;26:100–106.

7 Binswanger U: Calcium flux during hemodialysis. Semin in Dial 1990;1:1–2.
8 Malberti F, Surian M: Ionized calcium changes and parathyroid hormone secretion in haemodiafiltration in relation to substitution fluid calcium content. Nephrol Dial Transplant 1991;S2: 104–107.
9 Duncan PH, Savory J, Gitelman HJ: Effects of hemodialysis on protein-bound calcium. Kidney Int 1979;15:283–285.
10 Argiles A, Kerr PG, Canaud B, Flavier JL, Mion C: Calcium kinetics and the long-term effects of lowering dialysate calcium concentration. Kidney Int 1993;43:630–640.

Luciano A. Pedrini, Piazza Mascheroni, 8, I–24129 Bergamo (Italy)
Tel. +39 0338 5719480, Fax +39 035 237277, E-Mail la.pedrini@katamail.com

Ronco C, La Greca G (eds): Hemodialysis Technology.
Contrib Nephrol. Basel, Karger, 2002, vol 137, pp 350–356

Dialysate/Infusate Calcium and Magnesium

Corrado Vitale, Martino Marangella, Adriano Ramello

Nephrology and Dialysis Unit, Mauriziano Umberto I Hospital, Turin, Italy

The intestinal absorption of magnesium (Mg) is not impaired in end-stage renal disease (ESRD). Thus, serum Mg levels tend to increase progressively, and an adequate removal by dialysis must be provided. Conversely, there is a marked impairment of intestinal calcium (Ca) absorption in ESRD, which makes the physiological intestinal Ca loss of about 4 mmol/day worse. As a consequence, there is a risk of negative Ca balances with these patients, especially if they are on a phosphate-restricted diet without Ca and vitamin D supplements. It is difficult to estimate the whole Ca balance in ESRD patients. The net intestinal absorption of Ca is not easy to define, because, among other things, the Ca availability of phosphate binders and the whole effect of vitamin D supplements are poorly predictable. On the other hand, different dialysis protocols can produce either positive or negative Ca fluxes during the treatment. Thus, in ESRD a metabolic equilibrium for Ca depends on a correct balance between the net intestinal absorption of Ca and the net Ca fluxes during dialysis sessions. Either a positive or a negative imbalance of dietary and dialytic Ca fluxes may have detrimental effects, namely hypercalcemia, adynamic bone disease and ectopic calcifications result from sustained positive balances, severe hyperparathyroidism and bone disease, on the other hand, from sustained negative balances.

Ca and Mg Balances in Standard Hemodialysis

Dialytic Ca balance depends on the plasma and dialysate Ca concentrations, the convective removal of the diffusible Ca with ultrafiltration and the plasma phosphate concentration. In the 1970s, many authors suggested that in

Table 1. Ca and Mg balances in HD and HDF with Ca/Mg-free infusional fluids

	HD (7 patients)	HDF (14 patients)
UF rate, ml/min	14 ± 3	38 ± 9*
Predialysis diffusible Ca, mmol/l	1.22 ± 0.21	1.16 ± 0.25
Postdialysis diffusible Ca, mmol/l	1.33 ± 0.30	1.31 ± 0.25
Dialysate diffusible Ca, mmol/l	1.74 ± 0.07	1.75 ± 0.05
Ca balance, mmol	31.74 ± 10.63	22.56 ± 10.33
Predialysis diffusible Mg, mmol/l	0.78 ± 0.30	0.86 ± 0.26
Postdialysis diffusible Mg, mmol/l	0.53 ± 0.14	0.59 ± 0.17
Dialysate diffusible Mg, mmol/l	0.39 ± 0.13	0.43 ± 0.12
Mg balance, mmol	−4.69 ± 2.21	−6.95 ± 7.99

*$p < 0.001$.

standard hemodialysis (HD), a dialysate Ca concentration of 1.75 mmol/l provided sufficient Ca to offset the intestinal losses, prevented bone disease and hyperparathyroidism and reduced the risk of metastatic calcification. Moreover, skeletal Ca loss frequently occurred with dialysate Ca of 1.5 mmol/l and total body Ca increased with the use of a 2 mmol/l dialysate Ca [1].

In our experience, by comparing fresh and spent dialysate during bicarbonate HD (dialysate Ca 1.74 ± 0.07 mmol/l, Mg 0.39 ± 0.13 mmol/l), we observed a positive Ca balance of 31.7 ± 10.6 mmol and a negative Mg balance of 4.6 ± 2.2 mmol (table 1) [2]. Goldsmith et al. [3] described a slight but significant inverse correlation between serum phosphate levels and diffusive gain of Ca from the dialysate. They speculated that it could have been an effect of a higher Ca drag caused by the augmented phosphate flux through the membrane. Furthermore, it has been pointed out that Ca mass transfer depends on the gradient between the predialysis serum diffusible Ca concentration and the dialysate diffusible Ca concentration, the latter being affected by pH and buffer composition [4]. Moreover, many authors reported that the actual measured dialysate Ca concentrations were lower than predicted by the manufacturers.

Over the past two decades, calcium-containing phosphate binders progressively replaced aluminum-containing compounds and, currently, they are frequently used together with vitamin D. This therapy enhances Ca bioavailability, so that a dialysis Ca content lower than 1.75 mmol/l was recommended to avoid hypercalcemia. Thus, a dialysate Ca of 1.5 mmol/l in HD patients given adequate Ca and vitamin D supplements was reported as safe, provided a careful metabolic surveillance was done. Lower dialysate Ca, i.e. 1.25 mmol/l, was reported to be at risk for detrimental effects on bone metabolism [5].

In order to control hyperphosphatemia minimizing the risk of hypercalcemia, Mg salts were added to Ca salts as phosphate binders. Kelber et al. [6] observed that a 0.75 mmol/l Mg dialysate removed a negligible amount of Mg, and evaluated the effects of both 0.25 mmol/l and Mg-free dialysates in patients given $MgCO_3$ as a phosphate binder. They observed a poor clinical tolerance of a Mg-free dialysate (muscular cramps), whereas a 0.25 Mg dialysate was well tolerated and allowed a good Mg balance in patients given about 1 g $MgCO_3$ per day [6]. Thus, concentrations of about 0.25–0.50 mmol/l appear advisable, the lower values being more useful in patients taking significant amounts of Mg-containing phosphate binders.

More recently, a new phosphate binder was produced, which is both aluminum- and calcium-free, namely, sevelamer hydrochloride. It is generally used in patients with an exaggerated calcemic response to Ca-containing compounds in spite of low-dialysate Ca. It should be considered that the withdrawal of Ca-containing binders induces a sudden reduction of intestinal Ca absorption, and that it may be necessary to readjust dialysate Ca upwards to avoid negative balances. Similarly, if the noncalcemic vitamin D metabolites confirmed their theoretical advantages, patients who shifted from calcitriol to these compounds probably needed to have their dialysate Ca raised as well.

In conclusion, a dialysate Ca of 1.75 mmol/l should provide adequate balances for HD patients taking Ca-free phosphate binders, whereas a dialysate Ca of 1.50 mmol/l is advisable for patients taking Ca-containing binders and vitamin D supplements. Levels between 1.25 and 1.50 mmol/l should be used in selected cases and under thorough metabolic surveillance. A Mg dialysate content of 0.25–0.50 mmol/l provided both adequate Mg removal and Mg plasma levels in all patients on HD.

Ca and Mg Balances in Hemodiafiltration

In hemodiafiltration (HDF), diffusive and convective transports are coupled. In comparison with HD, the higher ultrafiltration (UF) rate counteracts the diffusive Ca gain from dialysate to blood and enhances the diffusive removal of Mg from blood to dialysate. Moreover, the variable Ca and Mg contents of the infusional fluids may further influence the electrolyte balances. In order to investigate this topic, we measured Ca and Mg balances in HD and in HDF patients with Ca- and Mg-free infusions; in both groups the same dialysate composition was used. Although it was not statistically significant, we observed a 50% reduction of the positive Ca balance and a 50% increase of the negative Mg balance in HDF (table 1). In accordance with others, we observed a negative Ca balance for UF rates over 70 ml/min [2].

In the last decade, safe techniques for on-line production of sterile infusate from dialysate were developed, so that HDF was more frequently performed by using infusional fluids of the same composition as dialysate. Argilés et al. [5], from instantaneous mass transfer measurements in on-line HDF, reported negative Ca balances only with dialysate Ca below 1.25 mmol/l. Malberti et al. [4], from a whole on-line dialysate collection, observed a nearly neutral Ca balance with dialysate Ca of about 1.75 mmol/l and negative Ca balances (6–9 mmol/session) with dialysate Ca of 1.5 mmol/l or lower. The main determinants of Ca balance were the dialysate Ca content and the dialysate to serum gradient of diffusible Ca, with negligible effects of UF rates ranging from 2.5 to 5 liters/h [4]. Thus, on-line HDF with a dialysate/infusate Ca of 1.75 mmol/l seems advisable in almost all patients, whereas Ca concentrations of 1.5 mmol/l or lower may induce negative Ca balances and should be used in patients given adequate amounts of Ca and vitamin D. On the other hand, if Ca-free substitution fluids are used along with 1.75 mmol/l Ca dialysate, a negative Ca balance may ensue, if the UF rate exceeds 70 ml/min.

Ca and Mg Balances in Hemofiltration

In hemofiltration, Ca and Mg balances depend on both their different concentrations between the removed plasma water and infusional fluids and their electrolyte losses with net UF. A negative Ca balance may occur despite an increase in plasma Ca levels. It has been reported that an infusate Ca concentration of 1.75 mmol/l provided positive Ca balances in the case of slight net fluid loss, whereas a 2 mmol/l infusate Ca was needed for net weight loss exceeding 4 liters [7]. As far as Mg is concerned, an infusate concentration of 0.25–0.5 mmol/l provided an adequate Mg removal and normal Mg plasma levels.

Ca/Mg Dialysate, Parathyroid Function and Bone Metabolism

As outlined above, neutral or even negative intra-HD/HDF Ca balances were used to allow a wider use of calcium-containing phosphate binders and vitamin D. In such cases, one must assume that the intestinal Ca absorption counterbalances the dialysis Ca losses. However, the Ca intake, intestinal bioavailability and absorption may vary significantly over time, so that the safety of a long-term use of low-Ca dialysate on bone metabolism must be carefully evaluated. The variations of bone mineral content over time should depend on similar variations of the net Ca balance. However, little data exists on this topic. During a 2-year observation, using an in vivo neutron activation analysis, a negative total body Ca balance was reported in patients on HD treated with a dialysate Ca concentration of 1.25 mmol/l and a nil or positive balance in those treated with a Ca concentration of 1.6 mmol/l [8]. Other authors observed an increase in bone mineral density (BMD) in HD only in patients with 1.75 mmol/l Ca dialysate [9]. Recently, BMD was determined by quantitative computerized tomography (QCT) in patients on HD with 1.50 mmol/l of dialysate Ca, given Ca-containing phosphate binders. Of these patients, one half had been switched to 1.25 mmol/l of dialysate Ca (group 2), the others had been left on the standard treatment (group 1). One year later, no significant variations in both BMD and parathyroid hormone (PTH) were observed in group 1. Conversely, a significant reduction of BMD and an increase of PTH were observed in group 2, despite an intake of 6 ± 3 g of elemental Ca, with a significant inverse correlation between PTH increases and the rate of BMD losses [10]. This data suggests that in patients without severe impairment of Ca sensitivity of parathyroid glands, plasma profiles of PTH are reliable markers of overall Ca balance. Moreover, it has been reported that the large intradialytic reduction of PTH and positive Ca balance using a standard Ca dialysate of 1.75 mmol/l are temporary events. Therefore, the interdialytic events, namely net Ca balance, are probably the strongest stimulus to physiological parathyroid activity.

As far as PTH levels are concerned, lowering standard Ca dialysate (1.75 mmol/l) to 1.50 mmol/l and raising oral Ca supplies provide a good control of both serum phosphate and PTH. The same effects were reported by means of a dialysate Ca of 1.25 mmol/l and very large doses of $CaCO_3$ or vitamin D [11–13]. A 2-fold increase of PTH was reported in HD patients 1 year after being shifted from 1.75 to 1.25 mmol/l Ca dialysate, with no concomitant serum ionized Ca or phosphate changes, thereby suggesting these are misleading indicators of Ca balance [14]. In patients on HDF, PTH showed a 40% reduction in those treated with a Ca dialysate of 1.50 mmol/l and who were given Ca-containing phosphate binders.

In the end, Ca dialysate composition should be tailored to each case. Many authors considered a dialysate Ca concentration of 1.50 mmol/l as the first choice in HD patients taking Ca-containing phosphate binders and/or vitamin D. This results in a continuous rather than intermittent and unphysiological intradialytic Ca load. A Ca concentration of 1.75 mmol/l could be temporarily used with Ca-depleted patients, if attention is paid to the occurrence of hypercalcemia and high serum Ca $\times$ P products, which can induce soft tissue calcifications. A dialysate Ca of 1.25 mmol/l may be used in patients with a high tendency to hypercalcemia who have good compliance with $CaCO_3$.

In the past two decades, some authors suggested that high Mg levels could suppress PTH and used high-Mg dialysate levels. However, these findings were not confirmed. Therefore, since both positive and negative Mg balances may have detrimental effects on bone and other organs, it appears advisable to adjust dialysate Mg to values yielding fluctuations across the normal range, namely 0.25–0.50 mmol/l [6].

Ca Dialysate and Cardiovascular Effects

In HDF patients, the changes in serum ionized Ca induced by a reduction of dialysate Ca from 1.75 to 1.25 mmol/l significantly impaired myocardial contractility and blood pressure [15]. On the other hand, Nappi et al. [16] reported that an HD with 1.75 mmol/l dialysate Ca reduced left ventricular relaxation when compared with HD with dialysate Ca of 1.50 mmol/l or lower.

The high plasma ionized Ca improves the vascular tone and blood pressure during HD. This reduction of vascular elasticity induces an increase in pulse pressure, which is an independent factor of cardiovascular mortality. A significant reduction in vascular elasticity was observed during HD with 1.75 mmol/l of dialysate Ca. No impairment was demonstrated during HD with 1.50 mmol/l dialysate Ca [17]. Ionized Ca levels may also play a role in the occurrence of ECG derangements and arrhythmias during HD. Taking the variations in QT interval length as a predisposing factor to heart ventricular arrhythmias, it has been demonstrated that HD increases QT dispersion if 1.25 mmol/l of dialysate Ca is used [18]. In order to correct intradialytic instability and simultaneously minimize the risk of developing hypercalcemia, an innovative approach with variable dialysate Ca concentrations has recently been proposed, namely 1.25 mmol/l for the first 2 h and 1.75 mmol/l for the last 2 h [19]. Further studies are required to confirm the safety and usefulness of dialysate Ca profiling during HD.

References

1 Denney JD, Sherrard DJ, Nelp WB, Chestnut CH, Baylink DJ: Total body calcium and long-term calcium balance in chronic renal disease. J Lab Clin Med 1973;82:226–240.

2 Vitale C, Marangella M, Petrarulo M, Cosseddu D, Tricerri A, Bianco O, Linari F: Studio del bilancio minerale in emodialisi e in emodiafiltrazione. Minerva Urol Nefrol 1990;42:173–176.

3 Goldsmith RS, Furszyfer J, Johnson WJ, Beeler GW Jr, Taylor WF: Calcium flux during hemodialysis. Nephron 1978;20/3:132–140.

4 Malberti F, Corradi B, Tetta C, Imbasciati E: Calcium balance and serum ionised calcium fluctuations in on-line hemodiafiltration in relation to ultrafiltration rate and dialysate calcium concentration. Nephrol Dial Transplant 1994;9:1759–1764.

5 Argilés A, Kerr PG, Canaud B, Flavier JL, Mion C: Calcium kinetics and the long-term effects of lowering dialysate calcium concentration. Kidney Int 1993;43:630–640.

6 Kelber J, Slatopolsky E, Delmez JA: Acute effects of different concentration of dialysate magnesium during high-efficiency dialysis. Am J Kidney Dis 1994;24:453–460.

7 Fuchs C, Dorn D, Henning HV, Matthaei D, McIntosh C, Kramer P, Ritter D, Schunemann B, Scheler F: Calcium and phosphate metabolism in hemofiltration. Klin Wochenschr 1978;56: 1163–1169.

8 Asad SN, Ellis KJ, Cohn SH, Letteri JM: Changes in total body calcium on prolonged maintenance hemodialysis with high and low dialysate calcium. Nephron 1979;23/5:223–227.
9 Van der Niepen P, Sennesael J, Louis O, Verbeelen D: Effect of treatment with 1.25 and 1.75 mmol/l calcium dialysate on bone mineral density in hemodialysis patients. Nephrol Dial Transplant 1995;10:2253–2258.
10 Sanchez Perales MC, Garcia Cortes MJ, Borrego FJ, Fernandez Martinez S, Borrego J, Perez de Barrio P, Liebana A, Perez Banasco V: Hemodialysis with 2.5 mEq/l of calcium in relative hypoparathyroidism: Long term effects on bone mass. Nefrologia 2000;20:254–261.
11 Argilés A, Mourad G: How do we have to use the calcium in the dialysate to optimize the management of secondary hyperparathyroidism? Nephrol Dial Transplant 1998;13(suppl 3):62–64.
12 Slatopolsky E, Weerts C, Norwood K, Giles K, Fryer P, Finch J, Windus D, Delmez J: Long-term effects of calcium carbonate and 2.5 mEq/liter calcium dialysate on mineral metabolism. Kidney Int 1989;36:897–903.
13 Moriniere P, El Esper N, Viron B, Judith D, Bourgeon B, Farquet C, Gheerbrant J, Chapuy M, Van Orshoven A, Pamphile R, Fournier A: Improvement of severe secondary hyperparathyroidism in dialysis patients by intravenous 1α (OH) vitamin D_3, oral $CaCO_3$ and low dialysate calcium. Kidney Int Suppl 1993;41:S121–S124.
14 Fernandez E, Borras M, Pais B, Montoliu J: Low-calcium dialysate stimulates PTH secretion and its long-term use worsens secondary hyperparathyroidism. J Am Soc Nephrol 1995;6/1:132–135.
15 van der Sande FM, Cheriex EC, van Kuijk WHM, Leunissen KML: Effect of dialysate calcium concentrations on intradialytic blood pressure course in cardiac-compromised patients. Am J Kidney Dis 1998;32/1:125–131.
16 Nappi SE, Saha HH, Virtanen VK, Mustonen JT, Pasternack AI: Hemodialysis with high-calcium dialysate impairs cardiac relaxation. Kidney Int 1999;55:1091–1096.
17 Kyriazis J, Stamatiadis D, Mamouna A: Intradialytic and interdialytic effects of treatment with 1.25 and 1.75 mmol/L of calcium dialysate on arterial compliance in patients on hemodialysis. Am J Kidney Dis 2000;35:1096–1103.
18 Nappi SE, Virtanen VK, Saha HHT, Mustonen JT, Pasternack AI: QTc dispersion increases during hemodialysis with low-calcium dialysate. Kidney Int 2000;57:2117–2122.
19 Kyriazis J, Glotsos J, Bilirakis L, Smirnioudis N, Tripolitou M, Georgiakodis F, Grimani I: Dialysate calcium profiling during hemodialysis: Use and clinical implications. Kidney Int 2002;61/1:276–287.

Dr. Corrado Vitale, U.O. Nefrologia e Dialisi,
Ospedale Mauriziano Umberto I, Largo Turati, 62, I–10134 Torino (Italy)
Tel. +39 011 5082424, Fax +39 011 5082425, E-Mail covitale@libero.it

Ronco C, La Greca G (eds): Hemodialysis Technology.
Contrib Nephrol. Basel, Karger, 2002, vol 137, pp 357–363

Dialysate/Infusate Buffer Modulation in Dialysis

Mariano Feriani

Department of Nephrology and Dialysis, Umberto I° Hospital,
Mestre-Venezia, Italy

In the search for the 'uremic toxin', metabolic acidosis is the one that clearly has been demonstrated to be toxic. In renal replacement therapy patients' serum bicarbonate value is often lower than the normal range for healthy subjects, while the pH is within the normal range or only very slightly reduced because of adaptive hypocapnia. However, it seems that the acids produced by the metabolism do not continually accumulate since metabolic production is compensated by replacement therapies [1]. Particularly, Uribarri et al. [2] demonstrated that patients in RRT were in day-to day acid balance. Nonetheless, this type of metabolic acidosis probably worsens metabolic bone disease and, even when only mild, has detrimental effects on protein and amino acid metabolism. Thus, it seems prudent to try to correct this acid-base disorder in patients with renal failure.

What is still matter of debate is the desired serum bicarbonate level.

In hemodialysis, two randomised studies examining the effect of increasing dialysate bicarbonate concentration on nutritional parameters have resulted in opposite conclusions: Brady and Hasbargen [3] did not find any effect on serum albumin and total lymphocyte count, taken as nutritional markers, in two groups of patients treated with a high and a low bicarbonate concentration despite a significant difference in predialysis arterialised bicarbonate (17.3 ± 3.2 and 20.2 ± 2.9). In contrast, Williams et al. [4] found a significant increase in triceps skinfold thickness associated with an increase in predialysis arterialized total CO_2 when patients were treated with the high bicarbonate dialysate (from 22.5 ± 3.2 to 26.7 ± 3.9 and from 19.8 ± 2.7 to 23.3 ± 2.8 in the two groups studied). This beneficial effect was then reversed by resuming the standard bicarbonate dialysate. The major differences in these two studies were the levels

Table 1. Pre-and postdialysis blood bicarbonate levels in different studies

Ref.	Predialysis	Postdialysis	Dialysis bicarbonate concentration mmol/l	Patients n
7	19.8 ± 0.29	24.2 ± 0.3	36	16
8	19.1 ± 0.85	24.7 ± 0.52	35	10
9	18.4 ± 3.0		33	34
10	22.0 ± 2.4		36	8
11	21.5 ± 2.0	27.3 ± 4.0	30	5
12	21.0 ± 4.0	26.0 ± 3.0	variable	5
13	17.4	25.7	32	9
13	18.0	26.7	36	9

of serum bicarbonate achieved: despite an improvement, the serum bicarbonate concentration in the study by Brady was far from the normal range (25.2 ± 1.0 for arterialised bicarbonate [5]), while in the second study a substantial number of patients achieved the normal range (26.4 ± 1.0 for arterialised total CO_2 [5]).

These data support the view that the target for the acid base correction in dialysis patients should be the normal value for the healthy population. This value is, however, difficult to achieve in the majority of patients treated with renal replacement therapies.

During continuous therapies (CAPD and CAVH), the continuous buffer flux towards the patient continuously offsets the metabolic acid production and consequently a stability of the patient's acid base status is normally recorded. In standard thrice-a-week intermittent therapies (HD, HF, HDF) the task of counterbalancing a 48-hour metabolic acid production during the interdialytic period should be accomplished during the few hours of dialysis. Consequently, acid base status fluctuates from a postdialytic alkalosis to a predialytic acidosis. Between these two periods and for a variable length of time a normal acid base status is generally achieved [6]. Thus, the best compromise between predialysis acidosis and postdialysis alkalosis should be searched.

Factors Influencing Predialysis Serum Bicarbonate

Table 1 reports the patient's predialysis blood bicarbonate of some series in which bicarbonate hemodialysis was performed. A large interpatient and interstudy variability could be noted [7–13].

The predialysis bicarbonate level is modulated by 3 variables: metabolic acid production, ultrafiltration and amount of buffer infusion dependent on dialytic procedure.

Table 2. Influence of dialysis schedule on predialysis blood bicarbonate

	Blood bicarbonate mmol/l [17]	Buffer flux mmol/min [18]
Bicarbonate HD	15.8 ± 2.7	1.05
Lactate HDF	18.6 ± 3.3	1.56
Bicarbonate HDF	21.0 ± 2.1	2.06

When dialysis procedure (blood flow, dialysate flow, bicarbonate bath concentration, filter) and ultrafiltration are constant, dialytic base gain depends on predialysis blood bicarbonate being increased when this latter parameter is low and decreased when it is high. This is due to the transmembrane concentration gradient that varies inversely with blood bicarbonate concentration. In turn, predialysis blood bicarbonate depends on metabolic acid production during the interdialytic period, being low when acid production is high and high when acid production is low. Thus, the feedback between dialytic base gain and metabolic acid production determines a steady predialytic blood bicarbonate at a given dialytic procedure [14, 15]. Since in a stable condition the metabolic acid production is rather constant, the equilibrium could be moved to a higher level of predialysis blood bicarbonate by changing the dialytic procedures.

Several studies have demonstrated that bicarbonate concentration in dialysate bath greatly influences the dialytic buffer gain. Seyffart et al. [13] demonstrated that by increasing the bicarbonate content in the dialysate from 32 to 36 mmol/l, a significant increase in predialysis blood bicarbonate could be achieved. In 75% of the dialytic population, a total $CO_2 > 23$ mmol/l was recorded by using a 42-mmol/l bicarbonate dialysis fluid [16].

This aspect is very important in mixed diffusive convective treatments since in these treatments the concentration of buffer and the administration rate of the replacement fluid could be easily changed.

Table 2 reports the predialysis blood bicarbonate changes in 11 patients treated consecutively for 3 months with 3 different dialysis schedules [17]. These changes were correlated with the buffer flux calculated for each dialytic schedule for the same blood bicarbonate [18].

Ultrafiltration reduces predialysis blood bicarbonate by reducing the dialytic base gain. It could be theoretically calculated that 1 liter of fluid removal reduces about 20 mmol/session of the dialytic base gain [19]. Although these convective losses do not change the blood bicarbonate concentration during dialysis, the subsequent retention of an equivalent amount of alkali-free fluid in the interdialytic period does.

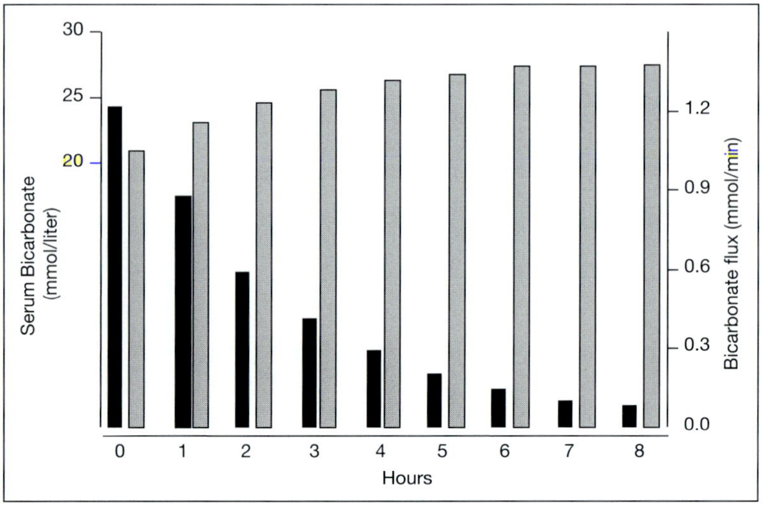

Fig. 1. Theoretical bicarbonate flux (black columns) and blood bicarbonate increase (grey columns) during dialysis

This theoretical phenomenon is demonstrated in clinical practice. In a cross-over study of 29 patients, Fabris et al. [20] found that by reducing the interdialytic weight gain of 1 kg, predialysis blood bicarbonate significantly increased by 1.6 mmol/l.

Factors Influencing Postdialysis Serum Bicarbonate

The postdialysis blood bicarbonate depends on distribution space for bicarbonate that is a function of both predialysis blood bicarbonate and body weight and on the bicarbonate concentration in the dialysate or on the amount of infused buffer with the replacement fluid [21].

During the session bicarbonate is transferred towards the patient following the concentration gradient between blood and dialysate. The gained buffer distributes into the bicarbonate space and increases the blood bicarbonate concentration. This increase in blood bicarbonate decreases the transfer of bicarbonate from dialysate by decreasing the concentration gradient across the membrane (fig. 1). When the blood bicarbonate concentration, tends to equal the dialysate bicarbonate concentration, no further bicarbonate flux from the dialysate occurs. This mechanism prevents severe alkalemia at the end of dialysis. In figure 2, the theoretical time course of blood bicarbonate during a standard

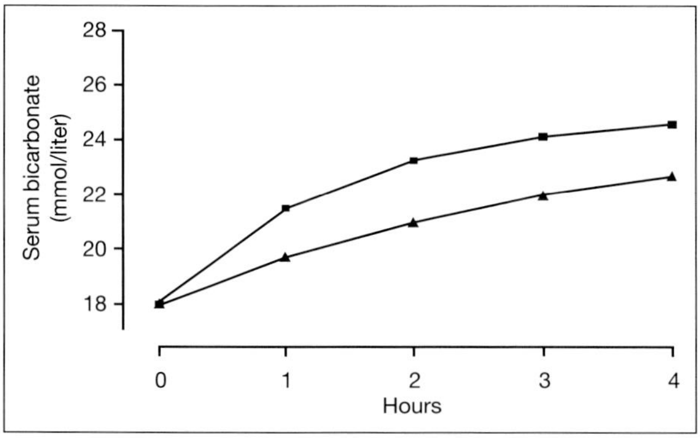

Fig. 2. Theoretical time course of blood bicarbonate levels during a standard hemodialysis (dialysate bicarbonate 35 mmol/l). Squares represent a 21.7-liter distribution space for bicarbonate, triangles represent a 43.5-liter distribution space for bicarbonate.

hemodialysis session is represented and two different distribution spaces for bicarbonate are compared. A linear increase in blood bicarbonate could be hypothesized for the high-distribution-space patients throughout the whole dialysis session, while, for the low-distribution-space patients the line could plateau during the session. In patients with a large distribution space, the dialytic bicarbonate flux during the session is diluted into a large distribution space, while the dialytic bicarbonate flux rapidly saturates the small distribution space in low-body-weight patients.

The large interpatient postdialysis variability was also confirmed in a clinical setting (table 1).

A further mechanism of the defence against alkalosis during the dialysis session has been hypothesized: the rapid addition of alkali could determine a production of organic acids, the hydrogen ion consumes the infused bicarbonate while the organic anion is lost with the dialysate. No studies have measured the size of this phenomenon.

Again, the dialytic procedure plays a basic role: probably, the concentration of bicarbonate in the dialysis fluid determines the level of equilibrium at which no more bicarbonate crosses the dialytic membrane and the organic acids production mechanism starts when the individual threshold for alkalosis is overcome. The clinical equivalent of these concepts are well illustrated by the data of Ottinger and Oliver [16]. When patients were shifted from a total base containing dialysis fluid of 39 mmol/l to a higher buffer containing fluid (42 mmol/l), postdialysis blood TCO_2 increased to around 29 mmol/l with a difference from total CO_2 at the beginning of the session of the same extent recorded for the lower-buffer-containing dialysate. In a subgroup of patients with a higher pre- and postdialysis serum total CO_2 during the low-buffer-dialysate treatment, the increase in dialysate concentration led to an increase in predialysis serum total CO_2 but the postdialysis values remained at the same level as in the low-buffer-containing dialysis solution.

There are very few data in the literature about the clinical consequences of alkalosis and no data about the clinical consequences of chronic intermittent alkalosis in dialysis patients.

Severe alkalosis depresses the central nervous system and increases neuromuscular excitability [22]. It causes hypokalemia, cardiac arrhythmias and enhances digitalis intoxication. Alkalosis also increases binding of oxygen to hemoglobin, preventing the release of oxygen to the peripheral tissues. These effects were described in acute alkalosis; however, the postdialysis alkalosis is also an acute alkalosis.

Conclusion

The acid base status of dialysis patients is determined by the dialytic schedule. The most physiological correction is achieved by continuous treatments because metabolic acid production is a continuous body function.

Acidosis and perhaps alkalosis have a clinical relevance even if they are mild and transient in dialysis patients. In intermittent treatments, certain degrees of acidosis and/or alkalosis are unavoidable because in a few hours of treatment the dialytic base gain should provide the buffer reservoir required for the long interdialytic period.

References

1 Gennari JF: Acid-base balance in dialysis patients. Semin Dial 2000;13:235–239.
2 Uribarri J, Zia M, Mahmood J, Marcus RA, Oh MS: Acid production in chronic hemodialysis patients. J Am Soc Nephrol 1998;9:114–120.
3 Brady JP, Hasbargen JA: Correction of metabolic acidosis and its effect on albumin in chronic hemodialysis patients. Am J Kidney Dis 1998;31:35–40.
4 Williams A, Dittmer I, McArley A, Clarke J: High bicarbonate dialysate in hemodialysis patients: Effect on acidosis and nutritional status. Nephrol Dial Transplant 1997;12:2633–2637.
5 Gennari FJ, Cohen JJ, Kassirer JP: Normal acid base values; in Cohen JJ, Kassirer JP (eds): Acid/Base Boston, Little, Brown, 1982, pp 107–110.
6 Feriani M: Behaviour of acid base control with different dialysis schedules. Nephrol Dial Transplant 1998;13(suppl 6):62–65.
7 Hakim RM, Pontzer MA, Tilton D, Lazarus JM, Gottlieb MN: Effects of acetate and bicarbonate dialysate in stable chronic dialysis patients. Kidney Int 1985;28:535–540.
8 Henrich WL, Woodard TD, Meyer BD, Chappel TR, Rubin LJ: High sodium bicarbonate and acetate hemodialysis: double-blind crossover comparison of hemodynamic and ventilatory effects. Kidney Int 1983;24:240–245.

9 La Greca G, Feriani M, Bragantini L, Petrosino L, Santoro A, Altieri P: Effects of acetate and bicarbonate dialysate on vascular stability: A prospective multicenter study. Int J Artif Organs 1987;10:157–162.
10 Bijaphala S, Bell AJ, Bennett CA, Evans SM, Dawborn JK: Comparison of high and low sodium bicarbonate and acetate in stable chronic hemodialysis patients. Clin Nephrol 1985;23:179–183.
11 Malberti F, Surian M, Colussi G, Minetti L: The influence of dialysis fluid composition on dialysis tolerance. Nephrol Dial Transplant 1987;2:93–98.
12 Heinechen FG, Brady-Smith M, Haynie J, Van Stone JC: Prescribing dialysate bicarbonate concentration for hemodialysis patients. Int J Artif Organs 1988;11:45–50.
13 Seyffart G, Ensminger A, Scholz R. Increase of body mass during long-term bicarbonate hemodialysis. Kidney Int 1987;32(suppl 22):S174–S177.
14 Gennari FJ, Rimmer JM: Acid base disorders in end-stage renal disease? Part I. Semin Dial 1990; 3:81–85.
15 Gennari FJ: Acid base balance in dialysis patients. Kidney Int 1985;28:678–688.
16 Oettinger CW, Oliver JC: Normalization of uremic acidosis in hemodialysis patients with a high bicarbonate dialysate. J Am Soc Nephrol 1993;3:1804–1807.
17 Biasioli S, Feriani M, Chiaramonte S, Cavallini L, Cesaro A, Fazion S, Petrosino L, Porena P, Zambello A: Different buffers for hemodiafiltration: A controlled study. Int J Artif Organs 1989; 12:25–30.
18 Feriani M, Ronco C, Biasioli S, Bragantini L, La Greca G: Effect of dialysate and substitution fluid buffer on buffer flux in hemodialfiltration. Kidney Int 1990;39:711–717.
19 Sargent JA, Gotch FA: Bicarbonate and carbon dioxide transport during hemodialysis. Am Soc Artif Intern Organs J 1979;2:61–72.
20 Fabris A, La Greca G, Chiaramonte S, Feriani M, Brendolan A, Bragantini L, Dell'Aquila R, Pellanda MV, Crepaldi C, Ronco C: The importance of ultrafiltration on acid base status in a dialysis population. Am Soc Artif Intern Organs 1988;34:200–201.
21 Santoro A, Spongano M, Ferrari G, Bolzani R, Augella F, Borghi M, Briganti M, Cagnoli L, Docci D, Feletti C, Fusaroli M, Gattiani A, Sanna G, Stallone C, Zucchelli P: Analysis of the factors influencing bicarbonate balance during acetate free biofiltration. Kidney Int 1993;43(suppl 41): S184–S187.
22 Bazilinsky NG, Dunea G, Ing TS: Treatment of metabolic alkalosis in renal failure. Int J Artif Organs 1987;10:284–286.

Mariano Feriani, Department of Nephrology and Dialysis,
Umberto I° Hospital, Via Circonvallazione, 50, I–30174 Mestre-Venezia (Italy)
Tel. +39 041 260 7383, Fax +39 041 260 7378, E-Mail mferiani@goldnet.it

Ronco C, La Greca G (eds): Hemodialysis Technology.
Contrib Nephrol. Basel, Karger, 2002, vol 137, pp 364–370

Chronic Inflammation: An Overview

Nathan W. Levin[a], *Claudio Ronco*[b]

[a] Renal Research Institute, New York, N.Y., USA
[b] Department of Nephrology, St. Bortolo Hospital, Vicenza, Italy

Inflammation

In a recent editorial Ridker [1] suggests that large parts of the human genome are devoted to responding to infection and trauma on the one hand and to maintenance of gluconeogenesis during starvation on the other. What was a successful response when lifestyle and diet encouraged atheroma-free arteries is far less useful with the high incidence of obesity and diabetes in our population. Insulin resistance and diabetes with low grade inflammation may be linked, e.g. adipocytes produce cytokines, incriminating obesity as a potential mechanism for atherogenesis. While a normal range for high sensitivity CRP (HSCRP) has been established it is not clear that any level can be considered normal. Increased mortality in the general population occurs at the higher end of the normal range [2]. In smaller studies the same has been described in dialysis patients. An underlining basis for increased CRP has been described in association with a wide variety of commonly encountered infective agents. These include herpes simplex, cytomegalovirus, E-B virus, *Haemophilus influenzae*, *Chlamydia pneumoniae*, *Mycoplasma pneumoniae* and *Helicobacter pylori* [3]. While CRP levels appear to be similar in dialysis patients in the US and Europe these appear to be lower in Japanese. Is this due to differences associated with genetic makeup or to earlier exposure to infective agents in the Japanese and Koreans with fewer disturbances in later life? (The relative absence of coronary artery disease in the Japanese population is well known.)

Ridker has emphasized the necessity for not assuming causation between infection and atherosclerosis since increased smoking, less access to care, and poverty are also associated with both infections and atherosclerosis. Prospective studies of *H. pylori* and *C. pneumoniae* infection have shown (in both cases) only a 15% increase in coronary death or myocardial infarction following these infections. Fully powered randomized trials of antibiotics to test the hypothesis relating CRP to infections above are underway.

To summarize Ridker's argument: in primeval times cytokines and inflammation were essential to overcome infection but now their involvement in atherosclerosis and its consequences have become major determinants of survival at least in the western world. There is a long list of papers testifying to the importance of inflammation as a major predictive and pathogenic factor in atherosclerotic vascular disease and in malnutrition, the major indication of which is hypoalbuminemia [4, 5]. Raised CRP levels are powerful independent risk factors for coronary artery disease, myocardial infarction, stroke and peripheral vascular disease. Increases in the level of other substances responding to inflammatory stimuli such as IL-6, α_1-glycoprotein or serum amyloid A have also been shown to be indicators of disease. In the US, routine laboratories use a less sensitive method for CRP, which has a lower limit of detection of 6.9 mg/dl. Even with this much higher range there are clearly continuing correlations of higher CRPs with increased mortality, hospitalization, and resistance to erythropoetin repeatedly demonstrated in dialysis patients. In the general population when the CRP concentrations are divided into quintiles, for such quintile increase in HSCRP, the adjusted relative risk of a future cardiovascular event increasing is 26%. The lowest quintile was 0.01–0.07 and the highest 0.38–1.50 (mg/dl). Ridker has previously shown that the combination of low HDL and high CRP is the most sensitive indicator of vascular disease compared to lipoproteins, homocysteine, total cholesterol and LDL cholesterol. CRP alone was the most significant single factor in a univariate analysis. In the multivariate analysis, only HSCRP and the HDL had independent predictive value after age, smoking status, obesity, hypertension, family history and diabetes were adjusted for. It is noteworthy that cerivastatin in doses of 0.4 or 0.8 mg resulted in a 24.5% reduction in mean levels of CRP in the population at risk [6]. Unlike the effect on LDL-C no dose dependence was noted with CRP. Surprisingly there was no substantive correlation between the magnitude of changes in CRP and in LDL-C decrease or HDL-C increase. This drug is no longer available. Previous studies with pravistatin and lovastatin have given similar results. In all studies $<2\%$ of the variance in the percent change in CRP was accounted for by the percentage change in LDL-C. This important finding suggests that the beneficial effects of statins exceed effects on lipids, and that the statins might be useful even when lipid concentrations are normal. The application to the dialysis population is obvious. This paper also suggests that statins impact several different components of the inflammatory cacade. For example cerivastin may suppress macrocyte growth and expression of matrix MPO and tissue factors. Other possibilities include anti-inflammatory effects at the level of vascular endothelium including the expression of several cellular adhesion molecules important in early atherogenesis. P-selectin levels have been reported to be indicative of future cardiovascular events in apparently healthy women, independent of other traditional risk factors [7]. This molecule appears to be involved as an adhesion receptor expressed on activated endothelial. P-selectin and CRP levels correlate, but they act separately from each other. There is strong experimental support for the hypothesis that early inflammatory processes of leukocyte rolling, tethering and attachment and transmigration across the vascular endothelium are critical initiating events in atheromatosis.

Oxidative Stress

There are many cross-relationships between oxidative stress and inflammation in their association with vascular disease. Oxidative stress and inflammation both coexist in health albeit at levels which do not occasion clinical (symptomatic) detection. Oxidative stress represents the effect of reactive oxygen species on a broad range of biological molecules and is detected by measurement of the resultant modified macromolecules. In dialysis patients factors such as the uremic state itself, diabetes, endotoxin exposure from water used for dialysate, membrane effects, transient bacteremia, bacterial DNA, and loss of antioxidants may all play a part in the pathogenesis of oxidative stress. Handelman et al. [8] have reported increased concentration of F2 isoprostanes in dialysis patients. This is useful since it is stable and a product of oxidation of arachidonic acid. Oxidation of low density lipoprotein is an integral step in atherosclerosis. Reactive molecules such as hydrogen peroxide can activate the NF-kappa pathway leading to an increased production of cytokines with consequences promoting inflammation. Alternatively CRP can enhance intracellular generation of reactive oxygen species.

Some Factors Involved in Inflammation

A major potential source of endotoxin exposure is through dialysate contamination. Different standards between the US and European countries and Japan in regard to recommended endotoxin levels are striking. The AAMI standard for endotoxin in water is <2 EU/ml while in Europe and Japan the figure is <0.25 EU/ml. Decreased activation of monocytes with consequent reduction in CRP levels is established when pyrogen-free dialysate is used [9]. The link between quality of water, hypoalbuminemia and survival in the US has yet to be convincingly proven. Canaud et al. [10] described the rationale for and the

Table 1. Mechanisms and factors involved in inflammation as a cause of atherosclerosis [adapted from 4]

CRP deposits in arterial wall	Increased oxidative stress
CRP causes tissue damage	Ceruloplasmin increase
SAA affects lipoprotein structure	Increased AGE formation
LP(a) promotes atherosclerosis	Malnutrition with hypoalbuminemia
Fibrinogen promotes atherosclerosis and thrombosis	Diabetes
Local increase in myeloperoxidase	Infection especially *C. pneumoniae*
Correlation of CRP with P-selectin and other adhesion molecules	Periodontal disease; antibodies to *P. gingivalis*
MSH	Dialysate ultrafiltrate stimulates α_1-glycoprotein

technology required for dialysate purity. Advanced glycation end products, advanced oxidation products and acute phase reactants are all increased in concentration in uremic patients [11]. Colocalizations of all three products in the arterial wall has been described. AGEs induce expression of adhesion molecules and attraction to leukocytes. However, clinical correlations are lacking (table 1).

Riegel et al. [12] investigated the effects of dialysate ultrafiltrate from low and high flux membranes on synthesis of the acute phrase reactant, α_1-acid glycoprotein (AGP) in cultured hepatic cells (HeHG 2). Ultrafiltrate from high flux dialysis stimulated more AGP synthesis suggesting that hepatotoxic substances having a role in cytokine stimulation are removed during dialysis. Malatino et al. [13] show prediction of survival by level of hepatic growth factor HGF particularly in HD. HGF correlated with CRP and intimal thickness. They suggest HGH as a major cytokine.

Don et al. [14] report a negative correlation of leptin with CRP and other APPs in hemodialysis (HD) patients. However in peritoneal dialysis patients studied by Stenvinkel et al. [15] serum leptin and CRP levels increased with loss of lean body mass. This occurred in the face of increased body fat content. Chronic *C. pneumoniae* infection increased the risk of cardiovascular mortality in patients with raised CRP [16]. CRP and IgA *C. pneumoniae* antibody levels were highly correlated. Similar results were observed in smokers among HD patients, but not in nonsmokers, which supports the role of this additional cause of inflammation.

Discussion of anti-inflammatory cytokines such as IL-10, IL-2 or IL-5 to limit host reactions is much less than that of the proinflammatory compounds. Airaghi et al. [17] compared HD and renal insufficiency patients and normal controls in regard to plasma α-melanocyte-stimulating hormone (α-MSH),

IL-6, TNF-α and neopterin before and after dialysis. α-MSH concentrations were increased (but not changed by dialysis) particularly in patients with detectable endotoxemia. Patients in renal failure had the same lower concentrations of α-MSH. Level et al. [18] describe in HD a positive correlation of procalcitonin levels with CRP and fibrinogen and a negative one with albumin concentrations. Procalcitonin and CRP concentrations were raised only during infections while IL-6 were elevated at all times.

Kaysen et al. [19] described the competing effects between inflammation and dietary protein intake on serum albumin and creatinine in HD patients. Increased CRP correlated with albumin decline which was attenuated by increased protein intake. Similar results with creatinine change suggest the need for a prospective trial of dietary protein intake on nutritional status in patients with inflammation.

Destructive periodontal disease has been associated with increased CRP levels, values and prevalence of atherosclerosis in the general population. Its role in ESRD patients is not clearly delineated but one study has shown elevated IgA antibodies to *Porphyromonas gingivalis* and CRP levels in HD patients [20].

Peritoneal Dialysis

Fewer studies have discussed the predictive values of serum CRP in peritoneal dialysis patients. Noh et al. [21] found that independent predictors of mortality were cardiovascular disease (RR = 8.96), increased CRP (RR = 1.19) and higher hematocrit (1.18).

Herzig et al. [22] followed a cohort of 50 patients for 3 years after initial determination of CRP. In a multivariate Cox model the CRP level was predictive of myocardial infarction (adjusted hazard ratio 4.8), but only tended to predict fatal myocardial infarction ($p \leq 0.07$). However CRP was not significantly associated with all-cause mortality. When combined with the examination of *C. pneumoniae* seropositivity, the value of a raised CRP in predicting the incidence of coronary artery disease was significantly increased. CRP and seropositivity were highly correlated. Ozdememir et al. [23] compared 109 HD and 65 age-, gender- and vintage-matched CAPD patients using ultrasonic measurement of carotid artery intimal thickness to identify atherosclerosis. Traditional risk factors, intact PTH, fibrinogen and CRP were determined. More atherosclerotic changes were seen in CAPD, but only total cholesterol, LDL-C and LP(a) levels were significantly higher and not CRP. Given the different types of exposure of peritoneal and HD patients it becomes important to understand if there are common features for CRP increase and the linkage between its effects in the two modalities of dialysis.

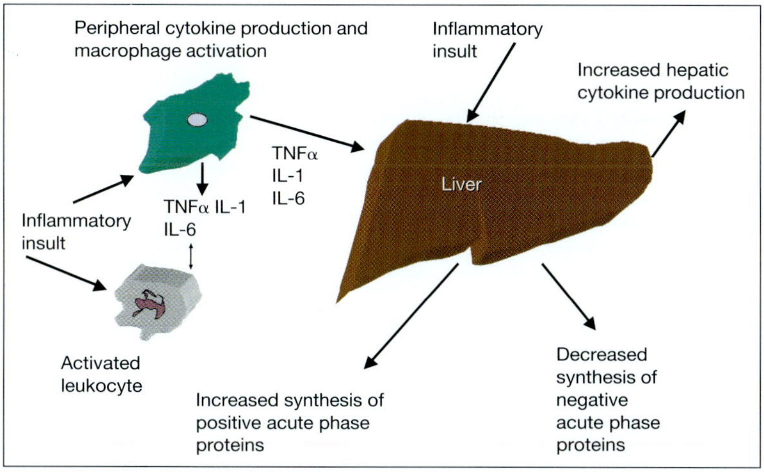

Fig. 1. Schema of factors involved in cytokine interactions [5].

Metabolic abnormalities in a wide variety of biological responses to known and unknown stimuli have been described in the general and dialysis populations with cardiovascular disease and hypoalbuminemia. Figure 1 is a schema of cytokine interactions. From the point of view of the general clinician a host of interrelated processes have been postulated which provide little understanding of their quantitative significance. The overall lesson is that atherosclerotic lesions are dependent on multiple mechanisms which have been identified, usually one by one, with their role in pathogenesis established by correlation with other mechanisms. Undoubtedly the list (table 1) of possible factors will grow and our understanding will deepen. From a therapeutic point of view dietary measures, statins, possibly antioxidants and aspirin are effective to varying degrees with antibodies to cytokines, and/or their receptors under investigation. Thalidomide, which increases the degradation rate of TNF mRNA, is also being studied. Understanding of causes of inflammation in uremic patients is poor. One mechanism is reduction in urinary clearance and in renal catabolic activity, which results in increased blood levels of oxidized and glycated proteins. Infection is common in dialysis patients especially from vascular access (catheters and grafts usually lined with biofilm) and exposure to endotoxin which may be a consequence of water standards that are too low. Are there hints from the findings that CRP concentrations are lower in the African American population (despite a higher incidence of diabetes) and in younger patients? It might be hypothesized that prior exposure to infections might limit the extent of an immune response later in life to exogenous stimuli but this relative protection is lost with increasing age.

References

1 Ridker PM: On evolutionary biology, inflammation, infection, and the causes of atherosclerosis. Circulation 2002;105/1:2–4.
2 Ridker P: High-sensitivity C-reactive protein, potential adjunct for global risk assessment in the primary prevention of cardiovascular disease. Circulation 2001;103:1813–1818.
3 Espinola-Klein C: Impact of infections burden on extent and long-term prognosis of atherosclerosis. Circulation 2001;105:15–21.
4 Malatino LS, et al: Hepatocyte growth factor predicts survival and relates to inflammation and intima media thickness in end-stage renal disease. Am J Kidney Dis 2000;36:945–952.
5 Kaysen GA: Role of inflammation and its treatment in ESRD patients. Blood Purif 2002;20/1: 70–80.
6 Ridker P, et al: Rapid reduction in C-reactive protein with cerivastatin among 785 patients with primary hypercholesterolemia. Circulation 2001;103:1191–1193.
7 Ridker P, et al: Soluble P-selectin and the risk of future cardiovascular events. Circulation 2001;103:491–495.
8 Handelman GJ, et al: Elevated plasma F2-isoprostanes in patients on long-term hemodialysis. Kidney Int 2001;59:1960–1966.
9 Lonnemann G: Chronic inflammation in hemodialysis: The role of contaminated dialysate. Blood Purif 2000;18/3:214–223.
10 Canaud B, et al: Microbiologic purity of dialysate in rationale and technical aspects. Blood 2000;18:210–213.
11 Stenvinkel P: Inflammatory and atherosclerotic interactions in the depleted uremic patient. Blood Purif 2001;19/1:53–61.
12 Riegel W, et al: Hepatotoxic substance(s) removed by high-flux membranes enhances the positive acute phase response. Kidney Int Suppl 2001;78:S308–S314.
13 Malatino LS, et al: Hepatocyte growth factor predicts survival and relates to inflammation and intima media thickness in end-stage renal disease. Am J Kidney Dis 2000;36:945–952.
14 Don BR, et al: Leptin is a negative acute phase protein in chronic hemodialysis patients. Kidney Int 2001;59:1114–1120.
15 Stenvinkel P, et al: Increases in serum leptin levels during peritoneal dialysis are associated with inflammation and a decrease in lean body mass. J Am Soc Nephrol 2000;11:1303–1309.
16 Haubitz M, Brunkhorst R: C-reactive protein and chronic *Chlamydia pneumoniae* infection – Long-term predictors for cardiovascular disease and survival in patients on peritoneal dialysis. Nephrol Dial Transplant 2001;16:809–815.
17 Airaghi L, et al: Plasma concentrations of alpha-melanocyte-stimulating hormone are elevated in patients on chronic haemodialysis. Nephrol Dial Transplant 2000;15:1212–1216.
18 Level C, et al: Procalcitonin: A new marker of inflammation in haemodialysis patients. Nephrol Dial Transplant 2001;16:980–986.
19 Kaysen GA, et al: Inflammation and dietary protein intake exert competing effects on serum albumin and creatinine in hemodialysis patients. Kidney Int 2001;60:333–340.
20 Craig R: Importance of periodontal disease in the kidney patient. Blood Purif 2002;20:113–119.
21 Noh H, et al: Serum C-reactive protein: A predictor of mortality in continuous ambulatory peritoneal dialysis patients. Perit Dial Int 1998;18:387–394.
22 Herzig KA, et al: Is C-reactive protein a useful predictor of outcome in peritoneal dialysis patients. J Am Soc Nephrol 2001;12:814–821.
23 Ozdememir FN, et al: Atherosclerosis risk is higher in continuous ambulatory peritoneal dialysis patients than in hemodialysis patients. Artif Organs 2001;25:448–452.

Nathan W. Levin, MD, Medical and Research Director, Renal Research Institute,
207 East 94th Street, Suite 303, New York, NY 10128 (USA)
Tel. +1 212 360 4954, Fax +1 212 996 5905, E-Mail nlevin@rriny.com

Ronco C, La Greca G (eds): Hemodialysis Technology.
Contrib Nephrol. Basel, Karger, 2002, vol 137, pp 371–378

Oxidant Stress in Hemodialysis Patients

F. Galli[a], *A. Floridi*[a], *U. Buoncristiani*[b]

[a] Department of Internal Medicine, Laboratory of Applied and Clinical Biochemistry, University of Perugia, and
[b] Nephrology and Dialysis Unit, 'R. Silvestrini' Hospital, Perugia, Italy

What is the Evidence for the Presence of Oxidant Stress in HD Patients?

Oxidant stress by definition is a biochemical condition in which oxidant species overwhelm antioxidant defenses ultimately leading to a given biological damage [1].

HD patients are considered at a high risk of oxidant stress because of the following factors:

(a) The uremic environment per se leads to the generation of low-molecular-weight free radicals (ROS) [2] and reactive free carbonyls [3].

(b) The repeated contact of blood cells with bioincompatible materials and possible endotoxiemia in HD patients leads to leukocyte activation and consequent increased formation of ROS, pro-inflammatory cytokine and pro-oxidant toxins [reviewed in 4],

(c) Chronic HD can lead to the release of catalytically active transition metals (such as iron-heme complexes) by blood cell lysis [5].

(d) Uremia modifies the expression and function of some antioxidant/detoxifying defenses such as the glutathione-related enzymes glutathione peroxidase (Gpx) and S-transferase (GST) [6, 7], the lipoprotein-associated paraoxonase [8].

(e) HD depletes blood antioxidants by several mechanisms including leakage through the dialysis membrane (fig. 1) and a higher consumption by oxidation and/or inadequate restoration [9–11].

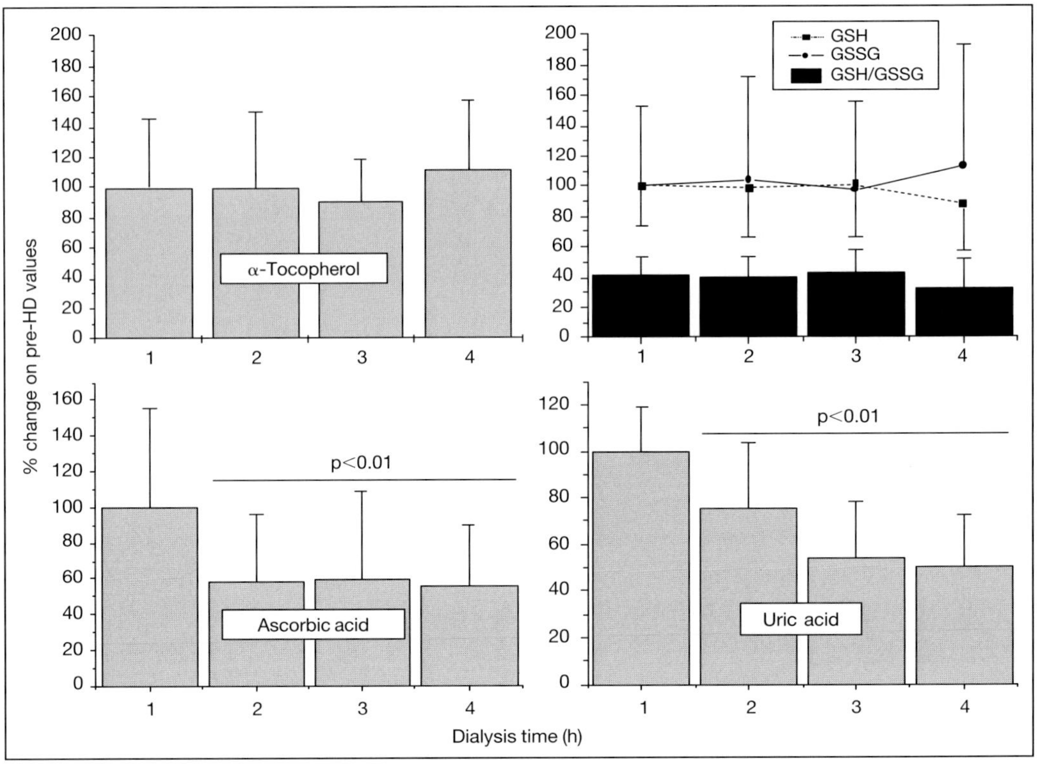

Fig. 1. Levels of the main nonenzymatic antioxidants in plasma during hemodialysis.

The clear-cut evidence of the presence of oxidant stress in advanced uremia and dialysis comes from studies that demonstrate how in the uremic blood accumulate byproducts of the chemical injury of reactive oxygen and nitrogen species (ROS and RNS, respectively) to biomolecules such as, oxidation and nitration products of amino acid residues of proteins [3, 12, 13], F_2-isoprostanes as lipid-oxidation byproducts [14] and the nucleic acid oxidation product 8-OH-dG [15].

A lot of evidence is accumulating on the role played by oxidant stress on the onset and progression of virtually the whole comorbidity of these patients (table 1), ultimately influencing morbidity and mortality scores in HD centers [reviewed in 4]. These aspects spurred nephrologists and dialysis technologists to boost their efforts in fighting oxidant stress in ESRD. The main aim of these efforts should be to improve dialysis quality and increase antioxidant defenses.

Table 1. Proposed pathogenic roles of the oxidant stress in the ESRD comorbidity

Disease state	Pathogenic role	References
Onset and progression of renal faillure	ischemia and reperfusion damage by inflammatory cells self-damage by an abnormal oxygen metabolism of kidney cells	27, 28
Atherosclerotic cardiovascular disease	endothelial cell damage and apoptosis impaired nitric oxide metabolism chemical modification of circulating and intraendothelia LDL leukocyte adhesion and chemotaxis	4, 5, 8, 9, 12, 20
Immune dysfunction and increased susceptibility to infectious diseases	challenges to mechanisms that regulate leukocyte function and viability (leukopenia) impairing effect on the cell-mediated response modified receptor function and antigen recognition	29–32
Malignancy	genotoxic activity of ROS and RNS	15
Diabetes	impaired function of insulin-secreting cells	33
Disorders of the peripheral and central nervous system	direct damage to neural components accumulation of protein and lipid oxidation products	13
Anemia	impaired erythropoietin function pro-oxidant activity of the supplemental EPO Reduced RBC survival	18, 24
Accelerated aging	impaired defense and repair processes increased molecular senescence in biological fluids and cells possible impairment of molecular mechanisms that regulate cell aging	34–36

Clinical Aspects of the Increased Susceptibility to Oxidant Stress in HD

Sooner or later, all HD patients develop signs of molecular damage related to the presence of oxidant stress. Among the clinical causes of this increased susceptibility to oxidant stress there is also that of the progression of the uremic comorbidity. Particularly important in this context is the persistence of chronic inflammation that sustains itself through proinflammatory cell activation and a defective feedback control. This pro-inflammatory loop ultimately contributes to the development of degenerative processes in target tissues such as the endothelium [4], to defective liver synthesis of albumin and malnutrition [16]. The latter aspects can be responsible for defective antioxidant function in that albumin is the main extracellular thiol. Furthermore, it possibly interferes with the bioavailability and metabolism of some naturally occurring antioxidants that are carried by albumin such as trace elements and liposoluble micronutrients. Again, the albumin can bind some pro-oxidant uremic toxins that in their free form could be more bioavailable and reactive, such as homocysteine and reactive carbonyls.

The tendency to develop severe anemia is another relevant clinical condition behind the oxidant stress of HD patients. In fact, the decrease of the red blood cell number can lead to an overall defective glutathione metabolism and impaired restoration of the ascorbic acid redox [17]. Again, supplementation of the hormone erythropoietin and iron has been demonstrated to favor oxidant stress [18, 19].

The role of an insufficient correction of uremic toxicity by current dialysis techniques is another possible factor in sustaining oxidant stress. Actually, some pro-oxidant toxins or oxidant-derived byproducts with pro-oxidant function are not removed by conventional dialysis. Among these toxins, modified proteins such as albumin, modified β_2-microglobulin, and lipoprotein ancillary proteins can sustain tissue oxidant stress by activation of receptor-mediated pathways in scavenger cells [20, 21].

Moreover, the uncontrolled use of poorly biocompatible materials and pro-oxidant drugs [18, 19] most likely remains the main support to the onset and progression of oxidant stress-related diseases in HD.

Antioxidant Therapy in HD

While sensible efforts have been made to improve materials and dialysis quality, antioxidant therapy has been only preliminarily approached and its potential remains largely unknown. Specific defects of the antioxidant defenses have been demonstrated in uremic patients [4, 6–8], which during HD can further exacerbate by depletion (fig. 1) and/or impaired restoration [9–11] of some antioxidant defenses.

Early results suggested a positive effect of antioxidant supplements in the prevention and/or slackening of some HD-related comorbidity and particularly atherosclerotic cardiovascular disease [23] and anemia [24]. However, some conflicting evidence has been obtained [4] and the probability of observing such a preventive effect of antioxidants on the oxidant stress-related pathologies in ESRD appears biased by: (1) small numbers of patients studied; (2) pre-existing severe lesions due to oxidant stress or confounding its possible correction; (3) absence of an appropriate biochemical diagnosis of the type of antioxidant defect and oxidant insult. Therefore, the demonstration of a role of antioxidant therapies to treat oxidant stress-related comorbidity in HD patients is still awaited.

Conceptually, antioxidant supplements should offer the safest and well-recognized way to set up prevention strategies against oxidant stress, but on the other hand they could be inappropriate both qualitatively and quantitatively. Therefore, to set up suitable antioxidant therapy, several aspects that characterize the biochemistry of the oxidant species responsible for a given oxidant insult should be considered [25]. These include their chemical identity, site of reactivity and rate of production. Furthermore, one should consider the biochemistry of the antioxidant(s) used and its specificity in scavenging these oxidant species. Therapeutic forms of natural antioxidants ought to be available in a reactive form exactly at the site where reactive species are formed or react, and in a suitable amount. Again, the byproducts of their reaction with oxidants should be safe and easily metabolized.

Unfortunately, several interventional studies including the most impressive ones [23] that reported on beneficial effects of increasing antioxidant protection in HD have been carried out without measuring antioxidant levels before and after the supplementation steps. And, most surprisingly, we still do not know exactly if uremia and HD might in some way limit the efficacy of the most used antioxidant drugs such as vitamin E, vitamin C and glutathione by affecting their absorption, metabolism and bioavailability.

Therefore, to develop an appropriate antioxidant therapy in HD some basic criteria should be adopted, these include:

(a) The specific neutralization of reactive species and pro-oxidants produced by the uremic environment and during HD.
(b) A suitable compensation of deficiencies in enzymatic and non-enzymatic antioxidants consequent to an increased demand, uremia-induced dysfunction, defects in the dietary intake and absorption of natural occurring antioxidants and trace elements.
(c) A timely and continuous treatment.
(d) The adaptation to specific needs related to interindividual differences in antioxidant defenses and susceptibility to ROS damage.

Altogether these aspects suggest that a proper biochemical diagnosis cannot be set aside while planning an antioxidant therapy in HD patients.

As conventional antioxidant therapies could not be sufficient per se to face the whole biochemical derangement sustaining oxidant stress in ESRD patients, new strategies combining antioxidant therapy with an improvement in dialysis biocompatibility and correction of uremic toxicity have recently been proposed and are still under investigation [discussed in 26].

Concluding Remarks

A range of severe disease states in which oxidant stress plays a key pathogenic role such as atherosclerotic cardiovascular disease, immune dysfunction, malignancy, anemia and neurological dysfunction strongly affect morbidity and mortality scores in HD centers [4]. Therefore, measures to prevent and/or reduce this comorbidity have been longed for since, but still appear largely insufficient.

Though it is a common belief that intradialysis generation of ROS is the main event leading to oxidant stress in HD, it could easily be foreseen that several other aspects can concur to different extents in its onset and progression. Therefore, assuming as primary measures to reduce the incidence of oxidant stress in HD those of improving biocompatibility and dialysis quality, one cannot disregard other strategies including those providing a better correction of uremia as well as specific anti-inflammatory and antioxidant therapies.

Antioxidant therapy is of course the most interesting one because of its low cost and overall innocuousness, not forgetting that in some HD patients it could be extremely important to face specific nutritional deficits.

Thus, while on one hand sensible progress has been made in the diagnosis of oxidant stress, on the other we are still far from understanding effective strategies to fight oxidant stress in ESRD.

References

1 Halliwell B, Gutteridge JMC: Free Radicals in Biology and Medicine, ed 3. Oxford, Oxford University Press, 1999.

2 Roselaar SE, Nazhat NB, Winyard PG, Jones P, Cunningham J, Blake DR: Detection of oxidants in uremic plasma by electron spin resonance spectroscopy. Kidney Int 1995;48:199–206.

3 Miyata T, van Ypersele de Sitrihou C, Kurokawa K, Baynes JW: Alterations in non-enzymatic biochemistry in uremia: origin and significance of 'carbonyl stress' in long-term uremic complications. Kidney Int 1999;55:389–399.

4 Galli F, Canestrari F, Bellomo G: Physiopathology of the oxidative stress and its implication in uremia and dialysis. Contrib Nephrol. Basel, Karger, 1999, vol 127, pp 1–31.

5 Ziouzenkova O, Sevanian A: Oxidative modification of low-density lipoprotein (LDL) in HD patients: role in electronegative LDL formation. Blood Purif 2000;18:169–176.

6 Niwa T, Tsukushi S: 3-Deoxyglucosone and AGEs in uremic complications: Inactivation of glutathione peroxidase by 3-deoxyglucosone. Kidney Int 2001;59(suppl 78):S37–41.

7 Galli F, Rovidati S, Buoncristiani U, Floridi A, Canestrari F: Erythrocyte glutathione S-transferase expression in the uremic syndrome. Clin Chem 1999;45:1781–1788.

8 Quaschning T, Krane V, Metzger T, Wanner C: Abnormalities in uremic lipoprotein metabolism and its impact on cardiovascular disease. Am J Kidney Dis 2001;38(suppl 1):S14–S19.
9 Clermont G, Lecour S, Lahet J, Siohan P, Vergely C, Chevet D, Rifle G, Rochette L: Alteration in plasma antioxidant capacities in chronic renal failure and hemodialysis patients: A possible explanation for the increased cardiovascular risk in these patients. Cardiovasc Res 2000;47:618–623
10 Clermont G, Lecour S, Cabanne J, Motte G, Guilland J, Chevet D, Rochette L: Vitamin E-coated dialyzer reduces oxidative stress in hemodialysis patients. Free Rad Biol Med 2001;31:233–241.
11 Peuchant E, Carbonneau M-A, Dubourg L, Thomas MJ, Perromat A, Vallot C, Clerc M: Lipoperoxidation in plasma and red blood cells of patients undergoing haemodialysis: Vitamins A, E and iron status. Free Rad Biol Med 1994;16:339–346.
12 Descamps-Latscha B, Witko-Sarsat V: Importance of oxidatively modified proteins in chronic renal failure. Kidney Int 2001;59(suppl 78):S108–S113.
13 Deng G, Vaziri ND, Jabbari B, Ni Z, Yan XX: Increased tyrosine nitration of the brain in chronic renal insufficiency: Reversal by antioxidant therapy and angiotensin-converting enzyme inhibition. J Am Soc Nephrol 2001;12:1892–1899.
14 Handelman GJ, Walter MF, Adhikarla R, Gross J, Dallal GE, Levin NW, Blumberg JB. Elevated plasma F_2-isoprostanes in patients on long-term hemodialysis. Kidney Int 2001;59:1960–1966.
15 Tarng DC, Huang TP, Liu TY, Chen HW, Sung YJ, Wei YH: Effect of vitamin E-bonded membrane on the 8-hydroxy 2′-deoxyguanosine level in leukocyte DNA of hemodialysis patients. Kidney Int 2000;58:790–799.
16 Parker TF 3rd, Wingard RL, Husni L, Ikizler TA, Parker RA, Hakim RM: Effect of the membrane biocompatibility on nutritional parameters in chronic hemodialysis patients. Kidney Int 1996;49:551–556.
17 May JM, Qu Z, Morrow JD: Mechanisms of ascorbic acid recycling in human erythrocytes. Biochim Biophys Acta 2001;1528:159–166.
18 Nemeth I, Turi S, Hasron I, Breczki C: Vitamin E alleviates the oxidative stress of erythropoietin in uremic children on hemodialysis. Pediatr Nephrol 2000;14:13–17.
19 Salahudeen AK, Oliver B, Bower JD, Roberts LJ 2nd: Increase in plasma esterified F_2-isoprostanes following intravenous iron infusion in patients on hemodialysis. Kidney Int 2001;60: 1525–1531.
20 Thornalley PJ: Cell activation by glycated proteins: AGE receptors, receptor recognition factors and functional classification of AGEs. Cell Mol Biol 1998;44:1013–1023.
21 Miyata T, Hori O, Zhang J, Yan SD, Ferran L, Ida Y, Schmidt AM: The receptor for advanced glycation end products (RAGE) is a central mediator of the interaction of AGE-beta2microglobulin with human mononuclear phagocytes via an oxidant-sensitive pathway: Implication for the pathogenesis of dialysis-related amyloidosis. J Clin Invest 1996;98:1088–1094.
22 Hashimoto H, Mio T, Sumino K: Lipid abnormalities of erythrocyte membranes in hemodialysis patients with chronic renal failure. Clin Chim Acta 1996;252:137–145.
23 Boaz M, Smetana S, Green MS: Secondary prevention with antioxidants of cardiovascular disease in endstage renal disease (SPACE): Randomised placebo-controlled. Lancet 2000;356: 1213–1218.
24 Usberti M, Bufano G, Lima G, Gazzotti RM, Tira P, Gerardi GM, Di Lorenzo D: Increased red blood cell survival reduces the need of erythropoietin in hemodialyzed patients treated with exogenous glutathione and vitamin E-modified membrane; in Ronco C, La Greca G (eds): Vitamin E-Bonded Membrane. A Further Step in Dialysis Optimization. Contrib Nephrol. Basel, Karger, 1999, vol 127, pp 208–214.
25 Rice-Evans CA, Gopinathan V: Oxygen toxicity, free radicals and antioxidants in human disease: biochemical implications in atherosclerosis and the problems of premature neonates; in Apps DK, Tripton KF (eds): Essays in Biochemistry. London, Portland Press, 1995, pp 39–63.
26 Galli F: Vitamin E-modified dialysers. Contr Nephrol. Basel, Karger, 2002, vol 137, pp 95–104.
27 Nath KA, Grande J, Croatt A, Haugen J, Kim Y, Rosenberg ME: Redox regulation of renal DNA synthesis, transforming growth factor-beta1 and collagen gene expression. Kidney Int 1998;53: 367–381.
28 Turi S, Nameth I, Torkos A, Saghy L, Varga I, Matkovics B, Nagy J: Oxidative stress and antioxidant defense mechanism in glomerular diseases. Free Rad Biol Med 1997;22:161–168.

29 Jaber BL, Cendoroglo M, Balakrishnan VS, Perianayagam MC, King AJ, Pereira BJ: Apoptosis of leukocytes: basic concepts and implications in uremia. Kidney Int 2001;78(suppl 78):S197–S205.

30 Galli F, Rovidati S, Benedetti S, Canestrari F, Ferraro B, Floridi A, Buoncristiani U: Lipid peroxidation, leukocyte function and apoptosis in hemodialysis patients treated with vitamin E-modified filters. Contrib Nephrol. Basel, Karger, 1999, vol 127, pp 156–171.

31 Ando M, Gafvels M, Bergstrom J, Lindholm B, Lundkvist I: Uremic serum enhances scavenger receptor expression and activity in the human monocytic cell line U937. Kidney Int 1997; 51:785–792.

32 Shurtz-Swirski R, Mashiach E, Kristal B, Shkolnik T, Shasha SM: Antioxidant enzymes activity in polymorphonuclear leukocytes in chronic renal failure. Nephron 1995;71:176–179.

33 Dypbukt JM, Ankarcrona M, Burkitt M, Sjoholm A, Strom K, Orrenius S, Nicotera P: Different prooxidant levels stimulate growth, trigger apoptosis, or produce necrosis of insulin-secreting RINm5F cells. J Biol Chem 1994;269:30553–30560.

34 Weiss MF, Erhard P, Kader-Attia FA, Wu YC, Deoreo PB, Araki A, Glomb MA, Monnier VM: Mechanisms for the formation of glycoxidation products in end-stage renal disease. Kidney Int 2000;57:2571–2585.

35 Amann K, Ritz E: Cardiovascular abnormalities in ageing and in uraemia – only analogy or shared pathomechanisms? Nephrol Dial Transplant 1998;13(suppl 7):6–11.

36 Grune T, Sommerburg O, Siems WG: Oxidative stress in anemia. Clin Nephrol 2000;53(suppl 1): S18–S22.

Francesco Galli, PhD, Department of Internal Medicine,
Section of Applied and Clinical Biochemistry
University of Perugia, Via del Giochetto, I–06100 Perugia (Italy)
Tel. +39 075 5857445, Fax +39 075 585 7441, E-Mail f.galli@unipg.it, fragalli@libero.it

Ronco C, La Greca G (eds): Hemodialysis Technology.
Contrib Nephrol. Basel, Karger, 2002, vol 137, pp 379–385

End-Stage Renal Disease: A Slowly Progressive Systemic Inflammatory Response Syndrome

Claudio Ronco[a], *Nathan W. Levin*[b]

[a] Department of Nephrology, St. Bortolo Hospital, Vicenza, Italy
[b] Renal Research Institute, New York, N.Y., USA

In the setting of intensive care, patients with acute renal failure often present a clinical picture of SIRS (systemic inflammatory response syndrome). SIRS can be caused by bacterial stimuli or by non microbiological stimuli that induce a significant inflammatory response. When this response is exaggerated, the patient experiences multiple organ system failure and a condition of sepsis also defined as a systemic malignant inflammation. This is mostly characterized by an invasion of cytokines and other pro-inflammatory mediators into the systemic circulation where major biological effects take place including vasopermeabilization, hypotension and shock [1].

In end-stage renal disease (ESRD) patients are less severely ill but they may still suffer from a condition of inflammation leading to cardiovascular complications, progressive malnutrition and death [2]. In these patients, however, inflammation is subclinical and chronic disorders of the cytokine system or acute phase proteins may be observed as the sole evidence of a proinflammatory disorder [3].

There are several reasons why hemodialysis patients are subject to chronic inflammation (fig. 1). The condition of uremia per se is characterized by a series of metabolic disturbances that produce an imbalance between immunostimulation and immunodepression. There is a disequilibrium between production of reactive oxygen species (ROS) and antioxidant defense of the organism. The hemodialysis membrane per se, together with several dialysis procedures and possible contamination of the hemodialysis fluid may lead to a condition of subclinical but progressive inflammation. This may also be exacerbated by other comorbid states including infections, periodontal disease and atherosclerosis [4–6].

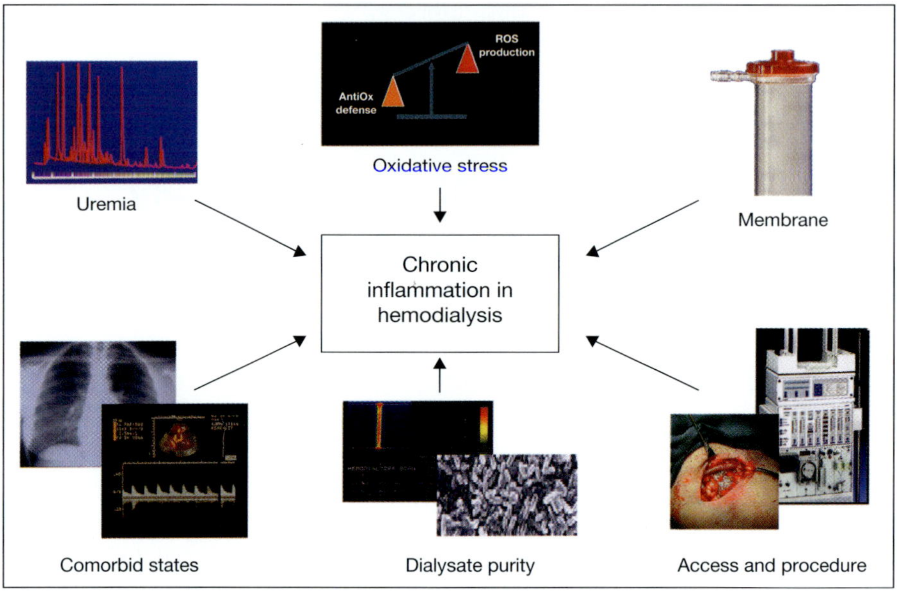

Fig. 1. Factors contributing to chronic inflammation in hemodialysis.

In spite of recent improvements in dialysis technology, cardiovascular disease still remains the main cause of morbidity and mortality in ESRD. Traditional risk factors include hypertension, chronic heart failure, dyslipidemia, obesity, tobacco smoking and diabetes. Further risks, however, have recently been shown to be involved including chronic inflammation, oxidative stress, AGEs formation, malnutrition, Ca-P product, endothelial dysfunction and hyperhomocysteinemia [7].

All these risks seem to combine their action to produce long-term clinical derangements. In particular, the production of proinflammatory cytokines as a response to a specific stimulus increase the level of acute phase reactants (CRP, fibrinogen, SAA, transferrin) causing a cascade of events including endothelial dysfunction, accelerated atherogenesis and cardiovascular disease [4–7]. Mortality, morbidity and hospitalization are positively correlated with the serum acute phase proteins (C-reactive protein (CRP) or serum amyloid A(SAA)) and with the cytokines that regulate them (IL-6) in ESRD and in the general population [3]. In particular, CRP seems to be an indicator of the amount and the activity of the inflammatory process but it could also be an active participant in the process. CRP tends to be higher in the ESRD population compared to the normal population (fig. 2). Furthermore, a variability within the so-called normal values can be observed when high-sensitivity assays are utilized to

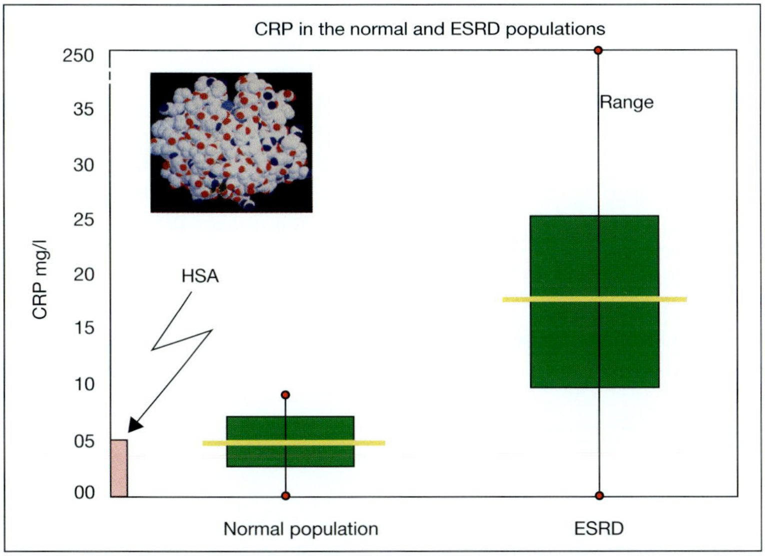

Fig. 2. CRP (C-reactive protein) levels studied in a sample of normal population (52 healthy subjects) and in a similar sample of ESRD patients.

measure CRP. Stevinkel et al. [8] have demonstrated significantly different outcomes in patients with CRP above or below 10 mg/l. Kaysen et al. [9] have also demonstrated that longitudinal variations in albumin concentration correlate with CRP levels, suggesting that malnutrition is a condition induced by chronic inflammation.

In conclusion, ESRD patients are at risk for cardiovascular disease and early atherosclerotic lesions seem to contribute to negative outcomes. A chronic status of inflammation has been demonstrated in patients undergoing chronic hemodialysis. Several factors may mediate biochemical and physical processes that activate an inflammatory response in the patient and influence outcomes. What are the factors involved in the initiation of this processes? What can we do to correct or prevent them and possibly improve outcome? The list of possible causes is reported in table 1. As can be noted, there are patient-related and treatment-related causes. While the latter can be addressed by an improvement in dialysis quality, most of the causes in the former can be addressed in the phase of pre-ESRD care.

As far as treatment-related causes are involved, AV fistulas are subject to repeated mechanical damage due to puncture. Further causes of local inflamation may be mechanical stress on the vessel wall due to jet lesions, pseudoaneurysms and thrombosis with infection. Grafts may present thrombotic lesions

Table 1. Chronic inflammation

Patient-related issues endogenous causes	Treatment-related issues hemodialysis-related
Age, sex and race	Repeated vascular access puncture
Decreased cytokine clearance	Indwelling temporary catheters
Reduced AGEs metabolism	Presence of prosthetic devices
Increased cytokine synthesis	Repeated contact with incompatible surfaces or biomaterials
Gene polymorphism (differences)	Backtransport of pyrogens from dialysate
Chronic heart failure, atherosclerosis	Oxidative and carbonyl stress
Chronic infections and localized infections in the atherosclerotic plaque	
Periodontal infections	

and pseudoaneurysms. Temporary catheters and prosthetic devices are subject to exit site infection and endothelial damage. A further cause of inflammation is the presence of biofilm on the artificial surface. The presence of contaminated dialysate together with bioincompatibility reactions due to the contact with artificial surfaces in dialysis, may contribute to a typical condition of monocyte activation and chronic inflammation. Hemodialysis may also impair the antioxidant protection system of the organism by losses of hydrophilic compounds such as vitamin C, trace elements and enzyme-regulatory compounds. Intravenous iron and other adjuvant treatments represent other components of the oxidant stress-mediated inflammation. In all these conditions, an improvement of the quality of treatment can definitely contribute to moderating the status of inflammation even though a complete normalization seems impossible.

At this point a clinical paradox becomes evident. Why is it that proinflammatory mediators and monocyte activation do not protect patients from infections and on the contrary patients are more infection prone than normal subjects?

A possible clinical and biological explanation is that, as in sepsis, the condition of ESRD does not lead only to a chronic inflammation state, but also stimulates a significant anti-inflammatory response. In subsequent moments of the patient's clinical history, pro-inflammatory mediators and anti-inflammatory mediators display peak levels in the circulation (fig. 3). This condition leads to a subclinical battle within the organism in which phases of inflammation are followed by phases of immunodepression and cell hyporesponsiveness. While the former phases increase cardiovascular abnormalities and malnutrition, the subsequent phases lead to an impaired response to bacterial invasion and easy occurrence of infections. These, in turn, result in subsequent phases of inflammation and the patient enters a slippery slope of progressive clinical impairment.

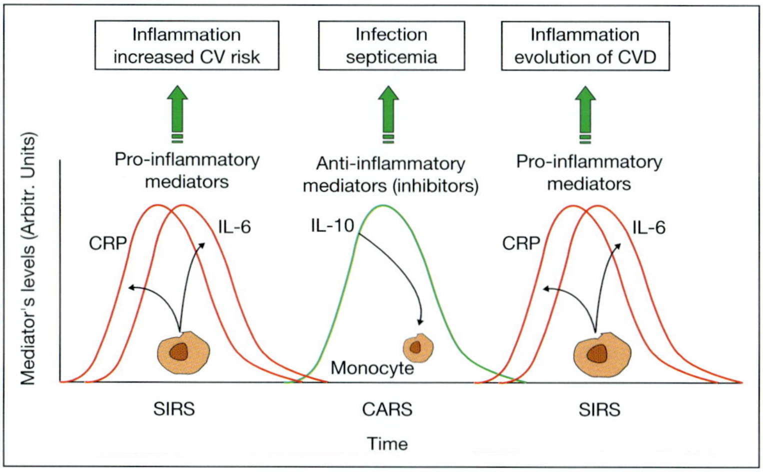

Fig. 3. Graphical representation of the SIRS-CARS hypothesis. Subsequent events in the life of a hemodialysis patient may occur: Inflammation and progression of CVD may be followed by periods of infection or septicemia corresponding to a state of cell hyporesponsiveness. Infection stimulates a new inflammatory response. In such circumstances alternate SIRS and CARS periods may occur.

This process may take several years but it is documented by subsequent episodes of acute inflammation and infections, cardiovascular events and hospitalization, malnutrition and progressive reduction in body mass.

The SIRS-CARS Hypothesis

In physiological conditions, the biological activity of inflammation-associated mediators is under the control of specific inhibitors that may act at different levels. In SIRS, the homeostatic balance is altered and a profound disturbance of relative production of different mediators may be observed (altered immuno-homeostasis). In severely ill patients with acute renal failure the spillover into the circulation of mediators intended to have autocrine or paracrine effects generates systemic effects including endothelial damage and loss of permselectivity, hemodynamic shock and vasoparalysis. On the other hand, monocytes present a profound depression of their capacity to respond to different stimuli with cytokine production as in the case of cell exhaustion or inhibition [10–13]. In ESRD patients, all these mechanisms are less evident and mostly subclinical but nevertheless present and dangerous in the long term. The paradoxical clinical condition in which chronic inflammation and tendency to infection coexist might be similar to that of SIRS eventhough it is in a different dimension of clinical evidence. We could therefore describe this clinical condition as a progressive and mild SIRS with a chronic imbalance of pro- and anti-inflammatory factors in the host. The concept of dialysis-induced chronic inflammation as being a simply proinflammatory event can be consequently challenged. SIRS and CARS (compensated anti-inflammatory response syndrome) might therefore coexist in patients on dialysis with alternate moments of inflammation and immunodepression. The clinical counterpart of these two entities could be an increased cardiovascular risk with progressive cardiovascular disease, and a series of infections that periodically stimulate a new inflammatory cycle. SIRS and CARS might even co-exist in different compartments of the body at the same time. SIRS could predominate within the inflamed tissues while blood leukocytes may simultaneously display a significant hyporeactivity.

This is a new hypothesis alternative to those proposed so far to explain chronic inflammation and its correlation with outcome in dialysis patients. Accurate longitudinal measurements of biochemical mediators of both pro- and anti-inflammatory states should therefore be undertaken in order to support this hypothesis. So far it could be a challenging and speculative theory that requires a solid and rigorous clinical validation.

References

1 Pinsky MR, Vincent JL, Deviere J, Alegre M, Kahn RJ, Duont E: Serum cytokine levels in human septic shock. Relation to multiple-system organ failure and mortality. Chest 1993;103:565–575.

2 Zimmermann J, Herrlinger S, Pruy A, Metzger T, Wanner C: Inflammation enhances cardiovascular risk and mortality in hemodialysis patients. Kidney Int 1999;55:648–658.

3 Bologa RM, Levine DM, Parker TS, Cheigh JS, Serur D, Stenzel KH, Rubin AL: Interleukin-6 predicts hypoalbuminemia, hypocholesterolemia, and mortality in hemodialysis patients. Am J Kidney Dis 1998;32:107–114.

4 Culleton BF, Larson MG, Wilson PWF, Evans JC, Parfrey PS, Levy D: Cardiovascular disease and mortality in a community-based cohort with mild renal insufficiency. Kidney Int 1999;56: 2214–2219.

5 Jungers P, Massy ZA, Khoa TN, Labrunie M, Lacour B, Descamps-Latscha B, Man NK: Incidence and risk factors of atherosclerotic accidents in predialysis chronic renal failure patients: a prospective study. Nephrol Dial Transplant 1997;12:2597–2607.

6 Sarnak MJ, MD Levey AS: Cardiovascular disease and chronic renal disease: A new paradigm. Am J Kid Dis 2000;35:S117–S131.

7 Harjai KJ: Potentially new cardiovascular risk factors: Left ventricular hypertrophy, homocysteine, lipoprotein(a), triglycerides, oxidative stress, and fibrinogen. Ann Intern Med 1999;131:376–386.

8 Stenvinkel P, Lindholm B, Heimburger M, Heimburger O: Elevated serum levels of soluble adhesion molecules predict death in pre-dialysis patients: Association with malnutrition, inflammation, and cardiovascular disease. Nephrol Dial Transplant 2000;15:1624–1630.

9 Kaysen GA, Chertow GM, Adhikarla R, Young B, Ronco C, Levin N: Inflammation and dietary protein intake exert competing effects on serum albumin and creatinine in hemodialysis patients. Kidney Int 2001;60:333–340.

10 Pinsky MR: Sepsis: A pro- and anti-inflammatory disequilibrium syndrome. Contrib Nephrol. Basel, Karger, 2001, vol 132, pp 354–366.

11 Adrie C, Pinsky MR: The inflammatory balance in human sepsis. Inten Care Med 2000;26: 364–375.
12 Casey LC, Balk RA, Bone RC: Plasma cytokine and endotoxin levels correlate with survival in patients with the sepsis syndrome. Ann Intern Med 1993;15:771–778.
13 Adib-Conquy M, Adrie C, Moine P, Ashnoune K, Fitting C, Pinsky MR, Dhainaut JF, Cavaillon JM: NF-κB expression in mononuclear cells of septic patients resembles that observed in LPS tolerance. Am J Respir Crit Care Med 2000;162:1877–1883.

Claudio Ronco, MD, Department of Nephrology,
St. Bortolo Hospital, Viale Rodolfi, I–36100 Vicenza (Italy)
Tel. +39 0444993869, Fax +39 0444993949, E-Mail cronco@goldnet.it

Ronco C, La Greca G (eds): Hemodialysis Technology.
Contrib Nephrol. Basel, Karger, 2002, vol 137, pp 386–395

LDL Modification during Hemodialysis

Markers for Oxidative Stress

Alex Sevanian, Liana Asatryan

University of California, School of Pharmacy, Los Angeles, Calif., USA

Introduction

The evidence linking LDL oxidative modification to atherosclerosis can now be found in several reviews. A review in 1996 [1] highlighted the major features of oxidatively modified LDL in terms of biological responses in vascular cells such as effects on vascular tone, recruitment and activation of inflammatory cells, smooth muscle cell migration and proliferation, platelet adherence and degranulation, inactivation of antioxidant and lipoprotein metabolic enzyme systems and stimulated deposition and accumulation of cholesterol. Recently, studies with uremic subjects following hemodialysis showed that LDL oxidation and modified LDL species are greatly increased [2]. LDL oxidation is strongly related to the extent of hemolysis, suggesting that release of hemoglobin (Hb) may result in a transient oxidative stress. This oxidative stress in blood/plasma can be manifested in specific ways, with formation of electronegative LDL particles (LDL^-) being a potentially useful indication.

Over the last 5 years, further details about LDL^- have been obtained, including features that impart its electronegative character and its effects on vascular cells. In attempts to identify subjects with high LDL^- levels, it was found that hemodialysis patients, particularly those experiencing hemolysis, had very high plasma LDL^- levels, irrespective of their total LDL content [2]. This revealed a potential mechanism for LDL oxidation in vivo, suggesting that oxidation occurs in the bloodstream (blood/plasma). LDL^- is readily measured in plasma by means of anion exchange chromatography which resolves LDL particles into three major fractions: native LDL (nLDL), representing ~90–99%

of plasma LDL, LDL^-, representing up to 8% of plasma LDL, and a more electronegative fraction (termed $LDL^=$), that usually comprises <1% of total LDL. The electronegative LDL are predominantly found in the small-dense LDL fraction which is widely regarded as an indicator of atherosclerosis risk [3]. A relationship between small-dense LDL and lipoperoxide enriched LDL^- suggests that denser LDL are heterogeneous and comprise an older population of particles [4] that contain low levels of peroxidation products. LDL^- behaves as an atherogenic lipoprotein analogous to minimally modified LDL containing a myriad of oxidized products that elicit lipid loading and pro-inflammatory responses.

Role of Heme Proteins in LDL Oxidation

Hemoglobin-dependent oxidation takes place by a mechanism similar to that described for heme peroxidases, such as myeloperoxidase (MPO), where attack of proteins by ferryl species is a common reaction with some well-characterized products [5]. In addition, considerable insights have emerged concerning mechanisms by which heme-peroxidase-mediated oxidation are modulated. LDL oxidation catalyzed by myoglobin (Mb), myeloperoxidase (MPO) or horseradish peroxidase (HRP) can occur in the absence of transition metals [6], utilizing higher oxidation states of heme as catalysts. The mechanism for heme-containing enzymatic oxidation of lipids and proteins is well understood, however, in the case of LDL the processes are complex and involve numerous reactions. This complexity is reflected by the pattern of reactions and products arising from MPO-mediated oxidation. The products generated by compound I- and compound II-mediated oxidations, as well as HOCl and nitrite, contribute to the modification of LDL [5, 7]. Nitrite reacts in two one-electron steps with MPO, resulting in a peroxidase cycle where compound I and compound II are formed [8]. The rapid oxidation rates account for the recent findings that MPO-mediated oxidation of LDL, and specifically macrophage oxidation of LDL, are enhanced in the presence of physiological concentrations of nitrite. This highlights the importance of NO products in the progress of LDL oxidation and the unique features of MPO-mediated oxidations that contribute to LDL modification during inflammation.

Recently, we confirmed the findings of Miller et al. [9] that apoB can be covalently modified via Hb-protein radical reactions [2]. A mechanism for peroxide-dependent oxidation of Hb to catalytically active metHb and ferryl-Hb was demonstrated in human blood that revealed a potent mechanism for LDL oxidation in vivo. A source of Hb may be hemolysis that occurs after local trauma and at intramural microhemorrhages arising in areas of high shear force and turbulent flow. The latter are reported to contain hemolyzed red cells and free hemin that may be in a form not immediately available to heme binding proteins. This is reported for diseases associated with high rates of atherogenesis, e.g. uremic patients undergoing hemodialysis. An important aspect of Hb-modified LDL is that radical-mediated binding of heme (as a part of Hb or a Hb-fragment) to LDL imparts pro-oxidant character to the particles. The conversion of LDL to HbLDL markedly increases the susceptibility of these particles to oxidation.

Characteristics of Hemoglobin-Modified LDL from Human Plasma

Figure 1 shows Western blots performed after SDS-PAGE of LDL apoB-100 that was isolated from human plasma before and after hemodialysis. The gels analyzed under these conditions show firstly that there are no differences in the patterns for protein migration under denaturing and nondenaturing conditions. Reducing-SDS-PAGE was used to confirm the stability of the bands and covalent nature of Hb association with apoB-100. Freshly isolated total LDL and LDL^- were separated by HPLC and used as standards and compared to bands derived from LDL isolated from HD patients. A standard of $HbLDL^-$ that was produced by reaction of Hb + H_2O_2 with LDL in 10% plasma, as described previously, [2] was also used. This HbLDL is virtually identical to LDL^- on the basis of HPLC and electrophoretic parameters. All bands cross-reacted with antibody to apoB-100 (not shown).

Two major bands (top panel) with molecular masses of 220 and 500 kD cross-reacted with the Hb antibodies; however, the 500-kD band showed a stronger reaction (e.g. lane 2). The middle panel shows another reducing SDS-PAGE blot where LDL^- and HbLDL had similar banding at 500 kD that reacted with Hb antibodies while normal LDL had protein fragments 220 kD or smaller that reacted by antibodies to Hb. The 4 columns on the right in the top panel are LDL from 4 uremic subjects prior to hemolysis. Mild reactivity was found suggesting different basal levels of the Hb-LDL adduct in these subjects – all associated with lower molecular weight proteins. Columns 4–7 in the two lower panels are LDL from the same uremic subjects after HD. A low and variable reactivity for the 220-kD band was seen with the migration of the protein to higher molecular weights in relation to the extent of hemolysis (columns to the right corresponding to higher hemolysis, i.e. 150 ng/ml free Hb, after 4 h). The increase in molecular mass from 220 to 500 kD may be due to Hb/protein adducts corresponding to the molecular weight for Hb molecules adducted to apoB-100. Since the same shift is seen for both reducing and nonreducing gels, it is more likely that the adducts are monomeric Hb; however, differing

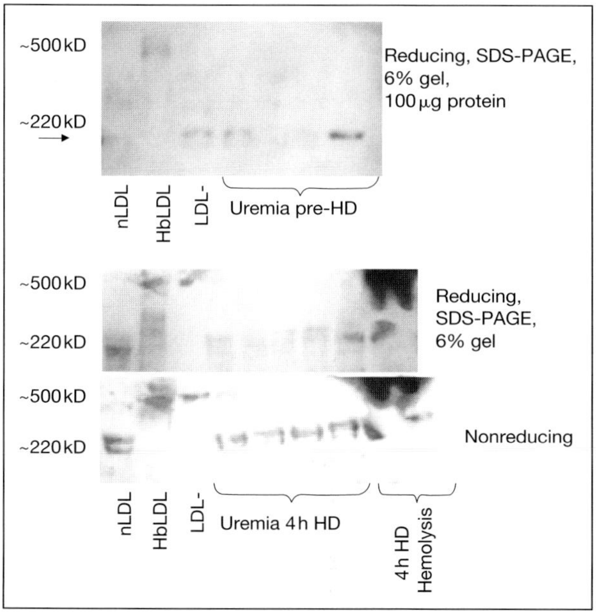

Fig. 1. HbLDL isolated from uremic subjects before and after hemodialysis. Lane 1 shows total fresh LDL, lane 3 is LDL^- standard separated from pooled LDL by HPLC. Lane 2 is $HbLDL^-$ isolated by HPLC after preparation by reaction of Hb + H_2O_2 with LDL in 10% plasma. IgG1 antibody (from Kamiya) that reacts specifically with human hemoglobin was used at dilutions of 1:2,000 and 1:15,000 antimouse IgG (from Jackson labs). All bands cross-reacted with antibody to apoB-100 (not shown). Two major bands (top panel) corresponding to 220 and 500 kD cross-reacted with the Hb antibodies; however, a 500-kD band showed the strongest reaction (e.g. lane 2). The middle panel shows reducing gel where LDL^- and HbLDL had similar banding at 500 kD using Hb antibodies while nLDL had proteins reacting at 220 kD and lower. The 4 columns on the right in the top panel are LDL from 4 uremic subjects prior to hemolysis. Columns 4–7 in the two lower panels are LDL from the same uremic subjects after HD followed by analysis using reducing and nonreducing conditions. The columns to the right correspond to subjects with the highest level of hemolysis (i.e. 150 ng/ml free Hb – after 4 h).

fragmentation patterns of apoB (due to degree of oxidation) could account for the various bands. The results suggest that ferryl species of Hb react with residues on apoB-100 to form covalent adducts and that the process is dependent on hemolysis and oxidation of apoB-100 and Hb.

The oxidative properties of HbLDL have been previously described and figure 2 demonstrates this in terms of the oxidation kinetics of various LDL preparations. In the presence of Cu^{2+}, HbLDL exhibits rapid propagation rates without an apparent lag phase. The rate of propagation is markedly reduced in

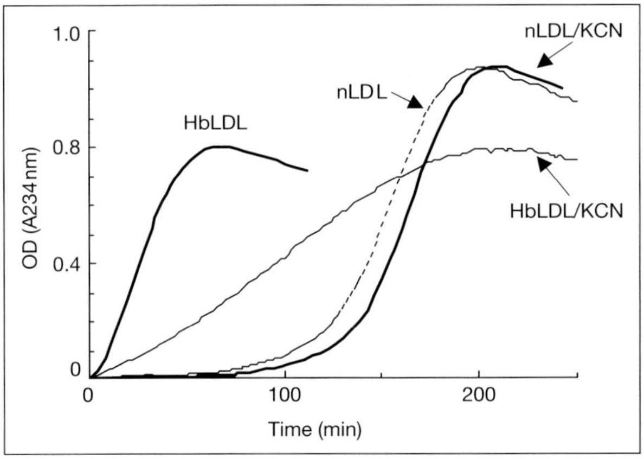

Fig. 2. Oxidation kinetics of LDL preparations monitored by conjugated diene levels (OD 234 nm). Samples (250 μg/ml) were monitored continuously in a temperature-controlled (24°C) spectrophotometer after addition of 1 μ*M* copper sulfate. The samples shown are: nLDL, normal LDL freshly isolated from plasma; HbLDL, generated by reaction of nLDL with Hb and H_2O_2 as described in the text; nLDL incubated in the presence of 50 μ*M* KCN; HbLDL incubated in the presence of 50 μ*M* KCN. The absence of lag phases are evident for HbLDL.

presence of KCN suggesting the participation of heme in this process. Although the products of lipid peroxidation (notably peroxides) are likely insufficient to account for the increased oxidizability of HbLDL, the rate at which they decompose and initiate a propagation phase may be adequate enough to account for the rapid oxidation kinetics. It was previously shown that plasma-derived LDL^- increases sensitivity of nLDL to oxidation [10] and HbLDL promotes the oxidizability of total LDL in a similar manner. However, the oxidation kinetics display two distinct propagation phases that differ from Cu^{2+}-mediated oxidation. The rapid decomposition of peroxides in the presence of heme and generation of ferryl species in lipids [11] suggest that HbLDL may undergo oxidation first and then facilitate the oxidation of the remaining nLDL through particle interactions. Interestingly, a biphasic type of oxidation can be found in native LDL containing small proportions of LDL^- when subjected to oxidation using very low concentrations of Cu^{2+} [12].

Pro-oxidant properties of LDL^- and HbLDL are thought to be responsible for the cytotoxicity of these particles, however, this is not due to increased uptake via receptors since the binding efficacy is lower than normal [13]. Figure 3 shows that HbLDL is assimilated by J774 cells at lower rates than normal LDL. Uptake of DiI-labeled nLDL, HbLDL and Cu^{2+}-oxidized LDL (Cu-oxLDL) added to cultures at 50 μg/ml showed that HbLDL was assimilated at lower rates

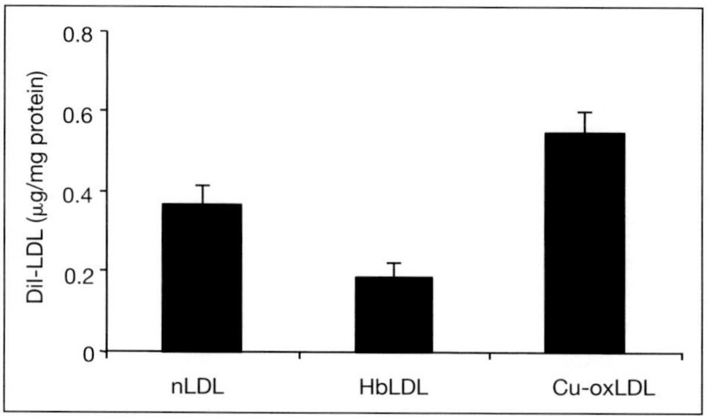

Fig. 3. LDL uptake by J774 cells using 1,1'-dioctadecyl-3,3,3',3'-tetramethylindo-carbo-cyanine perchlorate (DiI) as a fluorescent label. DiI-labeled-LDL were prepared by incubating 500 µg/ml of the respective LDL preparations with DiI in DMSO to achieve a final concentration of 50 ng DiI/µg LDL. Cells (2–3 × 10^5) were then incubated with 10 µg DiI-LDL/ml at 37°C for 3 h. The cell samples were extracted with isopropanol and fluorescent extract was measured in a fluorometer (Hitachi, CA) at Ex 523 nm, Em 563 nm. The amount of uptake was corrected on the basis of cell protein content and a calibration curve containing known amounts of DiI (referenced to the fluorescence content of the LDL added to the cell cultures) was used to compute the amount of DiI LDL assimilated by cells.

and Cu-oxLDL at higher rates than normal LDL. The enhanced rates of Cu-oxLDL uptake can be accounted for by scavenger receptors that are expressed predominantly in macrophages. The findings imply that HbLDL is not likely to be assimilated by scavenger receptors and is also not a good ligand for other lipoprotein receptors. The lower rates of uptake may account for the longer half-life for LDL^- in plasma.

Although LDL^- and HbLDL are assimilated at lower rates than normal LDL, previous studies showed that LDL^- is more cytotoxic and that at least part of this cytotoxicity is due to lipid peroxidation products. However, HbLDL does not show the same cytotoxic effects as LDL^- but contains similar levels of lipid peroxides. Figure 4 compares the cytotoxicity of normal LDL, HbLDL and Cu-oxLDL after a 24-hour treatment interval. A dose-dependent toxicity was found when J774 cells were treated with Cu-oxLDL; however, this was not found with HbLDL even at a high concentration (100 µg/ml) where LDL^- is highly toxic. Instead, a mild proliferative effect was found after treatments with HbLDL. These findings are at first inconsistent with previous studies showing that even minimally oxidized LDL is toxic when the treatment levels are high. However, it is possible that HbLDL may be inducing an oxidative stress response that evokes acute adaptation in cells. Although peroxides have been shown to induce antioxidant responses that are adaptive and protective, heme is

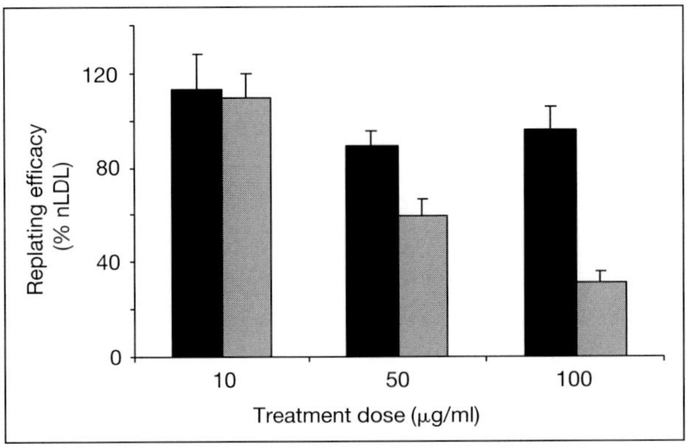

Fig. 4. Comparison of the cytotoxicity of HbLDL to Cu-oxLDL. The cytotoxicity of the LDL to J774 cells was determined by means of plating efficiency following a 24-hour treatment using the indicated concentrations of LDL. Plating efficiency was based on the number of growing cells measured 24 h after replating. The effect of HbLDL (solid bars) and Cu-oxLDL (slanted lines) are shown as a percent of the plating efficiency for cells treated with normal LDL (nLDL), and are expressed as the mean and standard error from 3 independent determinations. Similar effects were found for bovine aortic endothelial cells although the overall dose-related survival was approximately 10% lower for endothelial cells (data not shown).

also a potential candidate for inducing an antioxidant response [14]. An important protective response involves induction of heme-oxygenase-1 (HO-1) that is utilized for heme degradation with the formation of bilirubin and biliverdin, the former being an antioxidant. Hemin, H_2O_2, Cu-oxLDL and mildly oxidized LDL are reported to induce HO-1 in endothelial cells and macrophages [15] together with several acute-phase response genes.

When endothelial cells or J774 cells are treated with HbLDL, there is a rapid induction of HO-1 as part of an acute-phase response. This is described in figure 5 which shows a Western blot for HO-1. Treatment with HbLDL resulted in HO-1 induction in a dose-dependent manner with maximum induction by 12 h. No apparent induction was found with normal LDL. The response to HbLDL is comparable to the induction of HO-1 by 10 μM hemin and an induction of this magnitude is not seen after treatments with Cu-oxLDL despite the higher levels of lipid peroxidation products (data not shown). This pretreatment of cells with 50 μg/ml HbLDL for 12 h induced a subsequent resistance to an otherwise highly toxic doses of CuLDL (data not shown) whereas a comparable induction of resistance was not produced by pretreatments with 50 μg/ml CuLDL. Moreover, pretreatment of HbLDL with purified heme-oxygenase and subsequent addition of this pretreated HbLDL to cell cultures

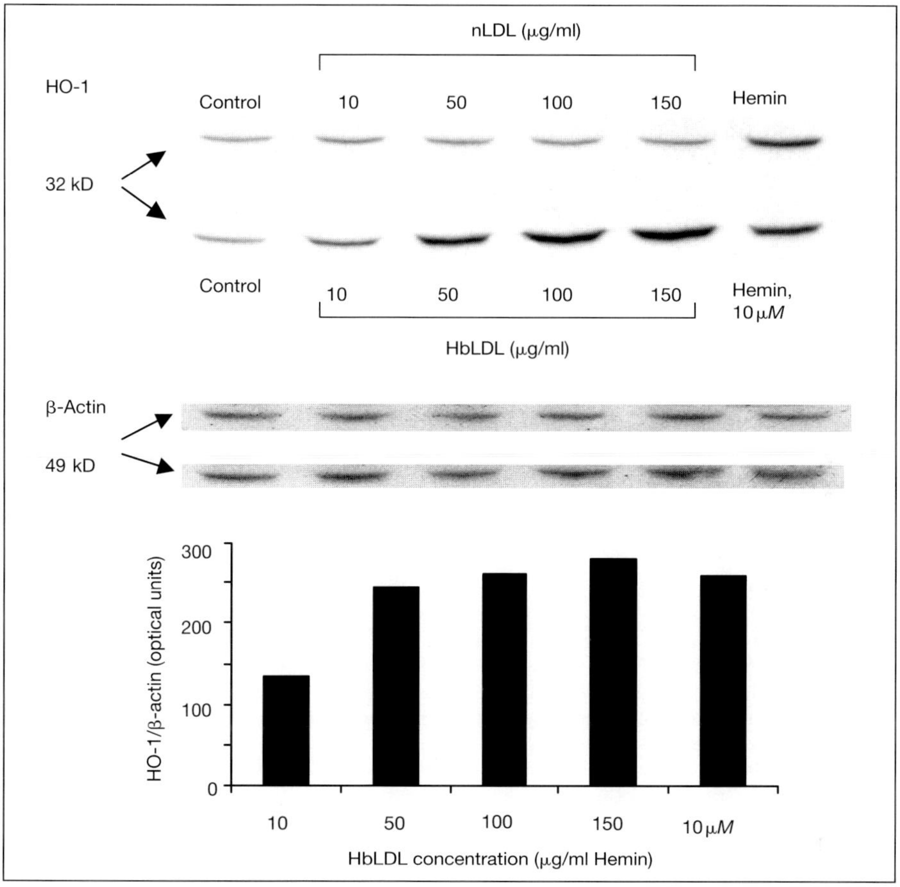

Fig. 5. The effects of HbLDL and nLDL on the induction of heme-oxygenase-1 (HO-1) in bovine endothelial cells. The figure shows Western blots for HO-1 that migrates on SDS-PAGE as a 32-kD band that was probed using a monoclonal antibody to HO-1. The concentration-dependent effects of HbLDL and nLDL are compared to the induction by 10 μ*M* hemin, where all samples were treated for 12 h. The level of sample loading was normalized to the content of β-actin, the levels of which are shown in the middle panel. The lower panel presents the results of induction graphically, where the levels of HO-1 are normalized to β-actin content.

resulted in a loss of the ability to induce HO-1. This suggests that an intact heme moiety associated with LDL is needed for the induction of HO-1, and perhaps other acute-response genes.

Taken together, these results show that oxidatively modified LDL can readily form under the hemolytic conditions that occur during hemodialysis.

The free hemoglobin acts as a potent catalyst LDL oxidation, especially in the presence of H_2O_2 which is a common product of activated vascular cells. Oxidation of LDL is also accompanied by radical-mediated modification of apoB-100, where one important reaction involves covalent binding of hemoglobin to apoB-100 – apparently via intermolecular bityrosine formation. The product – HbLDL – is part of the pool of LDL^- that can elicit a variety of oxidative stress responses in vascular cells. Despite the general toxicity of oxidized LDL, there is little cytotoxicity produced by HbLDL. Rather, exposure of vascular cells to HbLDL induces cell proliferation and an oxidative stress adaptation. Such a response when accompanied by other effects of LDL^- (notably induction of inflammatory cytokines and lipid loading) may create a highly atherogenic process where vascular cells continue to survive and proliferate while inducing influx and activation of inflammatory cells along with cholesterol accumulation.

References

1 Berliner JA, Heinecke JW: The role of oxidized lipoproteins in atherogenesis. Free Rad Biol Med 1996;20:707–727.

2 Ziouzenkova O, Asatryan L, Akmal M, Tetta C, Wratten M-L, Heinecke J, Sevanian A: Oxidative crosslinking of ApoB100 and hemoglobin results in low density lipoprotein modification in blood. J Biol Chem 1999;274:18916–18924.

3 Austin MA: Small, dense low-density lipoprotein as a risk factor for coronary heart disease. Intl J Clin Lab Res 1994;24:187–192.

4 Cazzolato G, Avogaro P, Bittolo-Bon G: Characterization of a more electronegatively charged LDL subfraction by ion exchange HPLC. Free Rad Biol Med 1991;11:247–253.

5 Carr AC, McCall MR, Frei B: Oxidation of LDL by myeloperoxidase and reactive nitrogen species: Reaction pathways and antioxidant protection. Arterioscler Thromb Vasc Biol 2000;20: 1716–1723.

6 Wieland E, Parthasarathy S and Steinberg D: Peroxidase-dependent metal-independent oxidation of low density lipoprotien in vitro: A model for in vivo oxidation. Proc Natl Acad Sci USA 1993; 90:5929–5933.

7 Anderson MM, Requena JR, Crowley JR, Thorpe SR, Heinecke JW: The meyeloperoxidase system of human phagocytes generates N^{ϵ}-(carboxymethyl)lysine on proteins: a mechanism for producing advanced glycation end products at sites of inflammation. J Clin Invest 1999;104: 103–113.

8 Burner U, Furtmuller PG, Kettle AJ, Koppenol WH, Obinger C: Mechanism of reaction of myeloperoxidase with nitrite. J Biol Chem 2000;275:20597–20601.

9 Miller YI, Altamentova SM, Shaklai N: Oxidation of low-density lipoprotein by hemoglobin stems from a heme-initiated globin radical: Antioxidant role of haptoglobin. Biochemistry 1997; 36:12189–12198.

10 Sevanian A, Hwang J, Hodis HN, Cazzolato G, Avogaro P, Bittolo-Bon G: Contribution of an in vivo oxidized LDL to LDL oxidation and its association with dense LDL subpopulations. Arterioscl Thromb 1996;16:784–793.

11 Kim E, Sevanian A: Hematin and peroxide catalyzed peroxidation of phospholipid liposomes. Arch Biochem Biophys 1991;288:324–330.

12 Ziouzenkova O, Sevanian A, Abuja PM, Ramos P, Esterbauer H: Copper can promote oxidation of LDL by markedly different mechanisms. Free Rad Biol Med 1998;24:606–623.

13 Demuth KI, Myara B, Chappey B, Vedie MA, Pech-Amsellem ME, Haberland M, Moatti N: A cytotoxic electronegative subfraction is present in human plasma. Arterioscl Thromb 1996;16: 773–783.
14 Ryter SW, Tyrell RM: The heme synthesis and degradation pathways: Role in oxidant sensitivity Free Rad Biol Med 2000;28:289–309.
15 Wang LJ, Lee TS, Lee FY, Pai RC, Chau LY: Expression of heme oxygenase-1 in atherosclerotic lesions. Am J Pathol 1998;152:711–720.

A. Sevanian, MD, University of Southern California, School of Pharmacy,
1985 Zonal Ave., Los Angeles, CA 90033 (USA)
Tel. +1(323) 442 1417, Fax +1(323) 224 7473, E-Mail asevan@hsc.usc.edu

Ronco C, La Greca G (eds): Hemodialysis Technology.
Contrib Nephrol. Basel, Karger, 2002, vol 137, pp 396–402

Erythropoietin Therapy in Europe: Results from the DOPPS

Ronald L. Pisoni

University Renal Research and Education Association (URREA), Ann Arbor, Mich., USA

Anemia has long been recognized as a major complication of renal failure. In the late 1980s, among patients receiving dialysis therapy for the treatment of end stage renal disease (ESRD), more than half had hematocrit values substantially below 30, and 12–14% required blood transfusions [1]. Since that time, numerous studies have indicated that quality of life, hospitalization rates, cardiovascular morbidity, exercise capacity, and endocrine, immune and sexual function are all improved both in predialysis patients and ESRD patients on dialysis if the hemoglobin concentration is increased to levels >10–11 g/dl [2, 3].

During the last 15 years, erythropoetin has played a major role as a standard treatment for partial correction of anemia, reducing the need for blood transfusions, and maintaining acceptable hematocrit and hemoglobin (Hb) levels in chronic renal failure (CRF) patients. Erythropoietin is an endogenous glycoprotein secreted by functioning kidneys in response to a decrease in tissue oxygenation. Secreted erythropoietin binds to specific receptors on the surface of red blood cell precursors in the bone marrow, inducing proliferation and differentiation of these cells, ultimately leading to increased red blood cell production and an increase in hemoglobin [4]. Since erythropoietin production is impaired or absent in kidneys of patients with end-stage renal disease (ESRD), recombinant human erythropoietin (Epo) is used as a therapeutic substitute for endogenous erythropoietin to stimulate red blood cell production. Since its introduction more than a decade ago, Epo has been shown to be very well tolerated and highly effective in managing anemia among dialysis patients.

This paper will summarize various aspects of Epo therapy among in-center hemodialysis patients (HD) in Europe. The results are shown in comparison to the European Best Practice Guideline (EBPG) on anaemia management which was published in September, 1999 [5]. Some of the results regarding Epo use are summarized from the European Survey on Anemia Management (ESAM) which was an observational study that included 13,121 HD patients from 14 European countries and was performed during a 6-month period beginning in September/October 1998 [6]. The results from ESAM serve as an indication of Epo use in Europe prior to publication of the EBPG on anemia management, with 60% of the HD patients living in either Germany or France, and nonrandom selection used in recruiting units into the study. Some of the other results presented on Epo use are from the Dialysis Outcomes and Practice Patterns Study (DOPPS) which is a prospective, observational and longitudinal study relating facility HD practices to patient outcomes [7, 8]. DOPPS data were collected from June 1998 through December 2000, spanning the time before and after publication of the EBPG on anemia management. DOPPS employs random selection of facilities and patients with stratification by region and unit type to provide nationally representative samples of HD patients. The European countries of France, Germany, Italy, Spain and the United Kingdom contributed to the current DOPPS results. These five countries represent approximately 84% of all HD patients in the European Union [9].

Epo Use During the Pre-ESRD Period

The EBPG on anemia management has recommended Epo treatment when the Hb concentration is consistently <11 g/dl for either CRF patients on dialysis, or not yet on dialysis [5]. Several studies have indicated that when new ESRD patients first start HD in Europe, 80% have Hb values <11 g/dl, 60% have Hb values <10 g/dl, and the mean Hb concentration of 9.5 g/dl when starting HD is approximately 1.3 g/dl lower than for prevalent HD patients [5, 8].

This level of anemia seen in new ESRD patients when starting HD is a reflection of inadequate anemia management during the predialysis phase. For patients enrolled in ESAM during September 1998 to March, 1999, only 11% received Epo during the pre-ESRD period [10]. For incident patients who enrolled in DOPPS in 1999 or 2000, a 3-fold higher rate of Epo use during the pre-ESRD period was seen compared to ESAM suggesting Epo use has increased for predialysis patients in Europe since early 1999. In addition, a recent Spanish survey on predialysis anemia management indicated that 37% of Spanish patients received Epo during the predialysis period [11], similar to that seen in DOPPS for Spanish HD patients.

The apparent increase in Epo use for CRF patients during the predialysis period is encouraging. However, these study results indicate that the great majority of CRF patients do not receive Epo therapy during the predialysis phase despite exhibiting levels of anemia in which Epo therapy is recommended by the EBPG. Anemia which is allowed to persist in CRF patients has been shown to cause cardiac abnormalities (e.g. left-ventricular hypertrophy, left-ventricular dilatation), and decrease exercise capacity and quality of life [2, 3, 12–14]. When Hb values are subsequently increased through Epo therapy, improvements are seen in patient quality of life and exercise capacity; however, left ventricular mass and exercise capacity do not return to normal levels. Recent studies have shown that partial correction of anemia by providing Epo therapy early during the predialysis phase allows reversal of left-ventricular hypertrophy and recovery of exercise capacity [14]. These studies suggest that important benefits may be gained by CRF patients if aggressive efforts are taken during the predialysis phase to prevent persistent anemia rather than waiting until patients begin dialysis.

Why do only one third of European CRF patients receive Epo during the predialysis phase? DOPPS [15] and a recent European survey by Lameire et al. [16] indicate that 70–84% of incident HD patients are seen by a nephrologist >1 month prior to ESRD, and with most of these patients having seen a nephrologist >4 months prior to initiating HD [15]. Therefore, there are many opportunities to initiate Epo therapy in the pre-ESRD period for the majority of CRF patients. However, two major impediments to providing Epo during the pre-ESRD period have been described: (1) some patients are not comfortable or skilled in self-administering Epo, and (2) costs for providing Epo therapy during the predialysis phase are often not reimbursed.

Epo Use among Incident and Prevalent HD Patients in EUR

In many regards, Epo use among prevalent HD patients in EUR follows the EBPG on anemia management, although the recommended target for the HD population has yet to be attained. The EBPG has recommended that the target Hb concentration (measured in a predialysis sample for those on HD) should be >11 g/dl for ≥85% of the patient population [5]. The EBPG recognizes that this guideline should not be applied for certain types of patients in whom high Hb concentrations could be harmful, such as patients with sickle cell disease for whom a total (HbF + HbS)Hb concentration between 7 and 9 g/dl is thought to be appropriate. Furthermore, Hb concentrations within the normal range were not recommended for patients with cardiovascular disease, diabetes mellitus, or chronic hypoxaemic pulmonary disease. For these patients, a target Hb concentration of 11–12 g/dl was suggested as a prudent guideline, although firm scientific evidence to support this latter guideline remains to be established. It is important to note that the above guideline is for Hb concentrations measured from blood samples taken prior to a dialysis session, since measured

Table 1. European best practice guideline 12 on anemia management: titration of Epo dosage

1	If the increase in Hb concentration after initiation of Epo therapy or after a dose increase has been <0.7 g/dl over a 2- to 4-week period, the dose of Epo should be increased by 50%
2	If the absolute rate of increase of Hb concentration after initiation of Epo therapy or after a dose increase is >2.5 g/dl per month, or if the Hb concentration exceeds the target Hb concentration, the weekly dose of Epo should be reduced by 25–50%
3	When the weekly Epo dose is being increased or decreased, a change may be made in the amount administered in a given dose and/or in the frequency of dosing (if given subcutaneously); it is preferable to round off the dose to the nearest whole vial to prevent wastage
4	The median maintenance dose of Epo in a nonselected population of patients given subcutaneous Epo will usually be <125 IU/kg/week; the lowest effective doses are likely to be about 50 IU/kg/week, with 90% of patients receiving <300 IU/kg/week.

Reproduced from ref. [5].

Hb concentrations often can differ by 1–2 g/dl depending upon whether the measurement is performed on a predialysis versus postdialysis blood sample and the amount of fluid removed during the treatment [5].

In terms of Epo dosing, EBPG recommends a starting Epo dose of 50–150 IU/kg/week; higher initial Epo doses are suggested if the patient has severe anemia (Hb conc. <8 g/dl) or has complicating disorders leading to anemia [5]. For the majority of patients this dosing strategy translates into 4,000–8,000 IU/week. When Epo is administered subcutaneously, doses in the lower part of this range are recommended by the EBPG at a frequency of 2–3 times per week. For intravenous Epo delivery, a starting dose in the upper part of the range is recommended at a frequency of 3 times per week. The subcutaneous (SC) route for administration of epoetin-alpha and epoetin-beta is given preference over the intravenous (IV) route by the EBPG since numerous studies have shown that the dose of Epo required to achieve a given Hb concentration may be lower for the SC route compared with the IV route in the case of epoetin-alpha and epoetin-beta. With the availability of darbepoetin-alpha in Europe there are no differences in recommended dose for SC versus IV administration. However, patient and physician preferences are an important consideration in determining the most suitable route for Epo administration.

Once Epo therapy has been initiated, EBPG recommends that the Epo dose should be titrated to a level which allows the patient to reach the desired Hb target range, with an acceptable rate of rise in Hb. These recommendations are indicated in table 1. In some cases, hyporesponsiveness to Epo therapy is

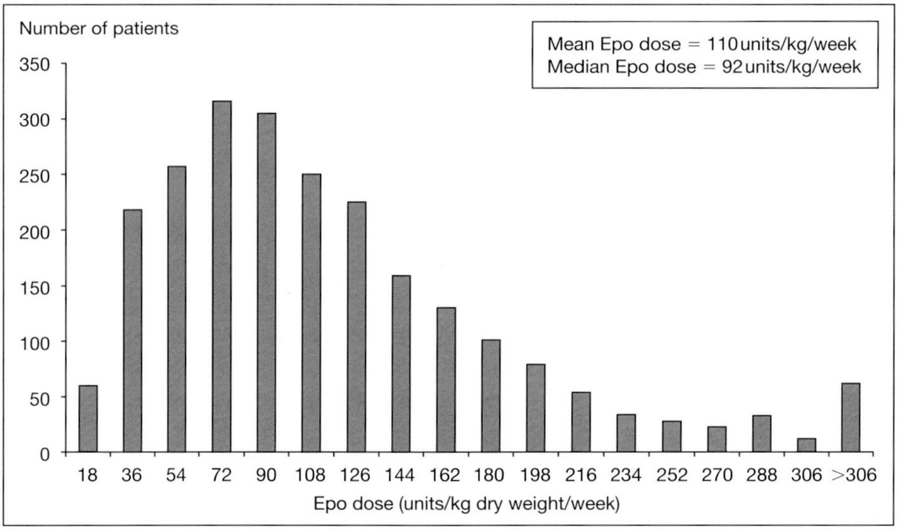

Fig. 1. Distribution of Epo dose among prevalent HD patients in DOPPS for year 2000. Epo dose is expressed as units/kg dry weight/week (n = 2,346).

encountered, which requires a comprehensive clinical evaluation to understand the underlying cause(s). Iron deficiency is the most common cause for Epo hyporesponsiveness [5].

The following are results of recent Epo use in Europe. Epo is prescribed for approximately 40% of new HD patients and 80% of prevalent HD patients in Europe [8]. Epo doses given to HD patients depend upon factors such as the patient's level of anemia, comorbidity profile, weight of the patient, route of Epo administration, and occurrence of hyporesponsiveness to Epo therapy. Because of these factors, a broad distribution in Epo dose is typically seen for prevalent HD patients, as shown in figure 1. At least three-fourths of patients receive Epo by the subcutaneous route in France, Italy, Spain, and the United Kingdom, with the opposite pattern observed in Germany [8]. However, there has not been a significant difference observed in the mean Epo dose or in the mean hemoglobin concentration in Europe for HD patients receiving Epo by the subcutaneous route versus the intravenous route [8].

In Europe, Epo is most often given 3 times per week. The mean and median Epo dose for HD patients in Europe lies well within the range of 50–150 IU/kg/week recommended by the EBPG. In ESAM, the mean Epo doses by country ranged from 93 to 161 IU/kg/week [17], and a similar range in mean Epo dose from 92 to 130 IU/kg/week observed for the countries participating in DOPPS [8]. However, despite this range of Epo therapy, slightly less than 50% of HD patients in Europe have a Hb concentration >11 g/dl [8]. Therefore, substantial gains yet are required to achieve the EBPG recommendation of ≥85% of HD patients with a Hb concentration >11 g/dl. The underachievement of this EBPG on anemia management does not appear to be due to dialysis facilities setting low target Hb ranges for their patients since the target Hb value for approximately 80% of patients in Europe has been reported to be >11 g/dl [18]. However, an important focus in trying to achieve the EBPG recommendation in Europe will be to examine the contribution of policies in many dialysis units which prohibit initiation of Epo therapy for patients until Hb concentrations fall to levels substantially below 10 g/dl. Furthermore, prescription of Epo use varies widely among European facilities in DOPPS, with some facilities prescribing Epo for 12% of prevalent patients while other units prescribe Epo for 100% of patients [8]. The relationship between Epo use within facilities, patient Hb levels, and outcome measures continues to be a very important area of investigation for ultimately understanding the many additional benefits to be gained for hemodialysis patients by programs aimed at achieving improvements in anemia management.

Acknowledgement

Funding for DOPPS was provided by an unrestricted scientific/educational grant from Kirin-Amgen.

References

1 US Renal Data System 1991: Annual Data Report. Bethesda, National Institutes of Health, National Institute of Diabetes and Digestive and Kidney Diseases, 1991, pp 77–81.

2 O'Riordan E, Foley RN: Effects of anaemia on cardiovascular status. Nephrol Dial Transplant 2000;15(suppl 3):19–22.

3 Macdougall IC: Higher target hemoglobin level and early anaemia treatment: Different or complementary concepts? Nephrol Dial Transplant 2000;15(suppl 3):3–7.

4 Egrie JC, Browne JK: Development and characterization of novel erythropoiesis stimulating protein (NESP). Nephrol Dial Transplant 2001;16(suppl 3):3–13.

5 Working Party for European Best Practice Guidelines for the Management of Anaemia in Patients with Chronic Renal Failure: European best practice guidelines for the management of anaemia in patients with chronic renal failure. Nephrol Dial Transplant 1999;14(suppl 5):1–50.

6 Valderrábano F, Hörl WH, Jacobs C, Macdougall IC, Parrondo I, Manhaeve D, Milisen K: Patients and methods. Nephrol Dial Transplant 2000;15(suppl 4):2–7.

7 Young EW, Goodkin DA, Mapes DL, Port FK, Keen ML, Chen K, Maroni BL, Wolfe RA, Held PJ: The Dialysis Outcomes and Practice Patterns Study (DOPPS): An international hemodialysis study. Kidney Int 2000;57(suppl 74):S74–S81.

8 Pisoni, RL, Port FK, Bragg JL, Greenwood RN, Combe C, Young EW, Wolfe RA, Held PJ, Locatelli F: Anemia management practices in Europe: Results from DOPPS. Nephrol Dial Transplant 2002;17:abstr, in press.

9 Berthoux F, Jones E, Gellert R, Mendel S, Saker L, Briggs D: Epidemiological data of treated end-stage renal failure in the European Union (EU) during the year 1995: report of the European Renal Association Registry and the National Registries. Nephrol Dial Transplant 1999;14:2332–2342.
10 Valderrábano F, Hörl WH, Jacobs C, Macdougall IC, Parrondo I, Cremers S, Abraham IL: European Best Practice Guidelines 1–4: Evaluating anaemia and initiating treatment. Nephrol Dial Transplant 2000;15(suppl 4):8–14.
11 Cruz JM: Estudio epidemiologico español sobre el tratamiento de la anemia en pacientes con insuficiencia renal progresiva. Nefrologia 2001;in press.
12 Macdougall IC: Present and future strategies in the treatment of renal anaemia. Nephrol Dial Transplant 2001;16(suppl 5):50–55.
13 Ritz E, Eisenhardt A: Early epoetin treatment in patients with renal insufficiency. Nephrol Dial Transplant 2000;15(suppl 3):40–44.
14 Portolés J: The beneficial effects of intervention in early renal disease. Nephrol Dial Transplant 2001:16(suppl 2):12–5.
15 Pisoni RL, Young EW, Dykstra DM, Greenwood RN, Hecking E, Gillespie B, Wolfe RA, Goodkin DA, Held PJ: Vascular access use in Europe and the United States: Results from the DOPPS. Kidney Int 2002;61:305–316.
16 Lameire N, Van Biesen W: The pattern of referral of patients with end-stage renal disease to the nephrologist: A European survey. Nephrol Dial Transplant 1999:14(suppl 6):16–23.
17 Jacobs C, Horl WH, Macdougall IC, Valderrabáno F, Parrondo I, Abraham IL, Segner A: European Best Practice Guidelines 9–13: Anaemia management. Nephrol Dial Transplant 2000;15(suppl 4): 33–42.
18 Jacobs C, Horl WH, Macdougall IC, Valderrábano F, Parrondo I, Segner A, Abraham IL: European Best Practice Guidelines 5: Target haemoglobin. Nephrol Dial Transplant 2000;15(suppl 4): 15–19.

Ronald L. Pisoni, PhD,
University Renal Research and Education Association,
315 W. Huron Street, Suite 260, Ann Arbor, MI 48103 (USA)
Tel. +1 (734) 665 4108 ext 223, Fax +1 (734) 665 2103, E-Mail rlpisoni@urrea.org

Ronco C, La Greca G (eds): Hemodialysis Technology.
Contrib Nephrol. Basel, Karger, 2002, vol 137, pp 403–407

Clinical Experience with Darbepoetin-Alfa (Aranesp®)

Francesco Locatelli, Lucia Del Vecchio, Paolo Marai

Divisione di Nefrologia e Dialisi, Ospedale A. Manzoni, Lecco, Italy

The majority of patients with chronic renal insufficiency (CRI) progress to end-stage renal disease, when the associated anaemia can have significant effects on quality of life, morbidity and mortality rate. Since this anaemia is under-recognised and under-treated, CRI is a crucial opportunity for early and aggressive prophylactic intervention to prevent the dangerous cardiac complications of chronic renal anaemia in patients with CRF [1].

Recombinant human erythropoietin (rHuEPO) has been the mainstay of treatment for renal anaemia since it was launched in the late 1980s. It is highly effective in correcting renal anaemia in the majority of patients. However, rHuEPO has a relatively short half-life (4–8 h) and patients need repeated administrations each week [2].

Development of Darbepoetin-Alfa

Darbepoetin-alfa (Aranesp®; Amgen Inc.) has been developed to simplify the management of renal anaemia with longer intervals between dosing [3]. Increased serum half-life and biological activity have been achieved by the addition of two carbohydrate side chains to rHuEPO to produce darbepoetin-alfa. The increased half-life of the new molecule predicts that it will have similar efficacy to rHuEPO but with less-frequent dosing.

Initial studies confirmed that the half-life of darbepoetin-alfa in humans is approximately three times longer than that of rHuEPO after intravenous (i.v.) administration (25.5 h compared with 8.5 h), allowing less frequent dosing. Darbepoetin-alfa can also be administered by subcutaneous (s.c.) injection, with

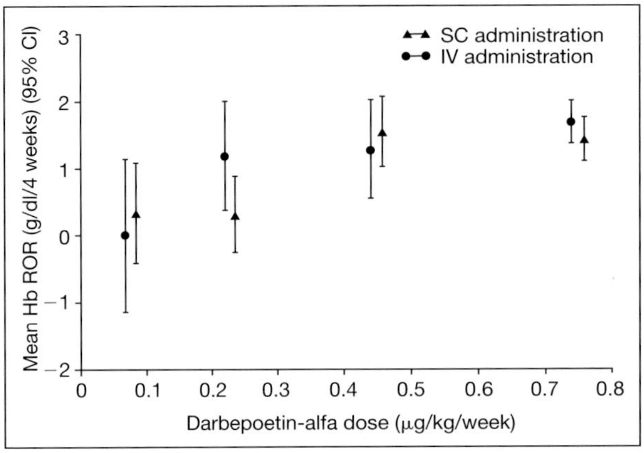

Fig. 1. Mean rate of rise in Hb concentration over the first 4 weeks of s.c. or i.v. darbepoetin-alfa treatment. ROR = Rate of rise. Reproduced with permission from the Oxford University Press from Macdougall [3].

a half-life twice as long as after i.v. administration. The mean bioavailability of darbepoetin-alfa (36.9%) is similar to the bioavailability of rHuEPO [4].

Thirteen studies involving more than 2,000 subjects in the USA, Europe, Australia and Canada have been reported. These address three phases of renal anaemia management: correction of anaemia, conversion of patients from rHuEPO to darbepoetin-alfa, and maintenance of haemoglobin levels.

Chronic Renal Failure

Correction of Anaemia in Patients with CRF

The optimal dosing schedule for darbepoetin-alfa was investigated in two multicenter studies with similar designs [5]. In one study, haemodialysis (HD) patients were treated with i.v. darbepoetin-alfa, while the other study included peritoneal dialysis (PD) patients treated with s.c. darbepoetin-alfa. Patients received open-label darbepoetin-alfa at the same total weekly dose. There was a dose-dependent increase in haemoglobin in both studies over the first 4 weeks (fig. 1) with no differences between once-weekly or three-times-weekly dose regimens. The optimal doses of darbepoetin-alfa (defined as Hb increase of 1–3 g/dl over 4 weeks) were 0.45 and 0.75 μg/kg/week and this was chosen as the starting dose range, administered either s.c. or i.v. once weekly.

In a further study to evaluate the efficacy of darbepoetin-alfa, 122 patients with CRF received 0.45 μg/kg/week darbepoetin-alfa (s.c. or i.v.) once weekly or rHuEPO 50 IU/kg three times weekly [6]. After 20 weeks of treatment, the Hb concentration in both groups was within the range 11–13 g/dl.

Switching Patients from rHuEPO to Darbepoetin-Alfa Therapy

Two studies involving more than 1,000 CRF patients have shown that darbepoetin-alfa is as effective as rHuEPO for maintaining Hb levels, and has the advantage of less frequent dosing [7, 8]. In both studies, the mean Hb concentrations remained stable from baseline to evaluation period and there were no significant differences between the two treatment groups. Nearly all patients were successfully managed at the reduced dose frequency (97% of patients treated with darbepoetin-alfa once weekly and 95% of patients treated with darbepoetin-alfa once every other week).

Maintenance of Hb Levels

In a 1-year study of efficacy and safety, 703 patients with end-stage renal disease (ESRD) receiving rHuEPO and with stable Hb were converted to darbepoetin-alfa at reduced dose frequency [8]. Mean Hb was maintained within the target range and at a stable level. Ninety-one percent of patients were within this range at week 36, and 96% of patients were managed at the reduced dose frequency.

Chronic Renal Insufficiency

A recent clinical trial has shown that darbepoetin-alfa is not only effective for the management of anaemia in patients with CRF, but also for those patients not yet receiving dialysis [10]. In an open-label study, 166 CRI patients were randomised to receive either darbepoetin-alfa (0.45 μg/kg once weekly) or rHuEPO (50 IU/kg twice weekly) administered s.c. for up to 24 weeks.

The majority of patients achieved an Hb response (93% in the darbepoetin-alfa group and 92% in the rHuEPO group). Hb concentrations increased over the first 12 weeks of the study, and after correction of anaemia Hb concentrations were maintained within the target range (fig. 2).

Safety and Tolerability

For the vast majority of CRF patients with anaemia, rHuEPO has proven to be a very well-tolerated treatment. The safety and tolerability of darbepoetin-alfa has been evaluated using an integrated database of more than 1,500 patients treated for up to 24 months [3]. The adverse events reported were mainly those

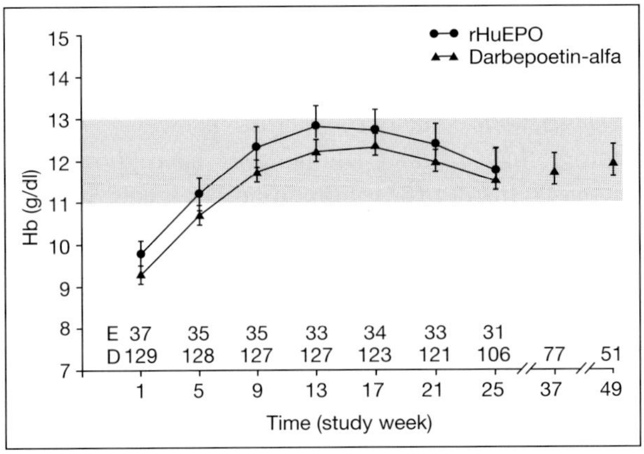

Fig. 2. Mean Hb concentrations after treatment with darbepoetin-alfa or rHuEPO in CRI patients. E = n-value for patients receiving rHuEPO; D = n-value for patients receiving darbepoetin-alfa. Reproduced with permission from Blackwell Science from Locatelli et al. [10].

normally seen in renal failure patients and were not attributable to treatment. In comparative studies with rHuEPO the adverse-events profile was similar. The overall proportion of patients who discontinued treatment due to an adverse event was 2% in the darbepoetin-alfa group and 4% in the rHuEPO group. The most common adverse events were hypertension, hypotension, myalgia and headache [3]. Importantly, the proportion of discontinuations due to death was the same in patients treated with darbepoetin-alfa or rHuEPO (6%) [2].

If Hb rises above target levels, the next dose of darbepoetin-alfa can be safely withheld to correct it, an important factor in patient management. In CRI and dialysis patients whose Hb exceeded 14 g/dl, withholding treatment caused a progressive decline in Hb concentration [4]. The rate of decrease was similar for patients treated with either darbepoetin-alfa or rHuEPO.

Conclusions

Darbepoetin-alfa is indicated for the treatment of anaemia associated with CRF in adults and paediatric subjects ≥11 years of age. It can be administered either s.c. or i.v. at a starting dose of 0.45 μg/kg once weekly. Dose should be titrated to achieve a target of 11–13 g/dl and therapy discontinued if Hb exceeds 14 g/dl.

All of the phase 3 studies confirm that darbepoetin-alfa achieves and maintains stable Hb levels with less frequent dosing than rHuEPO, regardless of route of administration. Trials designed to formally compare the two drugs are still lacking. If dose reductions are not made, higher Hb levels might be expected with i.v. darbepoetin-alfa.

Darbepoetin-alfa is effective for the treatment of anaemia associated with renal disease (both CRF and CRI) and has a similar safety profile to rHuEPO. This is of considerable clinical importance, as rHuEPO is an extremely well-tolerated drug. Darbepoetin-alfa represents a further improvement of care for patients with renal anaemia.

References

1 Besarab A, Levin A: Defining a renal anemia management period. Am J Kidney Dis 2000; 36(suppl 3):S13–S23.

2 Nissenson AR: Novel erythropoiesis stimulating protein for managing the anemia of chronic kidney disease. Am J Kidney Dis 2001;38:1390–1397.

3 Macdougall IC: An overview of the efficacy and safety of novel erythropoiesis stimulating protein (NESP). Nephrol Dial Transplant 2001;16(suppl 3):S14–S21.

4 Macdougall IC, Gray SJ, Elston O, Breen C, Jenkins B, Browne J, Egrie J: Pharmacokinetics of novel erythropoiesis stimulating protein compared with epoetin alfa in dialysis patients. J Am Soc Nephrol 1999;10:2392–2395.

5 Macdougall IC: Novel erythropoiesis-stimulating protein (NESP) for the treatment of renal anaemia. J Am Soc Nephrol 1998;9:258A–259A.

6 Coyne D, Ling BN, Toto R, et al: Novel erythropoiesis stimulating protein (NESP) corrects anemia in dialysis patients when administered at reduced dose frequency compared with recombinant-human erythropoietin (r-HuEPO). J Am Soc Nephrol 2000;1380A .

7 Nissenson AR, Swn SK, Lindberg JS, et al: Novel erythropoiesis stimulating protein (NESP) safely maintains Hb concentration levels in hemodialysis patients as effectively as r-HuEPO when administered once weekly. J Am Soc Nephrol 2000;11:1326A.

8 Vanrenterghem Y, Barany P, Mann J, on behalf of the European/Australian NESP 970200 Study Group: Novel erythropoiesis stimulating protein (NESP) maintains Hb in ESRD patients when administered once weekly or once every other week. J Am Soc Nephrol 1999;10:270A.

9 Graf H, Lacombe J-L, Braun J, Gomes da Costa AA: Novel erythropoiesis stimulating protein (NESP) for maintaining hemoglobin (Hb) at a reduced dose frequency compared with recombinant human erythropoietin (EPO) in ESRD patients. Nephrol Dial Transplant 2000;15:159A.

10 Locatelli F, Olivares J, Walker R, Wilkie M, Jenkins B, Dewey C, Gray SJ: Novel erythropoiesis stimulating protein for treatment of anemia in chronic renal insufficiency. European/Australian NESP 980202 Study Group. Kidney Int 2001;60:741–747.

Professor Dr. Francesco Locatelli, Divisione di Nefrologia e Dialisi,
Ospedale A. Manzoni, Via dell'Eremo 9/11, I–23900 Lecco (Italy)
Tel. +39 0341 489850, Fax +39 0341 489860, E-Mail nefrologia@ospedale.lecco.it

Ronco C, La Greca G (eds): Hemodialysis Technology.
Contrib Nephrol. Basel, Karger, 2002, vol 137, pp 408–411

Once-Weekly Epoetin-Beta in Renal Anemia: The Clinical Evidence

Alberto Albertazzi

Department of Nephrology Dialysis and Renal Transplantation,
General Hospital and University of Modena and Reggio Emilia, Modena, Italy

The standard recombinant human erythropoietin (rh-EPO, epoetin) maintenance regimen incorporates administration three times weekly. Data from trials of subcutaneous epoetin-beta (NeoRecormon®) indicate, however, that it is possible to reduce the number of doses required per week. This would provide an opportunity to individualize treatment regimens, which might help patients comply with therapy. Also, a simplified regimen may encourage patients to self-administer epoetin-beta treatment.

Clinical trial data have shown that once weekly epoetin-beta administration is as effective and well tolerated as the standard three-times-weekly regimen. This article reviews the evidence from studies conducted in chronic kidney disease (CKD) patients requiring dialysis, and in those not yet requiring dialysis.

Once-Weekly Regimen in Dialysis Patients

Several trials of patients receiving peritoneal dialysis or hemodialysis have shown that once weekly epoetin-beta is as effective as three times weekly administration. In one study, 33 anemic continuous ambulatory peritoneal dialysis (CAPD) patients with stable hemoglobin levels were randomly assigned to either three-times-weekly epoetin-beta, or once-weekly administration of the same weekly dose [1]. Three months later, analysis of hemoglobin levels showed no significant difference between the two treatment groups. Moreover,

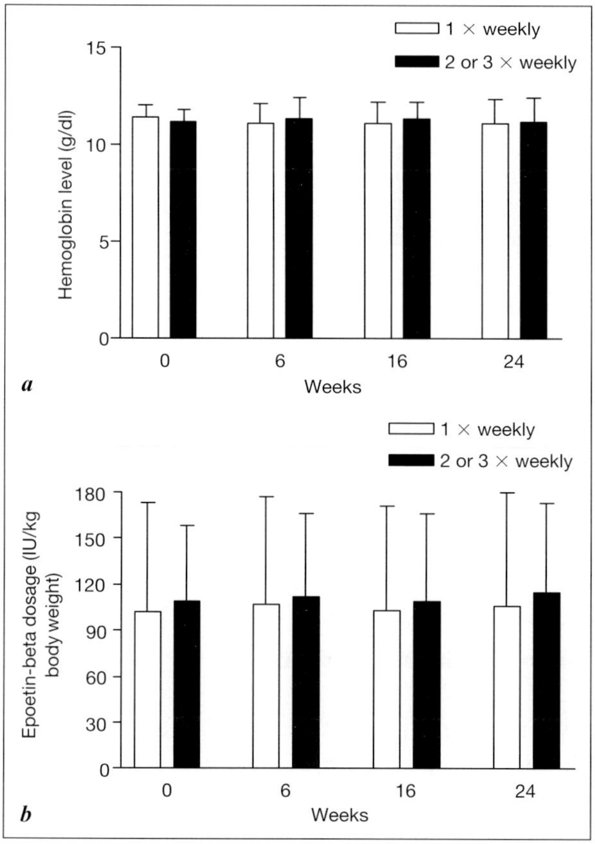

Fig. 1. Mean hemoglobin levels and epoetin-beta dose in hemodialysis patients receiving subcutaneous epoetin-beta once weekly (1 × weekly) and two or three times weekly (2 or 3 × weekly) [2]. For all timepoints, the difference between the once weekly and two or three times weekly groups was not statistically significant. ***a*** Mean hemoglobin levels (g/dl). ***b*** Mean epoetin-beta dosage (IU/kg body weight).

there were no statistically significant differences in weekly dose of epoetin-beta at any time during the study.

Once weekly subcutaneous epoetin-beta was also effective and well tolerated in two recent, large-scale, randomized studies of stable hemodialysis patients. A randomized trial of 158 patients showed no difference in hemoglobin levels and weekly doses between once-weekly and two- or three-times-weekly administration of epoetin-beta (fig. 1) [2]. Moreover, another recently reported trial (n = 173) used a statistically rigorous test to demonstrate that once-weekly and three-times-weekly administrations of epoetin-beta were therapeutically

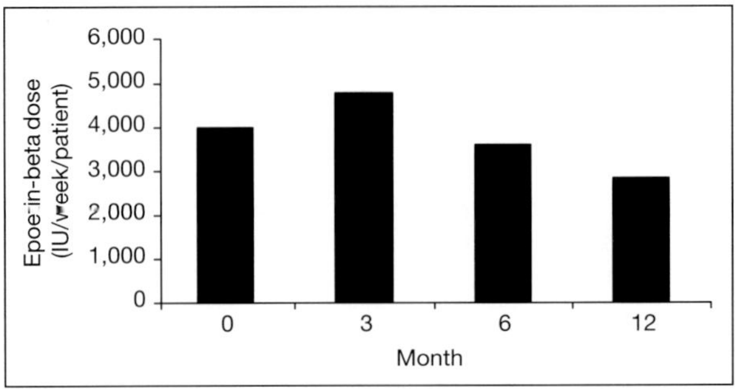

Fig. 2. Gradual reduction in mean epoetin-beta dose during a study of once weekly maintenance treatment in predialysis patients [4].

equivalent in maintaining hematocrit and epoetin-beta dose requirement [3]. Additionally, the incidence of adverse events was similar in both treatment groups.

Once-Weekly Regimen in Predialysis Patients

As well as being effective in patients already on dialysis treatment, once-weekly epoetin-beta has been shown to be efficacious in patients not yet requiring dialysis. In a multicenter study, 84 predialysis patients were administered epoetin-beta twice weekly until stable hemoglobin levels were achieved [4]. The epoetin-beta dose was then halved and administered once weekly. As the study progressed, the epoetin-beta dose gradually decreased (fig. 2), while the hemoglobin level increased significantly after the first 3 months ($p < 0.001$). After 12 months of once-weekly epoetin-beta treatment, the mean hemoglobin level had increased from the baseline value of 8–10 g/dl. Correspondingly, the mean weekly epoetin-beta dose decreased from 4,000 IU at baseline to 2,840 IU at the end of month 12.

Conclusions

Once-weekly subcutaneous epoetin-beta has been shown to be as effective and well tolerated as the standard three-times-weekly regimen in several studies conducted in CKD patients requiring or not yet requiring dialysis. The ability to administer epoetin-beta once weekly provides clinicians with another option, allowing greater opportunities to individualize treatment. Additionally, the convenience of once-weekly administration could encourage patients to self-administer and help them to comply with their treatment regimen. This is in line with the latest treatment guidelines for renal anemia, which recommend self-administration of epoetin where possible [5, 6]. Also, for patients unable to self-administer, once weekly injections of epoetin-beta free valuable time and resources for both clinic and patient.

References

1 Frifelt JJ, Tvedegaard E, Bruun K, Steffensen G, Cintin C, Breddam M, Dominguez H, Jørgensen JD: Efficacy of recombinant human erythropoietin administered subcutaneously to CAPD patients once weekly. Perit Dial Int 1996;16:594–598.
2 Weiss LG, Clyne N, Divino Fihlo J, Frisenette-Fich C, Kurkus J, Svensson B, on behalf of the Swedish Study Group: The efficacy of once weekly compared with two or three times weekly subcutaneous epoetin-beta: Results from a randomized controlled multicentre trial. Nephrol Dial Transplant 2000;15:2014–2019.
3 Locatelli F, Baldamus CA, Villa G, Martinez F, de Francisco ALM, on behalf of the Collaborative Group: Therapeutic equivalence of once versus thrice weekly subcutaneous epoetin-beta in patients with chronic renal failure. Nephrol Dial Transplant 2001;16:A136.
4 Albertazzi A, Di Liberato L, Daniele F, Battistel V, Colombi L: Efficacy and tolerability of recombinant human erythropoietin treatment in pre-dialysis patients: results of a multicenter study. Int J Artif Organs 1998;21:12–18.
5 NKF-K/DOQI Clinical Practice Guidelines for Anemia of Chronic Kidney Disease: Update 2000. Am J Kidney Dis 2001;37(suppl 1):S182–S238.
6 European Best Practice Guidelines for the Management of Anaemia in Patients with Chronic Renal Failure. Nephrol Dial Transplant 1999;14(suppl 5):1–50.

Professor Alberto Albertazzi, Department of Nephrology Dialysis and Renal Transplantation,
General Hospital and University of Modena and Reggio Emilia
Via del Pozzo, 71, I–41100 Modena (Italy)
Tel. +39 (0)59 4222485, Fax +39 (0)59 4222167, E-Mail albertazzi.alberto@unimo.it

Ronco C, La Greca G (eds): Hemodialysis Technology.
Contrib Nephrol. Basel, Karger, 2002, vol 137, pp 412–425

Iron Therapy in Hemodialysis Patients: How and When?

Carlo Crepaldi[a], *Valeria Bordoni*[a], *Maria Rosa Carta*[b]

[a] Nephrology Department, St. Bortolo Hospital and
[b] Clinical Chemistry and Hematology Laboratory, Vicenza, Italy

Iron supplementation has become an integral part of the management of patients receiving epoetin therapy, and clinicians have found it necessary to learn how and when to use it to the best advantage. Iron administration is particularly recommended in uremic patients undergoing regular hemodialytic treatment to correct a presumed iron deficiency due to impaired absorption and dialytic losses.

A number of factors have been shown to limit the response to recombinant human erythropoietin. One major factor appears to be an inadequate iron supply to the bone marrow. Erythropoiesis is dependent upon a continuous supply of iron to the bone marrow. The rate at which iron can be drawn from existing stores may easily limit the rate of delivery for hemoglobin synthesis.

Iron Kinetics

Iron is a critical body substance transporting oxygen to tissues via hemoglobin and functioning as a cofactor in a number of enzyme systems. In the healthy subject the iron losses are estimated at about 1 mg/day and happen by intestinal excretion. Because of this, under normal circumstances there is the need to absorb only approximately 1 mg iron from dietary sources per day [1]. The iron content of a normal diet in the western countries is significantly greater, amounting to about 6 mg of iron every 1,000 kcal. A normal diet contains about 10–20 mg of iron and, therefore, only 10% of this amount is absorbed by the gut. This percentage may increase after bleeding or during pregnancy. Iron is absorbed from the intestines mostly in the duodenum and early jejunum as ferric iron (Fe^{3+}) [2, 3]. Red meat contains primarily heme iron, which is more thoroughly absorbed. Ascorbate and citrate and a low pH of the stomach increase iron gut absorption. On the other hand, iron absorption is reduced by phytates (contained in vegetables), tannates (contained in tea) and phosphates all forming unabsorbable complexes with iron [4]. Intestinal iron absorption depends on both the amount and bioavailability of dietary iron and is controlled by the gut mucosal 'setting' which is responsive to the state of body iron stores [5]. Iron is stored in reticuloendothelial cells of liver, spleen and bone marrow bound to ferritin and hemosiderin. Ferritin is composed of a soluble (FeOOH)x core within an apoferritin protein shell, or as a part of insoluble hemosiderin. This storage iron constitutes one third of the 3–4 g of total body iron. The major part of the remaining iron is present in erythropoietic tissue or red blood cells [1]. The circulating red cell mass contains 3 g iron and is the major store. About 5% of body iron is in myoglobin and negligible amounts of iron are involved in nonheme iron-containing proteins such as metal cofactor for many enzymes (oxidases, peroxidase, catalases) and cytochromes. The transferring iron pool of the plasma contains only 3–4 mg of iron.

Mammals have specific iron-binding proteins that move iron from sites of absorption and storage to sites of use. The best characterized of these proteins are the transferrins: two-sided single-chain iron-binding proteins widely distributed in physiological fluid and cells. Two major types have been identified: serum transferrin and lactoferrin. Lactoferrins are found predominantly in tissue fluids and cells and seem to function in the body's defense against infection as well as in iron transport [6].

Transferrin, which transports iron in blood plasma, is a β-globulin with a relative molecular weight of about 79,500 daltons. This has two iron-binding sites which will pick up iron from and donate iron to cells surfaces. Cells which have a high demand for iron, particularly the proliferating erythropoietic tissue, have many binding sites on their surfaces. The economy of iron metabolism is dominated by the need to supply iron to the developing erythroid tissue. At the same time the reticuloendothelial system will hold a significant mass of iron in a storage form [7]. The uptake of iron is rapid, not only in erythroid progenitor cells but also to a large extent into the reticuloendothelial system cells (liver, spleen, lymph nodes), where it can be deposited as hemosiderin and is therefore not as easily accessible for erythropoiesis in the long term.

In uremic patients undergoing hemodialysis estimated iron losses are 1,500–3,000 mg/year [8].

It means that a uremic hemodialyzed patient needs this amount of iron plus 350 mg of iron normally lost by the gut. Several factors contribute to ongoing blood loss in dialysis patients: blood retained in the dialyzer and blood tubing, blood lost from vascular accesses, frequent blood testing.

In contrast, annual blood loss is only about 250 ml (100 mg iron) in patients with chronic renal failure or on peritoneal dialysis who have no dialysis-associated losses and generally have fewer blood samples taken [9].

Anemia is a common finding in dialysis patients and the most important factor for its development is represented by a decreased endogenous production of erythropoietin [10]. Many other factors are involved in the pathogenesis of renal anemia: inhibitors of erythropoiesis (uremic toxins, cytokines, drugs) reduced life span of erythrocytes, secondary hyperparathyroidism, aluminium intoxication and chronic blood loss. Absolute or functional iron deficiency plays a major role in the development of anemia as well as in the resistance to the therapeutic action of erythropoietin [11].

The distinction between absolute and functional iron deficiency is crucial to understand what constitutes adequate transferrin saturation (TSAT) and serum ferritin levels in epoetin-treated patients.

Absolute iron deficiency is defined in patients with chronic kidney disease as serum ferritin levels $<$100 ng/ml and TSAT levels $<$20% (or hypochromic red blood cells $>$10%).

Functional iron deficiency results when there is a need for a greater amount of iron to support hemoglobin synthesis than can be released from iron stores (reticuloendothelial cells). This situation, which can be produced by pharmacological stimulation of erythropoiesis by epoetin, can occur in the presence of adequate iron stores. As a result the percent TSAT or the hypochromic red blood cell count decreases to levels consistent with iron deficiency despite a normal or elevated serum ferritin. Patients with these conditions do not meet traditional laboratory criteria for absolute iron deficiency, but may demonstrate an increase in hemoglobin/Hct when intravenous iron is administered [9].

Iron: Ways of Administration

Oral Iron Administration

Oral iron has the advantage of being simple and cheap. Several iron salts are available in tablet or liquid form for oral ingestion: ferrous sulfate, ferrous fumarate, ferrous gluconate, ferrous succinate, iron polymaltose, and polysaccharide-iron complex. Ferrous sulfate, which for instance supplies 65 mg of elemental iron per 200 mg tablet, is the most widely used iron preparation.

In hemodialyzed patients oral iron is poorly absorbed [12], and it has been shown in a number of studies, including randomized controlled trials, to be incapable of maintaining iron balance in the long term. In addition, oral iron is often poorly tolerated with consequent poor compliance [13]. There are no clear data as to which preparation of oral iron should be used, and although ferrous sulfate or gluconate frequently give rise to side effects (especially gastrointestinal), neither ferrous fumarate nor iron polymers have been demonstrated to be superior insofar as side effects are concerned and both are poorly absorbed [14]. The absorption is increased by taking iron on an empty stomach, but the gastrointestinal intolerance increases with this way of ingestion. Tolerance can be improved by ingesting the iron tablets along with food, but this is associated with a corresponding decrease in iron absorption [15].

Intramuscular Iron Administration

Iron is available for intramuscular administration as iron sorbitol citrate. This way of administration is seldom used because of many disadvantages:

(1) The injections are painful and can leave a brownish discoloration on the skin that can persist for many weeks.
(2) There is a risk of bleeding into the muscle, especially in the hemodialyzed patients after having received heparin for the extracorporeal treatment.
(3) There are reports of muscle sarcoma developing at the site of injection.
(4) The absorption and bioavailability from this route can be highly variable.

For all these reasons [16] this route is rarely used in hemodialyzed patients receiving epoetin therapy.

Intraperitoneal Iron Administration

Iron dextran injected into the peritoneal cavity of rats penetrates the serosal surface of the small intestine and leads to an increase of ferritin in the liver and spleen [17]. Other studies performed in rats receiving iron dextran intraperitoneally, but at the time only one case of intraperitoneal iron dextran treatment in a erythropoietin-treated continuous ambulatory peritoneal dialysis patient has been reported [18]. A single dose of 500 mg elemental iron in the form of iron dextran was instilled into the peritoneal cavity during an overnight stay. The authors reported a significant increase of serum ferritin and hemoglobin after 4 weeks. Anyhow the risks related to this route of administration are not yet well known: the risk of peritoneal mesothelioma as reported after high-dose intraperitoneal iron administration in one animal study in rats [19] and the risk of damage (sclerofibrosis of peritoneum) of peritoneal membrane.

Intravenous Iron Administration

There are at least four different intravenous iron preparations available worldwide although each country may have access to only one or two of them: iron dextran, iron saccharate, iron gluconate or iron dextrin (polymaltose). All of these have very different molecular weights, physicochemical characteristics, degradation kinetics and side effect profiles [20, 21]. Complexes with lower molecular weight such as iron sodium gluconate (the only iron available in Italy for instance) may be released too rapidly and may overload the capacity of transferrin to bind it, leading to potential free iron reactions [22]. The advantage of a ready availability is counterbalanced by a risk of release of toxic amounts of free iron [12].

Iron gluconate and iron saccharate are the most frequent intravenous iron preparations used in Europe, while iron dextran had been the only iron available for parenteral use in the United States until 1999 (two different formulations).

Large molecules such as iron dextran are the most stable, and the tightly bound iron is released slowly. This molecule is removed from plasma by macrophage of the reticuloendothelial system with a half-life in plasma of between 5.9 h and 3 days. Iron dextran has a low but significant incidence of anaphylactic reactions due to the presence of antidextran antibodies. Anaphylactic reactions induced by the presence of antidextran antibodies are observed in a low (0.65%) but significant percentage. These reaction may range from immediate urticaria to hypotension, chest pain, bronchospasm, laryngospasm and angioedema.

On the other hand, preparations of iron-like iron saccharate and iron gluconate may produce hypotension and related manifestations of cardiovascular instability due to the accumulation of free iron in the blood circulation [22]. Iron dextrin (polymaltose) has been licensed for intravenous use in France for over 20 years and has an excellent safety records, particularly when given in small doses at every dialysis [23]. The intravenous route of iron administration is at the moment the most efficient way to restore a good iron status in hemodialyzed patients and iron saccharate is probably the most effective and the safest iron available for intravenous administration.

Markers of Iron Deficiency

Serum Iron

This parameter is not a reliable index to establish an iron deficiency. Iron is subjected to day-to-day biological variation [24], the measurement is affected by the dietary intake the days before the blood sampling and by an inflammatory status both chronic as well as acute [25]. Even when specimens are collected at the same time of day, variability in the same person on different days may be as much as 40% [26].

Serum Transferrin

An increase of transferrin levels in blood may indicate an iron deficiency. Unfortunately transferrin is a marker of nutritional status and very often the uremic patient is a malnourished subject with low transferrin levels. The transferrin concentration is also dependent upon the synthetic capacity of the liver [27].

For these reasons serum transferrin levels are not strongly predictive for iron deficiency in renal patients.

The Percentage TSAT with Iron

This test along with the serum ferritin represents the test used most frequently for the diagnosis of iron deficiency in patients with end-stage renal disease. TSAT is the ratio between iron/transferrin × 1.4 [28]. Transferrin × 1.4 is the total iron binding capacity, an indirect measure of both circulating unsaturated and saturated transferrin. A TSAT calculated as serum iron concentration/total iron binding capacity is an index of iron deficiency, but is limited by variability of serum iron concentration, particularly because of marked diurnal variation [26]. A TSAT <20% usually indicates iron deficiency, although many exceptions are encountered, in part because of variation in TSAT from day to day [9]. Actually the percentage of TSAT may be used as a substitute to detect iron deficiency if measurement of hypochromic red cells is not available [9].

Serum Ferritin

Although a significant proportion of iron stored in the reticuloendothelial system is present as ferritin, only trace quantities of ferritin enter the circulation. In nonuremic populations, the serum ferritin has been considered to be the most valuable diagnostic test for iron deficiency [29].

Just as serum ferritin is not totally sensitive, it is also not completely specific in patients with chronic kidney disease [9].

There are many limitations to the diagnostic value of the serum ferritin for iron deficiency in patients with end-stage renal disease. In clinical states associated with inflammation, such as infection, rheumatoid arthritis, malignancy, smoking, and liver disease, the serum ferritin concentration rises independently of iron stores [28]. An explanation of this behavior of ferritin during inflammation may be the following: interleukin-1 stimulates intracellular ferritin biosynthesis by a translational mechanism that is independent of iron status and results in intracellular trapping of iron and reduced iron availability for hemoglobin synthesis [30]. In addition interleukin-1 and tumor necrosis factor-α induce secretion by liver of serum ferritin, an iron-poor, glycosylated molecule with a different amino acid sequence from intracellular ferritin, which plays a negligible role in iron exchange [31].

A second problem in the use of a ferritin-like marker of iron deficiency or iron overload in renal patients during epoetin therapy is that the lower and mostly upper thresholds of ferritin are not yet clear. Serum ferritin should probably be maintained at greater than 100 ng/ml: many studies have shown the erythropoietic benefit of increasing serum ferritin to >100 ng/ml. No upper limit has been clearly established [9]. Some authors propose an upper threshold of 330 ng/ml, considering values higher than 331 ng/ml a moderate iron overload [32]. Nevertheless, serum ferritin levels between 300 and 800 ng/ml have been common in dialysis patients, and there is no evidence that such levels are associated with adverse iron-mediated effects [33].

Serum Transferrin Receptors

Cells that require iron express on their surface transferrin receptors (sTfR), which bind to transferrin and lead to the internalization of circulating iron. A truncated form of the receptor is released from cells into the circulation in trace quantities, with a concentration in plasma that is proportional to the amount of cellular receptor expression [28]. When iron deficiency is present, cells increase their production of transferrin receptors, and their serum levels increase [34]. Beguin et al. [35] have found that a small increase in soluble transferrin receptors circulating in plasma occurs with functional iron deficiency in hemodialysis patients. A matter of discussion could be the threshold of sTfR to detect an iron deficiency. In our population the normal range of sTfR is 8.8–28.1 nmol/l (advantage sTfR – BYK Gulden Italia) and we consider a marker of iron deficiency values of sTfR >28.1 nmol/l. Like serum iron and transferrin, sTfR shows a diurnal and seasonal pattern in its peak through differences [36] but many authors confirmed that measurement of sTfR in serum is a sensitive indicator for iron deficiency [37, 38].

Reticulocyte Hemoglobin Content

The automated flow cytometry technique has made possible an accurate analysis of reticulocytes. One parameter derived is the reticulocyte hemoglobin content (CHr). The CHr is a direct measure in that it evaluates iron status at the level of the erythrocyte or its precursor. Some studies in nonuremic patients treated with erythropoietin demonstrated the sensitivity of this test for detecting iron deficiency [39]. Fishbane et al. [40] were the first to use CHr as a parameter for evaluating the iron status of 164 hemodialysis patients. They found that the CHr was highly accurate for the diagnosis of iron deficiency in hemodialysis patients, with a value of less than 26 pg indicating the presence of iron deficiency. The sensitivity of 100% and the specificity of 80% were considerably higher than they found for the serum ferritin and TSAT.

Tessitore et al. [41] found for values of CHr >26 pg a sensitivity of 9.8% and a specificity of 100%. These percentages reach a sensitivity of 68.6% and a specificity of 78.4% for values of CHr <30 pg. The same authors consider CHr as a reliable marker of iron deficiency, but inferior to the percentage of hypochromic red cells, even at its best cutoff value of 29 pg [41].

Hypochromic Red Blood Cells

An ideal test of iron status would be one that directly measures iron at the level of the erythrocyte or one of its precursors. It should be inexpensive, and easy to use. Studies of red cells are insensitive in this respect, yielding information summed over the relatively long life span of these cells. Reticulocytes are the first circulating form of red blood cells, existing in circulation for only approximately 1 day. A test evaluating reticulocytes, therefore, would provide a 'snapshot' of the iron status on the day the test was performed [40].

The automated flow cytometry enables the accurate analysis of reticulocytes. In the last years a determination of the percentage hypochromic red blood cells has been advocated as a sensitive and early marker of functional iron deficiency [42]. Normally there are less than 2.5% of red cells with individual cell hemoglobin of less than 28 pg/dl. Iron deficiency promotes an increase in the percentage of hypochromic red blood cells. Values exceeding 10% are compatible with iron deficiency in erythropoietin-treated patients [36]. This percentage threshold is discussed by some authors: Tessitore et al. [41] considers the best combination of sensitivity and specificity a threshold of >6% instead of the currently accepted cutoff >10% (the recommended threshold by the NKF-DOQI Clinical Practice Guidelines) which shows absolute specificity but a low sensitivity.

Red Blood Cell Zinc Protoporphyrin

Red blood cell zinc protoporphyrin (ZnPP) is an abnormal end-product of heme synthesis, generated in the red blood cells by incorporation of zinc instead of iron [43, 44]. In patients with iron deficiency anemia zinc instead of iron is incorporated into the protoporphyrin IX ring of heme, leading to a rise in the concentration of red blood cell. ZnPP has been suggested to be a sensitive and specific parameter of absolute iron deficiency in hemodialysis patients. Its determination is simple, rapid and inexpensive, although its long elimination half-life limits its usefulness in detecting rapid changes in iron status [41]. In fact, the elimination half-life of ZnPP from the blood compartments is closely related to the half-life of erythrocytes and the production rate of new ZnPP from the blood compartment is closely related to the half-life of erythrocytes and the production rate of new ZnPP in the bone marrow compartment. Though the half-life of erythrocytes in uremic patients on chronic hemodialysis has been found to be shorter than in nonrenal patients, data obtained after a 6-month follow-up did not show a significant ZnPP decrease in patients who had been given generous iron supplementation.

In uremic patients data on the use of ZnPP have produced conflicting results. Inflammatory processes and the presence of uremic factors potentially inhibiting ferrochelatase could eventually lead to an increase in ZnPP levels which is not strictly related to the iron status in itself [43].

ZnPP levels do not seem to consistently predict an erythropoietic response to iron supplementation in maintenance hemodialysis patients, and thus, iron overload during intravenous iron supplementation cannot be detected by measuring ZnPP [45].

Bone Marrow Examination

It is an invasive procedure not acceptable in renal patients who need a repeated and periodical evaluation of their iron status.

DOQI Guidelines for Iron Administration

The DOQI 2000 update addresses the question of how to ensure that patients have sufficient iron to achieve and maintain a target of hemoglobin of 11–12 g/dl [9]:

(1) Serum ferritin should be maintained at greater than 100 ng/ml.

(2) Hypochromic red blood cells should be maintained at less than 10%. This measurement is presently performed as part of a routine full blood count sample that requires a Technicon H-1, H-2, H-3 automate cell counter, which is specialized equipment (Bayer Diagnostic) available in certain parts of Europe.

(3) TSAT should be maintained at greater than 20% in the United States and in other countries where the equipment to measure the percent of hypochromic red blood cells is presently not available in most medical centers.

The Use of Intravenous Iron Preparations

To reach the goals of a serum ferritin higher than 100 μg/l, of a TSAT >20% and/or a hypochromic red cell count <10%, nephrologists vary widely in the posology and frequency of the administration of intravenous iron to dialysis patients.

Some authors performed an intermittent administration of high doses of iron to restore iron-depleted stores in hemodialysis patients (i.e. iron dextran 1,000 mg over 10 dialysis sessions [46]. This common practice to administer either 1 or 2 g of intravenous iron dextran over 10 to 20 hemodialysis sessions can cause some problems:

(1) the deposition of iron in the reticuloendothelial system as hemosiderin not easily accessible for erythropoiesis, and

(2) this form of iron supplementation may not be sufficient for maintaining adequate hemoglobin, ferritin and TSAT for prolonged periods [2, 46].

A more physiological approach is to administer intravenous iron chronically in small doses with each hemodialysis session:

(1) 10–20 mg of iron saccharate at the end of each hemodialysis session [47],
(2) 25 mg of iron dextran together with heparin as a continuous infusion during each hemodialysis [2] and
(3) 100 mg of iron sucrose once a week as a bolus injection over 1–2 min into the venous limb of the patients' vascular access at the end of dialysis [48].

The protocol that the Anemia Work Group recommends for administering intravenous iron dextran or iron gluconate in adult hemodialysis patients with absolute iron deficiency is 100 mg of iron dextran or 125 mg of iron gluconate during each dialysis for 10 or 8 doses, respectively. For maintenance iron therapy, and treatment and prevention of functional iron deficiency, the recommendation is 25–100 mg of iron dextran every week for 10 weeks, or 31.25–125 mg of iron gluconate every week for 8 weeks with measurement of the hypochromic red cells or TSAT and serum ferritin no sooner than 2–7 days after the last dose [9]. The frequency of maintenance intravenous iron therapy can be thrice weekly (with every hemodialysis), twice weekly, weekly or every other week, but should provide 250–1,000 mg of iron within 12 weeks.

The only iron preparation that can be given as a single dose of 500–1,000 mg is iron dextran, which must be administered as a slow infusion over several hours [16]. This dose would be practical for patients on CAPD treatment who live at a considerable distance from the hospital and for patients with chronic renal insufficiency on conservative therapy treated with erythropoietin.

We approach the iron deficiency in hemodialyzed patients as follows:

(1) We reach the ferritin target of 100–150 ng/ml, administering iron at every dialysis (iron gluconate 62.5 mg thrice/week). Hemoglobin, ferritin, hypochromic red cells and serum transferrin receptors are measured every month.
(2) When the serum ferritin reaches the target of 100–150 ng/ml intravenous iron is administered once a week (iron gluconate 62.5 mg) to maintain the ferritin levels greater than 100 ng/ml.
(3) If serum ferritin levels are greater than 300 ng/ml and not related to an inflammatory status, we do not administer iron, monitoring every 2 weeks the ferritin levels till these levels are lower than 300 ng/ml.

In our clinical practice we consider TSAT an unreliable marker of iron deficiency. The hypochromic red cell count can help us consider the amount and the frequency of iron administration in patients with ferritin levels lower than 100 ng/ml.

Iron Overload-Related Risks

Iron overload should be defined as a clinical situation in which iron not needed or being used for erythropoiesis, that is stored iron, contributes to a pathological process. Iron overload has been defined as being present when the serum ferritin chronically remains above 1,000 ng/ml or above 500 ng/ml [49].

Burns and Pomposelli [32] consider a moderate iron overload if serum ferritin is between 331 and 1,000 ng/ml and a severe iron overload if ferritin is between 1,001 and 2,000 ng/ml. Iron overload is related to different diseases: infections, malignancies and cardiovascular disease.

Iron Overload and Infections

A number of studies have implicated iron overload as a risk factor for bacterial infections in hemodialyzed patients. Many mechanisms are involved in this increased susceptibility to bacterial infection: stimulation of bacterial growth, impairment of T lymphocytes function, and impairment of polymorphonuclear leukocytes (PMNL) [50, 51].

The antibacterial effect of cytokines is mediated by intracellular iron depletion. In response to several cytokines such as interferon-γ, interleukin-1 and tumor necrosis factor, the cell depletes its intracellular labile, metabolically active iron pool by

(1) enhancement of ferritin synthesis, resulting in a shift of cellular iron into the relatively inert ferritin storage compartment, and
(2) downregulation of transferrin receptor production, decreasing cellular iron uptake and limiting availability for the intracellular pathogen.

In addition, high levels of serum iron may promote replication and dissemination of bacterial pathogens that use iron as a growth factor. It has been showed that the antibacterial effect of cytokines may be reversed by iron therapy and potentiated by deferoxamine treatment [51].

The phagocytic capacity of PMNL is significantly decreased with increasing the PMNL iron concentration [52]. It has been shown that polynuclear iron complexes impair the function of PMNL.

T lymphocytes are thought to have a relatively limited capacity to store and detoxify excess iron [53]. In vitro studies have shown that low concentration of non-transferrin-bound iron can inhibit the cloning capacity of CD4+ T cells and CD8+ cytotoxic precursor cells, while enhancing the function of suppresser T cells [54].

Iron Overload and Cancer

During the past four decades, numerous research groups have reported, in prospective studies in animals, that administration of excessive amounts of injected or oral iron markedly increases the risk of adenocarcinomas, colorectal tumors, hepatomas, mammary tumors, mesotheliomas, renal tubular cell carcinomas and sarcomas [55]. In large groups of humans such a 0.5% of whites and 10% of sub-Saharan Africans, genetic defects result in assimilation of excessive dietary iron. In the white disease, hereditary hemochromatosis, the elevation in tissue iron is associated with an increase in hepatic carcinoma of as much as 200-fold; excessive frequency of nonhepatic malignancies is also observed [55]. In the African disease, African siderosis, the incidence of hepatic carcinoma likewise is quite high [56].

The higher risk of malignancies in patients with iron overload may be related to an impairment of PMNL and T lymphocyte activities [52, 53].

Iron Overload and Cardiovascular Disease

Most studies have not adequately assessed the relationship between iron, either circulating or in tissues, and coronary artery disease. As a result, there is currently no conclusive evidence that parenteral iron therapy is associated with an increased risk of coronary artery disease or death from myocardial infarction [57]. A recent study suggests that serum ferritin values over 50 ng/ml are associated with a marked increase in carotid atherosclerosis in men and women [58]. It has been shown in experimental studies that iron overload enhances [59] and iron depletion decreases formation of atherosclerotic plaque [60]. It is likely that free iron regularly occurs in plasma during and following intravenous iron therapy (mostly with iron gluconate). Cumulative damage to the heart and other tissues cannot be ruled out on the basis of available evidence.

References

1 Nissenson AR, Strobos J: Iron deficiency in patients with renal failure. Kidney Int suppl 1999;69: S18–S21.
2 Donnelly SM, Posen GA, All MA: Oral absorption in hemodialysis patients treated with erythropoietin. Clin Invest Med 1991;14:271–276.
3 Bridges KR, Seligman PA: Disorders of iron metabolism; in Blood: Principles and Practice of Hematology. Philadelphia, Lippincott, 1995.
4 Schaefer AI, Bunn FH: Anemias of iron deficiency and iron overload; in Harrison's Principles of Internal Medicine, ed 11. 1987, pp 1493–1498.
5 Hallberg L: Bioavailability of dietary iron in man. Annu Rev Nutr 1981;1:123–147.
6 NCCLS: Determination of Serum Iron, Total Iron Binding Capacity and Percent Transferrin Saturation; Approved Standard, NCCLD document H17-A. Waine, NCCLS, 1998.
7 Fishbane S, Lynn RI: The efficacy of iron dextran for the treatment of iron deficiency in hemodialysis patients. Clin Nephrol 1995;44:238–240.
8 Sakiewicz P, Paganini E: The use of iron in patients on chronic dialysis: Mistakes and misconceptions. J Nephrol 1998;11:5–15.
9 Guidelines for anemia of chronic kidney disease. Am J Kidney Dis 2001;37(suppl 1):S194–S206.
10 Erslev AJ, Besarab A: Erythropoietin in the pathogenesis and treatment of the anemia of chronic renal failure. Kidney Int 1997;51:622–630.

11 Gallieni M: Iron in treatment of anemia in dialysis patients: An important support to erythropoietin. Int J Artif Organs 1998;21:681–686.
12 Kooistra MP, Van Es A, Struyvenberg A, et al: Iron absorption in erythropoietin-treated haemodialysis patients: Effects of iron availability, inflammation and aluminium. Nephrol Dial Transplant 1998;13:82–88.
13 European best practice guideline for the management of anaemia in patients with chronic renal failure. Nephrol Dial Transplant 1999;14/S5:17–18.
14 Wingard RL, Parker RA, Ismail N, et al: Efficacy of oral iron therapy in patients receiving recombinant human erythropoietin. Am J Kidney Dis 1995;25:433–439.
15 MacDougall IC: Strategies for iron supplementation: Oral versus intravenous. Kidney Int 1999; 55(suppl 69):S61–S66.
16 Thirayothin P, Crosby WH: The distribution of iron injected intraperitoneally: Evidence of serosal absorption by the small intestine. J Clin Invest 1962;41:1206–1210.
17 Bastani B, Gulley S: Intraperitoneal iron-dextran as a potential route of iron therapy in CAPD patients (letter). Perit Dial Int 1996;16:646–648.
18 Okada S, Hamazaki S, Toyokuni S: Induction of mesothelioma by intraperitoneal injections of ferric saccharate in male Wistar rats. Br J Cancer 1989;60:708–711.
19 MacDougall IC: Intravenous administration of iron in epoetin-treated haemodialysis patients – Which drugs, which regimen? Nephrol Dial Transplant 2000;15:1743–1745.
20 MacDougall IC, Chandler G, Armstrong A, et al: Characterisation of iron availability from three different IV iron preparations in dialysis patients. J Am Soc Nephrol 1997;8:221.
21 Zanen AL, Adriaansen HJ, van Bommel, et al: 'Oversaturation' of transferrin after intravenous ferric gluconate (Ferrlecit) in haemodialysis patients. Nephrol Dial Transplant 1997;11:820–824.
22 Shaldon S: Intravenous administration of iron in epoetin-treated haemodialysis patients. Nephrol Dial Transplant 2001;16:1076–1077.
23 Horl WH, Cavill I, MacDougall IC, et al: How to diagnose and correct iron deficiency during r-huEPO therapy – A consensus report. Nephrol Dial Transplant 1996;11:246–250.
24 Tietz NW, Rinker AD, Morrison SR: When is a serum iron really a serum iron? The status of serum iron measurements. Clin Chem 1994;40:546–551.
25 Withold W, Neumayer C, Beyrau R, et al: Efficacy of transferrin determination in human sera in the diagnosis of iron deficiency. Eur J Clin Chem Clin Biochem 1994;32:19–25.
26 Statland BE, Winkel P: Relationship of day-to-day variation of serum iron concentrations to iron binding capacity in healthy young women. Am J Clin Pathol 1977;67:84–90.
27 European best practice guidelines for the management of anaemia in patients with chronic renal failure. Target Guideline 6: Assessing and optimizing iron stores. Nephrol Dial Transplant 1999; 14(suppl 5):14–15.
28 Fishbane S, Maesaka JK: Iron management in end-stage renal disease. Am J Kidney Dis 1997; 29:319–333.
29 Finch CA, Bellotti V, Stray S, et al: Plasma determination as a diagnostic tool. West J Med 1986;145:657–663.
30 Rogers J, Lacroix L, Durmowits G, et al: The role of cytokine in the regulation of cytokine expression. Progress in Iron Research. New York, Plenum Press, 1994, pp 127–132.
31 Tran TN, Eubanks SK, Schaffer KJ, et al: Secretion of ferritin by rat hepatoma cells and its regulation by inflammatory cytokine and iron. Blood 1997;90:4879–4986.
32 Burns DL, Pomposelli JJ: Toxicity of parenteral iron dextran therapy. Kidney Int Suppl 1999; 69:S119–S124.
33 NKF-DOQI Clinical Practice Giudelines for the Treatment of Anemia of Chronic Renal Failure. New York, National Kidney Foundations, 1997, pp 34–35.
34 Suominen P, Punnonen K, Rajamaki A, et al: Serum transferrin receptor and transferrin receptor-ferritin index identify healthy subjects with subclinical iron deficits. Blood 1998;92: 2934–2939.
35 Beguin Y, Loo M, R'Zik S, et al: Early prediction of response to recombinant human erythropoietin in patients with the anemia of renal failure by serum transferrin receptor and fibrinogen. Blood 1993;82:2010–2016.
36 Kaltwasser JP, Gottshalk R: Erythropoietin and iron. Kidney Int Suppl 1999;69:S49–S56.

37 Maes M, Bosmans E, Scharpe S, et al: Components of biological variation in serum soluble transferrin receptors: Relationship to serum iron, transferrin and ferritin concentrations, and immune and haematological variables. Scand J Clin Lab Invest 1997;57:31–41.
38 Punnonen K, Irjala K, Rajamaki A: Serum transferrin receptor and its ratio to serum ferritin in the diagnosis of iron deficiency. Blood 1997;89:1052–1057.
39 Brugnara C, Collela GM, Cremins J, et al: Effects of subcutaneous recombinant erythropoietin in normal subjects: Development of decreased reticulocyte hemoglobin content and iron-deficient erythropoiesis. J Lab Clin Med 1994;123:660–667.
40 Fishbane S, Galgano C, Langley RC, et al: Reticulocyte hemoglobin content in the evaluation of iron status of hemodialysis patients. Kidney Int 1997;52:217–222.
41 Tessitore N, Soler GP, Lippi G, et al: The role of iron status markers in predicting response to intravenous iron in haemodialysis patients on maintenance erythropoietin. Nephrol Dial Transplant 2001;16:1416–1423.
42 Bovy C, Tsobo C, Crapanzano C, et al: Factors determining the percentage of hypochromic red blood cells in hemodialysis patients. Kidney Int 1999;56:1113–1119.
43 Canavese C, Grill A, Decostanzi E, et al: Limited value of zinc protoporphyrin as a marker of iron status in chronic hemodialysis patients. Clin Nephrol 2000;53/1:42–47.
44 Braun J, Hammerschmidt M, Schreiber M, et al: Is zinc protoporphyrin an indicator of iron-deficient erythropoiesis in maintenance haemodialysis patients? Nephrol Dial Transplant 1996; 11:492–497.
45 Braun J: Erythrocyte zinc protoporphyrin. Kidney Int Suppl 1999;69:S57–S60.
46 Sunder-Plassman G, Horl WH: Importance of iron supply for erythropoietin therapy. Nephrol Dial Transplant 1995;10:2070–2076.
47 MacDougall IC, Chandler G, Elston O, et al: Beneficial effects of adopting an aggressive intravenous iron policy in a hemodialysis unit. Am J Kidney Dis 1999;34(suppl 2):S40–S46.
48 Borel MJ, Smith SM, Derr J, et al: Day-to-day variation in iron-status indices in healthy men and women. Am J Clin Nutr 1991;54:729–735.
49 Gokal R, Millard PR, Weatherall DJ, et al: Iron metabolism in haemodialysis patients: A study of the management of iron therapy and overload. Q J Med 1979;48: 369–391.
50 Hoen B: Iron and infection: Clinical experience. Am J Kidney Dis 1999;34(suppl 2):S30–S34.
51 Patruta SI, Horl WH: Iron and infection. Kidney Int Suppl 1999;69:S125–S130.
52 Boelaert JR, Cantinieaux BF, Hariga CF, et al: Recombinant erythropoietin reverses polymorphonuclear granulocyte dysfunction in iron overloaded dialysis patients. Nephrol Dial Transplant 1990;5:504–507.
53 Kronke M, Leonard WJ, Depper JM, et al: Sequential expression of genes involved in human T lymphocyte growth and differentiation. J Exp Med 1985;161:1593–1598.
54 Rudd MJ, Good MF, Chapman DE, et al: Clonal analysis of the effect of iron on human cytotoxic and proliferating T lymphocytes. Immunol Cell Biol 1990;68:317–324.
55 Weinberg ED: The role of iron in cancer. Eur J Cancer Prev 1996;5:19–36.
56 Gangaidzo IT, Gordeaux VR: Hepatocellular carcinoma and African iron overload. Gut 1995;37: 727–730.
57 Besarab A: Iron and cardiac disease in the end-stage renal disease setting. Am J Kidney Dis 1999; 34(suppl 2):S18–S24.
58 Kiechl S, Willeit J, Egger G, et al: Body iron stores and the risk of carotid atherosclerosis: Prospective results from the Bruneck Study. Circulation 1997;96:3300–3307.
59 Araujo JA, Romano EL, Brito BE, et al: Iron overload augments the development of atherosclerotic lesions in rabbit. Arterioscler Thromb Vasc Biol 1995;15:1172–1180.
60 Lee TS, Shiao MS, Pan CC, et al: Iron deficient diet reduces atherosclerotic lesions in apoE-deficient mice. Circulation 1999;99:1222–1229.

Carlo Crepaldi, MD, Nephrology Department,
St. Bortolo Hospital, Viale Rodolfi, I–36100 Vicenza (Italy)
Tel. +39 0444 993650, Fax +39 0444 920693, E-Mail crepaldi@goldnet.it

Ronco C, La Greca G (eds): Hemodialysis Technology.
Contrib Nephrol. Basel, Karger, 2002, vol 137, pp 426–430

Carnitine as Adjuvant Therapy in the Management of Renal Anemia

B. Cianciaruso, S. Torraca, A. De Blasio, M. Fiorillo, R. Marino

Division of Nephrology, School of Medicine, University of Naples 'Federico II', Naples, Italy

The introduction of erythropoietin (EPO) has been the major advancement achieved in the last two decades of treatment of uremia. This therapy had such a great impact on the quality of life and the morbidity and mortality of patients undergoing dialysis treatment that nephrologists often refer to a pre- and post-EPO 'era' of dialysis. The treatment of renal anemia in recent years aims to optimize epoietin therapy in terms of cost-effectiveness by extending the benefits of this treatment also to those patients that show resistance to epoietin. For both these goals the adjuvant therapy of anemia has become crucial. Under the name of adjuvant therapy of anemia are grouped all those therapeutic maneuvers that enhance the effectiveness of epoietin such as preventing the deficiency of iron and vitamins (vitamin C, D, B_6, B_{12} and folic acid) and/or administering compounds like *L*-carnitine, androgens and IGF-1 that have been shown to have a positive effect on hemoglobin levels. We review here the published evidence showing that *L*-carnitine administration allows the use of less epoietin to control renal anemia and the possibility that carnitine supplements may be useful in those patients that do not respond to epoietin.

Carnitine is a small water-soluble molecule with a molecular weight of 162 daltons that is derived from preformed dietary carnitine (75%) and is synthesized (25%) in the liver, kidney and brain from two essential amino acids, lysine and methionine. Dietary carnitine is absorbed rapidly from the intestinal tract and released into the bloodstream. Skeletal muscle cells that contain almost 97% of all carnitine in the body and are not able to synthesize it take up this molecule, across the cell membrane, from the bloodstream.

Carnitine Functions

In body fluids and inside the cells carnitine is present in different forms, and represents a true 'carnitine system' which consists of carnitine, carnitine esters, several intracellular enzymes and membrane transporters. This system is involved in several functions: (1) it participates in a series of reversible reactions that regulate the cell trafficking of short-, medium- and long-chain fatty acids utilized for β-oxidation and energy production at the mitochondrial level, (2) lipid oxidation at the peroxisomal level, not related to energy production, (3) acylation and deacylation of proteins, such as very low density lipoprotein at the endoplasmic reticulum level, (4) membrane phospholipid turnover, and (5) maintenance of cell osmotic balance [1]. Skeletal muscle and myocardium that preferentially use fatty acids as primary energy source need adequate carnitine concentrations in the intracellular compartment for normal fatty acid metabolism. Human red blood cells (RBCs), which do not possess mitochondria, also have substantial amounts of *L*-carnitine and its esters and, since erythrocyte carnitines do not freely exchange with plasma, it has been suggested that they may have been acquired when the cells were erythrocyte precursors [2]. In vivo and in vitro studies have shown that *L*-carnitine affects the stability of RBC membranes through several mechanisms and under various adverse conditions. Function of Na-K pump and phospholipid turnover of RBC membranes are crucial in keeping the biconcave disc shape of RBCs. It has been reported that the number and the activity of Na-K pump sites of RBCs are reduced in the uremic state, particularly in young erythrocytes [3]. Labonia et al. [4] noted an increase of Na-K pump activity of the erythrocyte membrane in uremic patients after supplementation of *L*-carnitine.

Donatelli et al. [5] suggested another mechanism by which *L*-carnitine may prolong the life span of RBCs; in fact, *L*-carnitine while increasing the delivery of free fatty acids to the mitochondria for oxidation decreases the circulating levels of free fatty acids that are endogenous inhibitors of the Na, K-ATPase.

Phospholipids are important constituents of the red cell membrane and there is enough evidence that carnitine plays an important role in the regulation of membrane phospholipid turnover improving the uptake of lipids which form the plasma membrane. Since RBC membrane phospholipids in uremia are injured by oxidative stress, *L*-carnitine and its acyl esters could be considered as part of the defensive mechanism against free radical toxicity. These considerations indicate that the deficiency of *L*-carnitine affects the life span of the red cell and may play an independent role in the determination of anemia in renal failure.

Carnitine in Uremia

A typical condition of acquired carnitine deficiency can be found in patients undergoing maintenance dialysis. In patients treated with continuous ambulatory peritoneal dialysis or maintenance hemodialysis serum levels of free carnitine have been reported as low, whereas concentrations of acyl-carnitine esters are elevated, thus leading to a significant increase in the acyl to free carnitine ratio (normal value <0.4); an analogous pattern has been found in muscle of these patients. In contrast to muscle, erythrocyte intracellular concentrations of free carnitine are increased whereas those of acyl-carnitine are normal. Mechanisms accounting for these changes in carnitine pattern in dialysis patients are not completely understood and include the following: (1) impaired acetyl-CoA oxidation, (2) enhanced carnitine acylation secondary to increased fatty acid availability due to heparin, and (3) reduced intake of carnitine and its precursors. The primary sources of carnitine are red meats and dairy products but renal patients have often a poor appetite for red meat and an increase of the assumption of dairy products would require an increase in phosphate binders.

Carnitine Administration and EPO-Sparing Effect

A beneficial effect of *L*-carnitine administration on hemoglobin was reported in several studies in the early 1980s, before epoietin treatment was available. In a placebo-controlled study Trovato et al. [6] observed a progressive increase of hematocrit during 12 months of follow-up in the carnitine-treated group as compared to the placebo group. The increase of the hematocrit in this group was paralleled by a persistent increase in the absolute reticulocyte count by 40–60%, indicating that carnitine may have a different effect from the improved stability of the erythrocyte membrane.

On the basis of these observations several authors suggested that carnitine supplements in hemodialysis patients permit a more efficient use of epoietin. Only two prospective, randomized, placebo-controlled studies are available concerning the EPO-sparing effect of *L*-carnitine. Labonia [7] studied 24 hemodialysis patients for 6 months, administering 1 g *L*-carnitine i.v. after each dialysis session. In the carnitine-treated group (13 patients) the mean weekly EPO dose was 102 $\pm$ 52.6 U/kg/week at T0 and 63.3 $\pm$ 37.8 U/kg/week at T6, representing a 38.1% reduction in the total EPO requirement ($p < 0.02$), while the mean value for the hematocrit was 29.8 $\pm$ 2.6% at T0 and 29.1 $\pm$ 2.1% at T6. In the placebo group, the mean weekly dose of EPO was 78.6 $\pm$ 32.1 U/kg/week at T0 and 79.9 ± 46.7 U/kg/week at T6 with no significant variation, while the mean hematocrit value went from 29.5 ± 2.3% at T0 to 27.9 ± 1.9% at T6 ($p < 0.05$).

Kletzmayr et al. [8] conducted a placebo-controlled, double-blinded study in 40 patients on maintenance hemodialysis. Twenty patients received *L*-carnitine intravenously after each dialysis session (dose 5–15 mg/kg) and 20 received placebo for 8 months. Twenty-eight patients finished the study (12 carnitine, 16 placebo). Eight of 19 (42%) patients evaluable in the carnitine group responded to carnitine supplementation, reducing their EPO dose significantly ($p < 0.001$) from 183.7 ± 131.7 U/kg/week at T0 to 126.6 ± 127.9 U/kg/week after 4 months (T4), with a reduction of the EPO dose of 36.9 ± 23.3%. After 8 months, only two responders were evaluable, and in both patients, the EPO requirement was lower at T8 compared with T0, indicating an ongoing beneficial effect of *L*-carnitine. The authors did not find significant differences in free or total carnitine plasma concentrations between responders and nonresponders or a significant correlation of plasma carnitines with EPO requirement.

The mechanisms by which carnitine may have reduced the EPO requirement are still uncertain. Both studies, in contrast to previous clinical and experimental data, did not find any significant change of global osmotic fragility after carnitine treatment. It is worth stressing, however, that these studies had a small number of patients, the choice of control patients may not have been appropriate and finally have shown the existence of subgroups of patients responding to carnitine supplementation.

Carnitine Administration in EPO-Resistant Patients

The definition of a poor response to epoietin is arbitrary and a patient is defined as resistant to EPO when the hemoglobin does not increase to the expected level for the EPO dose given. Resistance to EPO treatment is generally due to aluminum toxicity, hyperparathyroidism, hemolysis and hypersplenism, an infectious or inflammatory state, or malignancy. In the recent years several case reports and a few noncontrolled studies have suggested that *L*-carnitine supplements, either orally or intravenously, have improved the response to epoietin treatment in patients with refractory anemia [9, 10].

Even if further studies are necessary to clarify the role of *L*-carnitine as adjuvant therapy of anemia in renal failure, several working groups suggest that carnitine supplementation should be recommended for selected dialysis patients who do not adequately respond to standard therapy.

References

1 Peluso G, Nicolai R, Reda E, Benatti P, Barbarisi A, Calvani M: Cancer and anticancer therapy-induced modifications on metabolism mediated by carnitine system. J Cell Physiol 2000;182: 339–350.

2 Di Donato S, Cornelio F, Storchi G, Rimoldi M: Ketogenesis and muscle carnitine deficiency. Neurology 1979;29:780–785.

3 Cheng JT, Kahn T, Kaji DM: Mechanism of alteration of sodium potassium pump of erythrocytes from patients with chronic renal failure. J Clin Invest 1984;74:581–588.

4 Labonia WD, Morelli JR, Gimenez MI, Freuler PV, Morelli OH: Effect of *L*-carnitine on sodium transport in erythrocytes from dialyzed uremic patients. Kidney Int 1987;32:754–759.

5 Donatelli A, Terrizzi C, Zummo G, Russo V, Bucalo ML, Scarpinato A: Effects of *L*-carnitine on chronic anemia and erythrocyte adenosine triphosphate concentration in hemodialysis patients. Curr Ther Res 1987;41:620–624.

6 Trovato GM, Ginardi V, Di Marco V, Dell'Aira A, Corsi M: Long-term *L*-carnitine treatment of chronic anemia of patients with end-stage renal failure. Curr Ther Res 1982;31:1042–1049.

7 Labonia WD: *L*-Carnitine effects on anemia in hemodialyzed patients treated with erythropoietin. Am J Kidney Dis 1995;26:757–764.

8 Kletzmayr J, Mayer G, Legenstein E, Heinz-Peer G, Leitha T, Horl WH, Kovarik J: Anemia and carnitine supplementation in hemodialyzed patients. Kidney Int Suppl 1999;69:S93–S106.

9 Kawabata M, Kasuga S, Hara H, Suyama S, Moriyama K, Takabatake T: Erythropoietin-resistant refractory renal anemia: Effects of oral *L*-carnitine supplementation. Clin Nephrol 2001;55: 265–266.

10 Matsumoto Y, Amano I, Hirose S, Tsuruta Y, Hara S, Murata M, Imai T: Effects of *L*-carnitine supplementation on renal anemia in poor responders to erythropoietin. Blood Purif 2001;19: 24–32.

Bruno Cianciaruso, MD, Cattedra di Nefrologia, Facoltà di Medicina,
Università di Napoli 'Federico II', Via Pansini 5, I–80131 Napoli (Italy)
Tel. +39 081 7462023, Fax +39 081 7462149, E-Mail cianciar@unina.it

Ronco C, La Greca G (eds): Hemodialysis Technology.
Contrib Nephrol. Basel, Karger, 2002, vol 137, pp 431–435

Erythropoietin Therapy and the Cardiovascular System

Antonio Santoro

Malpighi Nephrology and Dialysis Department, Policlinico S. Orsola-Malpighi, Bologna, Italy

Cardiac diseases are the major causes of mortality in dialysis patients, accounting for about 50% of deaths. The risk of cardiovascular diseases is 10–20 times greater in patients with chronic renal diseases than in the general population and the prevalence of left ventricular hypertrophy is approximately 75% while that of coronary artery disease is 40% [1, 2].

Arterial hypertension is the primary cause of pressure overload, while the expansion of the extracellular volume, AV fistula and anaemia are responsible for cardiac volume overload. Hypertrophy is typically eccentric in response to volume and concentric in response to pressure overload.

The coexistence of atherosclerotic/ischaemic disease may lead to the development of cardiomyopathies with systolic and diastolic dysfunction. Progressive LV dilation with compensatory hypertrophy appears to be the typical evolution of cardiomyopathy in dialysis patients (fig. 1). With the progressive death of the myocytes, the natural evolution is LV dilation that foreshadows cardiac failure and an increased risk of death [2, 3].

The pathogenetic cardiovascular disease factors in patients with an impaired renal function are complex and include factors relevant to the general population (smoking, lipids abnormalities, obesity, etc.), factors related to renal diseases (diabetes, hypertension, etc.), and factors associated to the uraemic condition per se, such as oxidized LDL, free radicals, hyperhomocysteinaemia, infections (herpes, chlamydia), acidosis, microinflammation, toxins [2]. Besides these complex factors, a particular role is played by anaemia which is very common in the course of uraemic status and may represent an independent risk factor for cardiac complications in patients with renal failure [4].

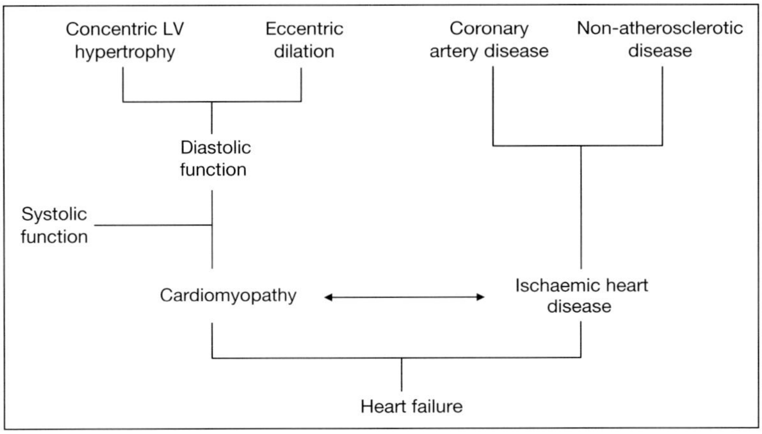

Fig. 1. Complexity of the myocardial damage in uraemia.

Acute and Chronic Cardiovascular Adjustments to Anaemia

In dogs, acute anaemia may induce an increase in cardiac output which in animals with high heart rate control is obtained with an increase in stroke volume rather than a further increase in heart rate [5]. In animals with a low heart rate control the acute increase in cardiac output was achieved entirely with a heart rate increase. As anaemia is maintained for several weeks, the stroke volume gradually increased and after 5 weeks it is 14% higher than in acute anaemia. The higher stroke volume presumably enhances the heart's capacity to deliver blood and oxygen to the peripheral tissues. Sympathetic system inhibition by different methods, including inhibition of β-adrenergic receptors, failed to block the increase in cardiac output in anaemia. Furthermore, an increase O_2 consumption and a higher basal metabolism occurs during anaemia. Two factors which would be expected to contribute to a higher basal metabolism: increase in red cell formation and an increased myocardial workload.

In humans an uncorrected pernicious or sickle-cell anaemia induces a hyperdynamic state and, in the course of time, cardiac hypertrophy [3, 6].

Cardiac anaemia results in cardiac dilation as a result of an increased cardiac output and determines a left-ventricular re-modelling. The concomitant presence of other deleterious factors related to uraemia, such as oxidative stress, toxins, phosphate retention and PTH increase may favour the appearance of a maladaptive LV hypertrophy (fig. 2). On the other hand, anaemia induces a significant increase in regional blood flows and in arterial wall tension. The addition of typical uraemic factors worsens the arterial damage and

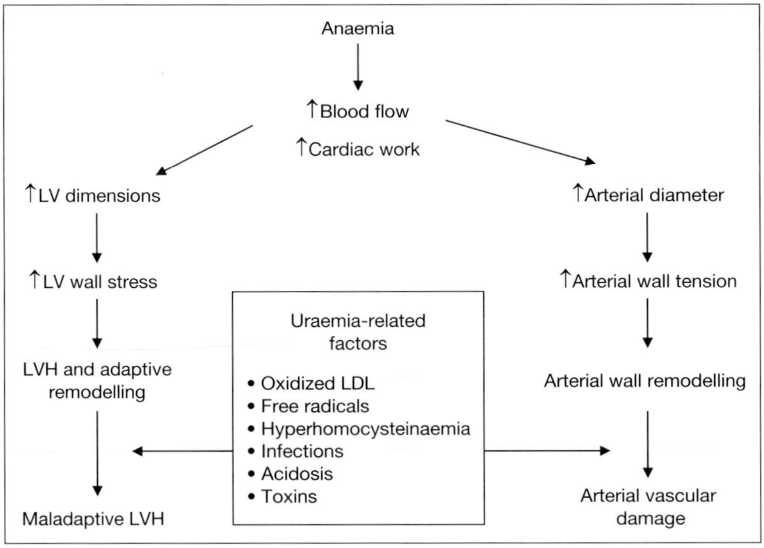

Fig. 2. Impact of anaemia on heart function and vascular damage.

can result in an accelerated atherosclerosis reduction in cardiac perfusion and thus in the oxygen supply. Finally, in addition to disturbances in the vasculature bed and a limitation in the blood's oxygen-carrying capacity, the oxygen utilization of cardiomyocytes may be disturbed further adding to insufficient oxygenation [7].

Association between Anaemia, Cardiac Diseases and Uraemia

The risk of developing cardiac hypertrophy is proportional to the decreased level of hemoglobin in predialysis patients, and an inverse relationship exists between left ventricular mass and the degree of anaemia. A prospective Canadian study, including 430 patients from the start of dialysis therapy, demonstrated that a 1-g/dl decrease in mean haemoglobin level was associated with a significantly increased risk for the development of left-ventricular dilation, cardiac failure and mortality [7].

A large retrospective study in the USA [8] on almost 22,000 patients in renal replacement therapy (RRT), showed a double odds death ratio in the presence of a haemoglobin concentration <8 g/dl compared with conditions of 10–11 g/dl.

A New Zealand study [9] also demonstrated that anaemia is a strong independent risk factor for left-ventricular hypertrophy.

Table 1. Reduction in LVM after Epoietin therapy

Study	N.	% reduction in LV mass	Follow-up
Goldberg et al. [12]	15	30	6
Pascual et al. [13]	15	34	12
London et al. [14]	11	18	6
McMahon et al. [15]	14	5	18

Effects of Anaemia Correction on Cardiovascular Function

Patients with anaemia tend to have a reduced peripheral vascular resistance and an elevated cardiac output. Treatment of anaemia with epoietin produces beneficial haemodynamic effects: the peripheral vascular tone tends to normalise, the cardiac index is reduced. As regards the patient symptoms, an increase in the patient's maximum workload and anaerobic threshold has been observed in patients treated with r-HuEPO [10].

In some patients treatment of anaemia was associated with an increase in total peripheral resistances. The latter effect may be beneficial in patients with chronic hypotension although it also can aggravate pre-existing hypertension or favour the development of hypertension in a previously normotensive patient. The blood pressure increase is the result of peripheral vasconstriction as whole blood viscosity increases and peripheral oxygenation improves. The hypertension is very rarely severe and in my experience can be prevented by a gradual correction of the haematocrit, and it is less evident with subcutaneous administration than with the intravenous route. An additional concern for haemodialysis patients with significant ischaemic heart disease may derive from a sudden correction of anaemia, rapid achievement of haematocrit over 42–45%. In these patients with severe cardiac diseases and several coexisting diseases (diabetes, hypertension, etc.) an increased mortality can be observed in the short-run [11].

However, in the majority of the treated patients a substantial improvement in echocardiographic parameters is observed [4]. The reduction regards the cardiac output and left ventricular diastolic diameter. Over time a consistent reduction in left-ventricular mass and a less consistent risk of congestive heart failure have been observed [12–15]. At least 3–4 months are required before a reduction in LV mass can be demonstrated following a haemoglobin correction by epoietin.

Table 1 summarises some studies showing a reduction in LV mass after epoietin therapy. There is no consensus as to the optimal haemoglobin concentration to be aimed for in dialysis patients to obtain a reduction in LVH.

Increases in left-ventricular mass in the renal population are both due to the hypertrophy of the myocytes and myocardial fibrosis [14]. Strategies to prevent the development and progression of LVH, including an optimal control of blood pressure, correction of anaemia and the calcium/phosphorus balance may be the right way to reduce the burden of cardiovascular illness in renal patients.

References

1 The USRDS Dialysis Morbidity and Mortality Study: Wave 2 US Renal Data System. Am J Kidney Dis 1997;30(suppl 1):567–586.
2 London M, Fabiani F, Marchais SJ, et al: Uremic cardiomyopathy: An inadequate left ventricular hypertrophy. Kidney Int 1987;31:973–980.
3 Katz AM: The cardiomyopathy of overload: An unnatural growth response in hypertrophied heart. Ann Intern Med 1994;121:363–371.
4 Levin A, Thompson CR, Ethier J, et al: Left-ventricular mass index increase in early renal disease: Impact of decline in hemoglobin. Am J Kid Dis 1999;34:125–134.
5 Neil WA, Oxendine JM, Moore SC: Acute and chronic cardiovascular adjustments to induce anemia in dogs. Am J Physiol 1969;217:710–714.
6 Roy SB, Bhatia ML, Mathur VS, et al: Hemodynamic effects of chronic severe anemia. Circulation 1963;28:346–356.
7 Foley RN, Parfrey PS, Harnett JD, et al: Clinical and echocardiographic disease in patients starting end-stage renal disease therapy. Kidney Int 1995;47:186–192.
8 Madore F, Lowrie EG, Brugnara C, et al: Anemia in hemodialysis patients: Variable affecting this outcome predictor. JASN 1997;8:1921–1929.
9 Greaves Sc, Gamble GD, Collins JF, et al: Determinant of left ventricular hypertrophy and systolic dysfunction in chronic renal failure. Am J Kid Dis 1994;24:768–778.
10 Mayer G, Thum J, Cada EM, Stumvol HK, Graf H: Working capacity is increased following recombinant human erythropoietin treatment. Kidney Int 1988;34:525–528.
11 Besarab A, Bolton WK, Browne JK, et al: The effects of normal as compared with low hematocrit values in patients with cardiac disease who are receiving hemodialysis and epoietin. N Engl J Med 1998;339:584–590.
12 Goldberg N, Lundin AP, Delano B, Friedman El, Stein RA: Changes in left ventricular size, wall thickness and function in anemic patients treated with recombinant human Erythropoietin. Am Heart J 1992;124:424–427.
13 Pascual J, Teruel JL, Moya Jl, et al: Regression of left ventricular hypertrophy after partial correction of anemia with erythropoietin in patients on hemodialysis: A prospective study. Clin Nephrol 1991;35:280–287.
14 London GM, Zins B, Pannier B, et al: Vascular changes in hemodialysis patients in response to recombinant human erythropoietin. Kidney Int 1989;36:878–882.
15 McMahon LP, Mason K, Skinner SL: Effects of hemoglobin normalization on quality of life and cardiovascular parameters in end-stage renal failure. Nephrol Dial Transplant 2000;15:1425–1430.

Dr. Antonio Santoro, UO Nefrologia e Dialisi Malpighi,
Policlinico S. Orsola-Malpighi, Via P. Palagi 9, I-40138 Bologna (Italy)
Tel. +39 051 6362430, Fax +39 051 6362511, E-Mail santoro@orsola-malpighi.med.unibo.it

Author Index

Albertazzi, A. 317, 408
Albright, R. 170
Aljama, P. 138, 325
Alper, A. 287
Asatryan, L. 386
Atti, M. 111

Bellomo, R. 181
Bordoni, V. 158, 412
Bosch, J.P. 60, 287, 300
Bowry, S.K. 85
Brady, J.A. 170
Brendolan, A. 120
Bruno, S. 54
Bruns, S. 78
Buoncristiani, U. 371

Cappelli, G. 317
Carracedo, J. 325
Carraro, G. 181
Carta, M.R. 412
Cheung, A.K. 129
Choquette, M. 170
Cianciaruso, B. 426
Cianciavicchia, D. 212
Clark, W.R. 70
Clemmer, J. 170
Cohen, G. 170
Colzani, S. 338
Cowgill, L.D. 170
Crepaldi, C. 120, 412

Davankov, V. 170
Day, M. 293
De Blasio, A. 426
De Cristofaro, V. 254, 344
Delfino, P. 146
De Nitti, C. 212
Del Vecchio, L. 403
Di Filippo, S. 193, 338
Donald, L.L. 311

Ene-Iordache, B. 54

Feriani, M. 357
Ferramosca, E. 317
Filippini, M. 254
Fiorenzi, A. 212
Fiorillo, M. 426
Floridi, A. 371
Folden, T. 272
Fontanazzi, F. 260
Formica, M. 181
Forneris, G. 46

Galli, F. 95, 371
Gao, D. 70
Gastaldon, F. 120
Gatti, E. 293
Gavioli, G. 78
Gennari, M. 78
Gervasio, R. 212

Ghezzi, P.M. 146, 212
Gotch, F.A. 170, 268

Hegbrant, J. 287
Hoenich, N.A. 146, 165, 189
Hörl, W. 170

Inguaggiato, P. 317

Kirchgessner, J. 293
Konner, K. 20
Kooman, J.P. 245

La Greca, G. XII, 1
Ledebo, I. 221
Leunissen, K.M.L. 245
Levin, N.W. 120, 158, 170, 272, 279, 364, 379
Leypoldt, J.K. 31, 129
Livigni, S. 181
Locatelli, F. 193, 338, 403
Lonnemann, G. 332

Mancini, E. 233, 260
Manzoni, C. 193, 338
Marai, P. 403
Marangella, M. 350
Marcelli, D. 293
Mariano, F. 181
Marino, R. 426

Martín-Malo, A. 138, 325
Masuda, T. 106
Milan, M. 279
Mitteregger, A. 293
Moscardó, V. 293

Orlandini, G. 293

Pagliari, B. 254, 344
Paolini, F. 260
Passlick-Deetjen, J. 201
Pavlov, M. 170
Pavlova, L. 170
Pedrini, L.A. 254, 344
Pisoni, R.L. 13, 396
Pohlmeier, R. 201
Polaschegg, H.-D. 227
Pozzato, M. 46
Pozzoni, P. 193, 338

Quarello, F. 46

Ramello, A. 350
Ramírez, R. 325
Remuzzi, A. 54
Remuzzi, G. 54
Renaux, J.-L. 111
Rodríguez, M. 325
Rodríguez-Benot, A. 138
Ronco, C. XII, 1, 70, 120, 146, 158, 170, 181, 272, 279, 364, 379
Ruggiero, P. 254, 344

Salsberg, J. 170
Sande, F.M. van der 245
Santamaría, R. 138
Santoro, A. 233, 260, 431
Sevanian, A. 386
Steil, H. 293

Tetta, C. 181, 212
Torraca, S. 426
Tsyurupa, M. 170

Vitale, C. 350

Walters, B.A.J. 60, 300
Wee, P.M. ter 38
Weijmer, M.C. 38
Winchester, F.J. 170
Wratten, M.L. 181

Yousha, E. 170

Zhu, F. 272

Subject Index

Access flow
measurement
accuracy 34
clinical guidelines 34
dilution without
intravenous injections 32, 33
reversed dialysis lines 33
overview of techniques 31, 32
precautions 35
precision 34, 35
ultrasound (saline) dilution with
reversed dialysis lines 32
variable flow Doppler without reversed
dialysis lines 33
stenosis evaluation rationale 31
Acetate-free biofiltration
benefits 207
potassium dialysate profiling
cardiac arrhythmia reduction 264–266
measurements 261, 262
patient features 262
removal rates 263–265
Acute renal failure
continuous renal replacement therapy
182–184
coupled plasma filtration adsorption for
sepsis
cytokines 182, 186, 187
immune cell responsiveness
restoration 185, 186
overview 182, 183
rationale 184, 185
sepsis pathophysiology 181, 182
Adsorbents
acute renal failure prevention with
coupled plasma filtration adsorption
for sepsis
cytokines 182, 186, 187
immune cell responsiveness
restoration 185, 186
overview 182, 183
rationale 184, 185
adsorption isotherms 163
biocompatibility
cellular and humoral immunity
activation 167, 168
definition 166, 167
particle embolization leaching and
hemolysis 167
prospects for improvement 168, 169
capacity 171
clinical applications 166
definition 165
efficiency 161–164, 171
historical perspective 159, 165, 170
materials 159, 160, 165, 166, 170
mechanisms of solute adsorption 161
principles 158, 159
prospects 164
rationale for use 159
requirements 161
specific vs nonspecific 171
structure 161
systems for dialysis augmentation

hemodialysis
charcoal hemoperfusion 175
MARS system 176
metal chelators 175
plasma filtration system 175
REDY system 176
resin hemoperfusion 176, 177
ultrafiltrate regeneration 175, 176
HemoTherapies Unit 172
peritoneal dialysis 172
table of types 173, 174
Advanced glycation end products, inflammation role 366, 367
AN69ST
contact phase activation reduction 114
electrical properties 114
fabrication 114
heparin adsorption 114, 115, 117
heparinization studies 115–118
physical properties 114
sterilization 114
Anemia
cardiac complications 431, 433
cardiovascular adjustments 432, 433
correction effects on cardiovascular function 434, 435
high-flux dialysis and hemodiafiltration correction 195, 196
incidence in dialysis patients 396
oxidative stress role 374
treatment, *see* Carnitine, Darbepoetin-alfa, Epoetin-beta, Erythropoietin, Iron
Angiography, arteriovenous fistula 26, 27
Anticoagulation
bleeding risks 111, 113
CLE membrane effects 111
heparinization
alternatives 113
complications 113
dosing 112
unfractionated heparin 111, 112
importance in hemodialysis 111
Aranesp, *see* Darbepoetin-alfa
Arteriovenous fistula
development 1, 2
diabetics 21, 22
Dialysis Outcomes and Practice Patterns Study
creation soon after referral for surgery 16, 17
facility characteristics yielding high use 15
factors affecting use 16
graft survival 15
needling skill development 17
nephrologist visit history in use 16
new patient utilization 14
prevalence for vascular access in Europe and United States 13, 14
surgical success rate 17
geographic distribution of use for vascular access 54, 55, 61
hemodynamics
assessment
computer simulation 57, 58
direct measurement 56, 57
geometry of anastomosis 56
wall shear stress in failure 55, 56, 58
histology of failure 55
inflammation 381
interventional vs surgical repair 28
maintenance 26–29
maturation 55
native vs constructed 20
surgery
arm selection 22
construction 23–25, 28
failure incidence 55
graft material and revisions 24, 25
planning 22, 23, 28
timing 23
ultrasound 22, 23, 57
venography 23
Atherosclerosis
CLE membrane prevention 99, 100, 102, 103
epidemic of cardiovascular disease in dialysis patients 212
inflammation and cardiovascular disease risks 325, 364–369
mortality in dialysis patients 431
Atomic force microscopy, Helixone 89

Atrial natriuretic peptide, fluid overload
indicator 274, 275

BetaSorb, resin hemoperfusion 176, 177
Bicarbonate
dialysate concentration effects on
nutrition 357, 358
history of use 2, 3
on-line hemodiafiltration,
dialysate/infusate composition and
infusion mode 346, 347
serum levels
postdialysis factors
alkalosis 361, 362
blood bicarbonate flux 360, 361
dialysate concentration 361, 362
predialysis factors
dialysate concentration 359
dialysis schedule 359
ultrafiltration 358–360
values 358
Biofeedback
blood volume control
adaptive controller 240, 241
clinical validation 241–243
control problem formulation 239, 240
control variables 240
effectors 240
prospects 243
system components 239
body temperature control 239
dialysis monitoring overview 7, 8
transmembrane pressure control
256–258
Blood flow
access flow, *see* Access flow
blood pump speed relationship 132
dialysate distribution 124
distributors 5
Newtonian behavior at high shear
rates 122
optimization 134–136
parabolic distribution in dye bundle 123
protein deposition effects on
membranes 122
rate effects on solute clearance 129, 130
urea clearance effects 132–134
Blood temperature
dialysate temperature and intradialytic
hypotension 246, 247, 251
dialysis-induced hypotension role
245, 246
heat and energy transfer rate in
hypotension control 247–250
monitoring 251
Blood volume
biofeedback control
adaptive controller 240, 241
clinical validation 241–243
control problem formulation
239, 240
control variables 240
effectors 240
prospects 243
system components 239
calculation of change over time 235
intradialysis hypotension 233, 234
monitoring
continuous monitoring 236–238
hematocrit relationship to blood
volume 235
hemodynamic monitoring
importance 234
hemoglobin optical absorbance
235, 236
hypovolemia threshold 237
radiodilution techniques 234, 235
ultrafiltration
effects 233
rate relationship 238
vascular refilling dynamics, factors
affecting 236
Body temperature, dialysate temperature
relationship 247–249
Bone, calcium dialysate effects on
metabolism 353, 354
Brain natriuretic peptide, fluid overload
indicator 274, 275

Calcium
dialysate effects
bone metabolism 353, 354
cardiovascular effects 355
parathyroid hormone status 354

hemodiafiltration balances 352, 353
hemodialytic balances 350–352
hemofiltration balances 353
metabolism in end-stage renal disease 350, 353
on-line hemodiafiltration, dialysate/infusate composition and infusion mode 347, 348
phosphate binders 351, 352
Cardiovascular stability, *see also* Blood volume
arrhythmias during dialysis 260
calcium dialysate effects 355
dialysis fluid temperature effects 205, 206
epidemic of cardiovascular disease in dialysis patients 212
high-flux dialysis and hemodiafiltration outcomes 193, 194
inflammation and cardiovascular disease risks 325, 364–369
low-flux dialysis outcomes 191
mortality in dialysis patients 431
on-line hemofiltration 224, 225
Carnitine
deficiency in uremia 428
functions 427
metabolism 426
sources 426
supplementation
erythropoietin-resistant patients 429
erythropoietin-sparing effect 428, 429
hematocrit response 428
Catheter
bacteremia prevention 43, 44
hospitalization and mortality risks 17, 18, 38, 46
inflammation 382
insertion sites 39, 40
jugular catheter design 40, 41
materials and coating 42, 43
new patient use 15, 16, 38
NKFF-DOQI guidelines 38, 39
prosthetic replacements, *see* Dialock, LifeSite
tip design 41, 42
trisodium citrate for locking 43, 44
tunneled vs temporary catheters 39, 40, 46
Cellulose triacetate membrane
blood interactions 109
hydrophobicity 108
mass transfer properties 108, 109
safety 109
spinning of hollow fibers 106, 107
sterilization 108
structure 106
Central venous catheter, *see* Catheter
Chronic inflammation
cardiovascular disease risks 325, 364–369
C-reactive protein levels
hemodialysis 364–368
peritoneal dialysis 368, 369
mechanisms and factors 366–368, 379, 380
oxidative stress role 366
Chronic kidney disease
epidemiology 311
erythropoietin therapy 397, 398
goals of management 313
provider-based disease management benefits 311–313
stages 311, 312
systematic care
administration 313
approaches 313
cost-effectiveness 316
databases 314, 315
education program 315
multidisciplinary team 314
CLE membrane, *see* Vitamin E-modified dialyzers
Compensated anti-inflammatory response syndrome
features 384
SIRS-CARS hypothesis 383, 384
Computational fluid dynamics, arteriovenous fistula hemodynamics 57, 58
Computer hemodialyzer searching, *see* Hemodialyzer
Computer information technology, *see* Data collection and management

Continuous quality improvement
Fresenius Medical Care 296, 299
Gambro Healthcare
databases 303–305
facility comparison 307, 308
monitoring of quality benchmarks 309
outcome quality markers 305, 307
overview 309, 310
quality objective components 306
Six Sigma theory 301, 303
statistical analysis 309
team 306–308
quality assurance comparison 303
vascular access, *see* Vascular access
Convection
convective flux of solute 120, 121
factors affecting 122
interference between diffusion and convection 124, 125
optimization for hemodiafiltration
biofeedback module for transmembrane pressure control 256–258
rationale 254
Costs, *see* Health care costs
C-reactive protein
hemodialysis levels and cardiovascular risks 364–368
inflammation marker 380, 381
peritoneal dialysis and cardiovascular risks 368, 369
Cuprophan, properties 3, 4
Cytokine-inducing substances
adverse effects 74
backfiltration 74, 75

Darbepoetin-alfa
anemia correction
chronic renal failure patients 404, 405
chronic renal insufficiency 405
dosing 405, 406
bioavailability 404
half-life 403, 404
safety and tolerability 405–407
Data collection and management
acquisition
approaches 280, 281
sources for input 281, 287, 294
computer underutilization in hemodialysis 279, 280
management
domains for management system 282, 284
principles 281, 282
tasks 284, 285
quality assurance, *see* Quality assurance
Databases, *see* Hemodialyzer, Quality assurance
Dialock
clinical experience
Canaud study 49, 50
German study 50
Italian multicenter study 51
Turin experience 50, 51
design 48, 49
implantation and use 49
safety 52
Dialysate
bicarbonate dialysate, *see* Bicarbonate
calcium dialysate effects
bone metabolism 353, 354
cardiovascular effects 355
parathyroid hormone status 354
distribution in fibers 124
flow rate
optimization 134–136
urea clearance effects 132–134
magnesium dialysate effects 354, 355
sodium content 339
temperature and intradialytic hypotension 246, 247, 251
water treatment, *see* Water treatment
Dialysis Outcomes and Practice Patterns Study
arteriovenous fistula for vascular access in Europe and United States
creation soon after referral for surgery 16, 17
facility characteristics yielding high use 15
factors affecting use 16
graft survival 15
needling skill development 17
nephrologist visit history 16

new patients 14
prevalence 13, 14
surgical success rate 17
catheters
hospitalization and mortality risks 17, 18
use in new patients 15, 16, 38
design 13
international scope 13
Dialysis-induced hypotension, *see* Blood volume, Blood temperature
Diffusion
interference between diffusion and convection 124, 125
resistance 121, 122
shear rate effects 123
solute diffusive flux 121
solute size effects 121
Dose, dialysis
Kt/V 268
prescribed vs delivered doses 269
Dry weight
definition 272
determination
bioimpedance analysis of extracellular fluid 275, 276
table of methods 273
extracellular fluid depletion during dialysis 274
fluid overload indicators 274, 275
overhydration in dialysis 272, 274

Electron beam radiation, sterilization of membranes 80
Electron microscopy, Helixone 89, 90
Endotoxin
adverse effects 74
backfiltration 74, 75
cellulose triacetate membrane permeation 108, 109
macrophage apoptosis prevention 328–330
on-line hemodiafiltration patient cytokine response 206
Epoetin-beta
anemia correction with once-weekly regimen
dialysis patients 408–410
predialysis patients 410
dosing 408, 410
self-administration 411
Erythropoietin
cardiovascular function effects 434, 435
carnitine supplementation and sparing effect 428, 429
European experience
anemia correction efficacy 400, 401
best practice guidelines 398, 399
dosing 399, 400
pre-end-stage renal disease use 397, 398
study sources 396, 397
half-life 403
on-line hemodiafiltration patient response 205
receptors 396
Ethylene oxide, sterilization of membranes
efficacy 82, 139
hypersensitivity reactions and prevention 139, 140
mechanism of action 139
mutagenicity 140, 141
standards 81, 82
EuCliD, *see* Quality assurance
Evidence-based medicine, components 301, 302

Fresenius Medical Care, *see* Quality assurance

Gambro Healthcare, *see* Continuous quality improvement, Quality assurance
Gamma rays, sterilization of membranes 79, 80, 141
GENIUS, system features 228

Hagen-Poiseuille equation 72, 126
Health care costs
dialysis machine heating energy cost savings 230
end-stage renal disease 311
hemodiafiltration 201
hemodialysis technology prospects 8, 9
vascular access complications 54, 60, 61

Heat sterilization, membranes
biocompatibility considerations 141, 142
dry heat 80
wet steam 80, 81, 141, 142
Helixone
atomic force microscopy 89
electron microscopy and image analysis 89, 90
β_2-microglobulin sieving 85, 86, 90
nanocontrolled spinning technology 87, 88, 92
nanostructure effects on performance 90–93
pore size and distribution 88, 90
sieving coefficient profile 88
surface elemental composition 90, 93
Heme oxygenase-1, induction by hemoglobin-modified low-density lipoproteins 392, 393
Hemodiafiltration
acetate-free biofiltration 207
advantages 201
anemia correction 195, 196
calcium and magnesium balances 352, 353
cardiovascular stability outcomes 193, 194
convection optimization
biofeedback module for transmembrane pressure control 256–258
rationale 254
costs 201
definition 4
features 193
HEMO study 199
β_2-microglobulin removal 197
morbidity and mortality outcomes 198, 199
MPO study 199
nutritional status effects 196
on-line hemodiafiltration, *see* On-line hemodiafiltration
push/pull hemodiafiltration 208
residual renal function preservation 194, 195
ultrafiltration control system 255, 256
Hemodialysis machine
bedside station complexity reduction 231
concentrate consumption reduction 231
conventional dialysis unit improvements
heat exchangers 229, 230
implementation 232
limitations 228, 229
redundant components 229
GENIUS system features 228
heating energy cost savings 230
ideal criteria 227
system approach to design 227, 228
Hemodialyzer, *see also* Hollow fiber membrane
blood flow 5
computer database
applications 156
dialysis simulator 153, 155
dialyzer searches
membrane type 149
producers 149
sterilization type 149
target Kt/V 155
usage 149, 151, 153
information sources 147, 148
maintenance 157
configurations, historical perspective 5, 70–72
ideal requirements 147
market 70
processes during dialysis 146
Hemofiltration
calcium and magnesium balances 353
definition 4
features 190
on-line hemofiltration, *see* On-line hemofiltration
Hemoglobin-dependent oxidation, *see* Low-density lipoprotein
Hemolipodialysis, rationale 96
HemoTherapies Unit, dialysis augmentation 172
Heparin
AN69ST adsorption 114, 115, 117
anticoagulation
alternatives 113

AN69ST membrane effects 115–118
complications 113
dosing 112
unfractionated heparin 111, 112
High-flux hemodialysis
anemia correction 195, 196
cardiovascular stability outcomes 193, 194
double high-flux dialysis 208
features 4, 5, 189, 190, 193
HEMO study 199
β_2-microglobulin removal 197
morbidity and mortality outcomes 198, 199
MPO study 199
nutritional status effects 196
on-line hemodiafiltration comparison 203, 204
residual renal function preservation 194, 195
Historical perspective, hemodialysis 1–5, 70–72, 222
Hollow fiber artificial kidney, development 71, 72
Hollow fiber membrane, *see also* specific membranes
adsorptivity of membranes 74, 75
backfiltration 125–127
composition and structure
modified cellulosic membranes 75
synthetic membranes 75, 76
unmodified cellulosic membranes 75
computer hemodialyzer searching, *see* Hemodialyzer
depuration properties 73–75
dimensions 72
fabrication, *see* Spinning, membranes
internal filtration 125–127
principles 125–127
solute-removing requirements of high-flux membranes 86
sterilization, *see* Sterilization, membranes
toxins 74, 75
vitamin E modification, *see* Vitamin E-modified dialyzers
water permeability 72, 73
Hypersensitivity reactions
ethylene oxide sterilization and prevention 139, 140
reused dialyzers 142, 143
Hypertension
hemodialysis patients 338
prevention 338, 339

Inflammation, *see* Chronic inflammation, Systemic inflammatory response syndrome
Information technology, *see* Data collection and management
Iron
deficiency
definition 413
markers
bone marrow examination 420
ferritin 417, 418
hypochromic red blood cells 419
red blood cell zinc protoporphyrin 419, 420
reticulocyte hemoglobin content 418
transferrin levels and saturation 416, 417
transferrin receptors 418
serum sampling 416
metabolism 411–413
overload-related risks
cancer 422, 423
cardiovascular disease 423
infection 422
supplementation with hemodialysis
DOQI guidelines 420
intramuscular administration 415
intravenous administration 415, 416, 420, 421
oral administration 414, 415
rationale 412

Kt/V
computer database of target Kt/V 155
customization of individual treatment 6
dialysis dose definition 268

Kt/V (continued)
on-line hemodiafiltration vs hemodialysis 204

Left ventricular hypertrophy
anemia correction effects 434, 435
uremia patients 431–433
Leukocyte activation
adsorbents 167, 168
CLE membrane prevention 100–102
LifeSite
clinical experience 47, 48
design 47
implantation and use 47
safety 52
Lipopolysaccharide, *see* Endotoxin
Low-density lipoprotein
electronegative particles
cytotoxicity 391
measurement 386, 387
hemoglobin-dependent oxidation
cytotoxicity 391, 392, 394
heme oxygenase-1 induction by lipoproteins 392, 393
kinetics 389, 390
mechanisms 387, 388
pro-oxidant properties of lipoproteins 390, 391
Western blot analysis 388, 389
oxidation and atherogenesis 386
Low-flux hemodialysis
cardiovascular stability outcomes 191
features 4
on-line hemodiafiltration comparison 204
prospects 191, 192
solute removal efficiency 190, 191

Macrophage, inflammatory response 325, 326
Magnesium
dialysate effects 354, 355
hemodiafiltration balances 352, 353
hemodialytic balances 351, 352
hemofiltration balances 353
metabolism in end-stage renal disease 350
phosphate binders 351, 352
MARS, adsorbent system 176
Membranes, *see* AN69ST, Cellulose triacetate membrane, Helixone, Hollow fiber membrane, Spinning, membranes, Sterilization, membranes, Vitamin E-modified dialyzers
Metabolic acidosis, renal failure 357, 362
β_2-Microglobulin
adsorbents 176, 177
AN69ST sieving 114
cellulose triacetate membrane sieving 108
Helixone sieving 85, 86, 90
high-flux dialysis and hemodiafiltration removal 197
on-line hemodiafiltration removal 203–206
toxic properties 171
Middle-molecule hypothesis, dialysis adequacy and prescription 2
Monitoring
biofeedback utilization, *see* Biofeedback
blood volume, *see* Blood volume
body temperature, *see* Blood temperature
on-line 7
Monocyte, hemodialysis membrane interactions
apoptosis induction by cellulose membranes 327
bacterial contamination and activation 328–330
inflammatory response 326, 327

Nutritional status
bicarbonate dialysate concentration effects 357, 358
high-flux dialysis and hemodiafiltration effects 196

On-line conductivity clearance
clinical application 271
effective conductivity clearance 270, 271
sodium control and interdialytic weight reduction 277, 278
urea clearance relationship 270

On-line fluid preparation, *see* Water treatment
On-line hemodiafiltration
circuit 201, 202
clinical benefits 209, 210
dialysate/infusate composition and infusion mode
bicarbonate 346, 347
calcium 347, 348
sodium 344–346
dose-dependent effects 204–207
erythropoietin response 205
hemodialysis comparison 203, 204
mortality outcomes 209, 210
on-line endogenous reinfusion of ultrafiltrate
advantages 214, 215
features 208, 212, 213
historical perspective 213, 214
rationale 215, 216
paired filtration dialysis 207, 212, 213
paired hemodiafiltration
advantages 216–218
definition 212, 213
double chamber hemodiafiltration 208, 217, 218
reinfusion rate 218
safety 217
prospects 210
safety 202, 203
substitution fluid infusion, predilution vs postdilution modes 203
substitution volumes 206, 207
On-line hemofiltration
hemodialysis comparison 222, 223
hemodynamic stability benefits and mechanisms 224, 225
historical perspective 221, 222
quantification of therapy 223
solute removal 223–225
Oxidative stress
anemia role 374
antioxidant therapy 374–376
causes in hemodialysis patients 371
chronic inflammation role 366
CLE membrane prevention, *see* Vitamin E-modified dialyzers
comorbid condition pathogenesis 372, 373
risks in dialysis 95, 373, 374
toxin induction 96

Paired filtration dialysis
benefits 207, 213–216
chambers 215
sodium kinetic model 341, 342
Paired hemodiafiltration, *see* On-line hemodiafiltration
Parathyroid hormone, calcium dialysate effects on status 354
Peritoneal dialysis
adsorbents 172
CRP levels 368, 369
Phosphate
binders 351, 352
cellulose triacetate membrane clearance 108
hemodiafiltration removal 203
Polysulfone membrane, *see* Helixone
Potassium
acetate-free biofiltration dialysate profiling
cardiac arrhythmia reduction 264–266
measurements 261, 262
patient features 262
removal rates 263–265
removal rates in hemodialysis 260, 261
Pre-end-stage renal disease, *see* Chronic kidney disease
Profiling, treatment session 6, 7

Quality assurance
continuous quality improvement comparison 303
data acquisition importance 287, 288
definition 295
Fresenius Medical Care EuCliD
data sources and collection 294, 295, 298
guideline creation and implementation 295, 296, 298
Gambro Healthcare International dialysis outcome reporting
Excel file format 288, 289

Quality assurance (continued)
International Renal Information Management System 290, 292, 304
Internet access to data 289, 290, 292
vascular access, *see* Vascular access
water treatment 321–323

REDY, adsorbent system 176
Resistance
dialysis system 121, 122, 135
solute removal rate comparison with Ohm's law 131
Reverse osmosis, *see* Water treatment

Sepsis
continuous renal replacement therapy 182–184
coupled plasma filtration adsorption
cytokines 182, 186, 187
immune cell responsiveness restoration 185, 186
overview 182, 183
rationale 184, 185
pathophysiology in acute renal failure 181, 182
Sieving coefficient
estimation 122
wall shear rate effects 123
Simulator, hemodialysis 153, 155
Sodium
clearance equivalence with urea clearance 270, 271
dialysate
content 339
levels and fluid intake 276, 277
hypertension role 38
kinetic model for hemodialysis 341, 342
on-line clearance detection 277, 278
on-line hemodiafiltration, dialysate/infusate composition and infusion mode 344–346
profiling 339, 340
Solute clearance, equations 129, 130
Solute removal rate, equation 131
Sorbents, *see* Adsorbents
Spinning, membranes
cellulose triacetate membranes 106, 107
convective transport optimization 85, 86
nanocontrolled spinning technology 87, 88, 92
pore size control 87
Square meter hypothesis, dialysis adequacy and prescription 2
Steam, *see* Heat sterilization, membranes
Sterilization, membranes
biocompatibility considerations 138, 139
computer database 149
dialyzer reuse 142, 143
ethylene oxide sterilization
efficacy 82, 139
hypersensitivity reactions and prevention 139, 140
mechanism of action 139
mutagenicity 140, 141
standards 81, 82
heat sterilization
dry heat 80
wet steam 80, 81, 141, 142
irradiation
electron beam radiation 80
gamma rays 79, 80, 141
standards 78, 79
validation 82, 83
verification of influence 83
Systemic inflammatory response syndrome
causes 379
immunohomeostasis alterations 383, 384
SIRS-CARS hypothesis 383, 384

Total quality management, components 301, 302
Transmembrane pressure
biofeedback module for transmembrane pressure control 256–258
ultrafiltration flow rate relationship 255
Trisodium citrate, catheter locking 43, 44

Ultrafiltration, historical perspective 3
Ultrafiltration coefficient
determination 254, 255
transmembrane pressure relationship to flow rate 255
Ultrasound
access flow measurements

dilution with reversed dialysis lines 32
variable flow Doppler without reversed dialysis lines 33
arteriovenous fistula
maintenance 26, 27
planning 22, 23, 57
Urea clearance
caveats in calculation 132
equations 129–132
equivalence with sodium clearance 270, 271
optimization 134–136
predictions 132–134

Vascular access
access flow assessment, *see* Access flow
arteriovenous fistula access, *see* Arteriovenous fistula
costs of complications 54, 60, 61
geographic distribution of modalities 54, 55, 61
prosthetic devices, *see* Dialock, LifeSite
quality control
continuous quality improvement process
analysis 66
countermeasure institution 66, 67
current situation assessment 65, 66
defining reason for improvement 64, 65
future plans 67, 68
goals 63, 64
results objective 67
standardization 67
quality assurance steps 63
team 62, 63, 68
venous catheter access, *see* Catheter
Vitamin C, dialysate infusion 95, 96
Vitamin E-modified dialyzers
CLE membrane
anticoagulation and antianemic function 102
antioxidant properties 97–99
clinical experience 96
endothelial protection and antiatherogenic function 99, 100, 102, 103
leukocyte function and activation 100–102
oxidative stress risks in dialysis 95
rationale 95, 96

Water treatment
costs 321, 322
deionization 319, 320
failure cases of water delivery systems 318
importance for hemodialysis 317
microbiological quality of dialysis water 332–334
on-line fluid preparation
double cascade filtration 335, 336
rationale 332
standards 333, 334
ultrafiltration through pyrogen-adsorbing high-flux membranes 334, 335
piping materials 321
plants 319–321
quality control 321–323
reverse osmosis 319, 320, 332, 333
standards 318–320
tap water contaminants 317, 318
Weight gain, interdialytic
fluid intake factors 276, 277
reduction methods
sodium control 277, 278
table 273